Adaptive Mentalization-Based Integrative Treatment (AMBIT) for People with Multiple Needs

Adaptive Mentalization-Based Integrative Treatment (AMBIT) for People with Multiple Needs

Applications in Practice

Edited by

Peter Fuggle
Laura Talbot
Chloe Campbell
Peter Fonagy
Dickon Bevington

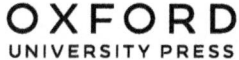

OXFORD
UNIVERSITY PRESS

OXFORD
UNIVERSITY PRESS

Great Clarendon Street, Oxford, OX2 6DP,
United Kingdom

Oxford University Press is a department of the University of Oxford.
It furthers the University's objective of excellence in research, scholarship,
and education by publishing worldwide. Oxford is a registered trade mark of
Oxford University Press in the UK and in certain other countries

© Oxford University Press 2023

The moral rights of the authors have been asserted

First Edition published in 2023

Published in the United States of America by Oxford University Press
198 Madison Avenue, New York, NY 10016, United States of America

British Library Cataloguing in Publication Data

Data available

Library of Congress Control Number is on file at the Library of Congress

ISBN 978–0–19–885591–0

DOI: 10.1093/med-psych/9780198855910.001.0001

Printed in the UK by
Ashford Colour Press Ltd, Gosport, Hampshire

Oxford University Press makes no representation, express or implied, that the
drug dosages in this book are correct. Readers must therefore always check
the product information and clinical procedures with the most up-to-date
published product information and data sheets provided by the manufacturers
and the most recent codes of conduct and safety regulations. The authors and
the publishers do not accept responsibility or legal liability for any errors in the
text or for the misuse or misapplication of material in this work. Except where
otherwise stated, drug dosages and recommendations are for the non-pregnant
adult who is not breast-feeding

Links to third party websites are provided by Oxford in good faith and
for information only. Oxford disclaims any responsibility for the materials
contained in any third party website referenced in this work.

Contents

Acknowledgements	xiii
Contributors	xv
Abbreviations	xix

1. Why has AMBIT come about?   **1**
Laura Talbot and Peter Fuggle
1.1 Introduction   1
1.2 Many clients have multiple needs   3
    1.2.1 Problems are often highly interconnected   4
1.3 Multiple needs attract multiple helpers   5
    1.3.1 Collaboration between agencies is hard to achieve   8
    1.3.2 Involving multiple services does not necessarily mean better help   9
    1.3.3 The limitations of service redesign in addressing these problems   10
1.4 The helping process is crucial   10
    1.4.1 The fragility of the helping process   11
    1.4.2 The role of attachment theory   12
1.5 The worker's state of mind is fundamental to help   14
1.6 Conclusion   15
1.7 The plan for the book   16

2. An introduction to AMBIT   **19**
Liz Cracknell and Dickon Bevington
2.1 Setting the scene   19
2.2 Introduction   19
2.3 Mentalizing: AMBIT as a mentalization-based approach   21
    2.3.1 The fragility of mentalizing: a great power leveller   25
    2.3.2 Mentalizing in four directions: balancing the wheel   27
2.4 Working with your Team   28
    2.4.1 Mentalizing and non-mentalizing in teams and workers   28
    2.4.2 Working with your Team: stance features   31
       2.4.2.1 Individual keyworker relationship   31
       2.4.2.2 Keyworker well connected to the team   32
    2.4.3 Working with your Team: basic practice   33
       2.4.3.1 Helping processes in teams   33
       2.4.3.2 'Ripples in the pond'   34
       2.4.3.3 'Who's got your rope?'   35
    2.4.4 Tools and techniques for Working with your Team   35
2.5 Working with your Client   36
    2.5.1 Mentalizing and non-mentalizing in working with clients   36

2.5.2   Working with your Client: stance features   39
   2.5.2.1   Scaffolding relationships   39
   2.5.2.2   Managing risk   39
2.5.3   Working with your Client: basic practice   40
   2.5.3.1   Epistemic trust   40
   2.5.3.2   The mentalizing stance   40
   2.5.3.3   Scaffolding relationships   41
   2.5.3.4   'Active Planning'   41
2.5.4   Tools and techniques for Working with your Client   42
2.6   Working with your Network   43
2.6.1   Mentalizing and non-mentalizing in networks   43
2.6.2   Working with your Network: stance features   45
   2.6.2.1   Meeting multiple needs   46
   2.6.2.2   Integrating the help   46
2.6.3   Working with your Network: basic practice   47
   2.6.3.1   Team around the Worker   47
   2.6.3.2   Taking a mentalizing approach to addressing dis-integration   48
2.6.4   Tools and techniques for Working with your Network   49
2.7   Learning at Work   51
2.7.1   Mentalizing and non-mentalizing in relation to learning   51
2.7.2   Learning at Work: stance features   53
   2.7.2.1   Respect for evidence   53
   2.7.2.2   Respect for local practice and expertise   54
2.7.3   Learning at Work: basic practice   55
2.7.4   Tools and techniques for Learning at Work   56
2.8   Implications   58

3. Epistemic trust and mistrust in helping systems   61
Peter Fonagy and Chloe Campbell
3.1   Setting the scene   61
3.2   Mentalizing in real-world settings   61
3.3   Mentalizing: a strength and a vulnerability   65
3.4   Mentalizing and collaboration within helping systems   67
3.4.1   Joint attention and the 'we-mode'   68
3.4.2   The we-mode and epistemic trust   69
3.4.3   Co-mentalizing and an epistemic match   70
3.5   What do we mean by non-mentalizing helping systems?   73
3.6   Why focus on mentalizing in systems?   74
3.7   AMBIT and non-mentalizing working contexts   77
3.8   Implications   79

4. Working out what is going on: Using the AIM cards with clients   83
Laura Talbot
4.1   Setting the scene   83
4.2   Introduction   83
4.3   What are the AIM cards?   85
4.3.1   A recap on mentalizing   86

4.4 Using the AIM cards with a client   87
    4.4.1 Step 1: worker introduces the cards   87
    4.4.2 Step 2: worker seeks agreement from client about using the cards   88
    4.4.3 Step 3: client decides how to look through the cards   89
    4.4.4 Step 4: client chooses labels for the piles of cards   90
    4.4.5 Step 5: client sorts the cards into piles   91
    4.4.6 Step 6: worker attunes to the client as they sort the cards   93
    4.4.7 Step 7: worker and client explore how they have sorted the cards   94
    4.4.8 Step 8: exploring whether there is anything the client might want
           to be different   97
    4.4.9 Step 9: exploring who can help with the chosen cards   100
    4.4.10 Other ways of using the cards when there is more significant
           ambivalence about help-seeking   101
    4.4.11 Summary   102
4.5 What do clients say about using AIM cards?   103
4.6 Implications   104

5. **Getting started with AMBIT: The ECID project in Barcelona**   **107**
Mark Dangerfield
5.1 Setting the scene   107
5.2 Introduction   108
5.3 Working with your Client   110
    5.3.1 Understanding adverse relational experiences as an impediment to
           relationships   112
    5.3.2 Implications of adverse relational experiences in our work: what
           AMBIT offers with our clients   116
    5.3.3 ECID goes live   119
    5.3.4 Professional's stance   124
5.4 Working with your Team   126
    5.4.1 Design of the ECID team   127
5.5 Working with your Network   130
5.6 Learning at Work   132
5.7 Implications   134

6. **Connecting psychotherapy to the streets: The Malmö approach**   **139**
Ernst Dahlquist
6.1 Setting the scene   139
6.2 The team today   139
6.3 How it started   140
6.4 The first meeting   142
6.5 How our thinking developed   144
6.6 The beginning   145
6.7 Our first clients   146
6.8 We become a team   147
6.9 AMBIT   148
    6.9.1 Theoretical aspects   149
    6.9.2 Working with your Client   149

6.9.2.1 Create contact: establishing epistemic trust	150
6.9.2.2 Care planning and linking to the network	152
6.9.2.3 Concrete targeted support	153
6.9.2.4 Emotional support	154
6.9.2.5 Coexistence	154
6.9.2.6 Reflective conversations	155
6.9.2.7 Parent work	158
6.9.2.8 Psychological assessment	162
6.10 Evaluation	163
6.11 Final reflection	164
6.12 Implications	164

7. AMBIT for adults with severe personality disorders: Experience from Utrecht, the Netherlands — **167**
Saskia Knapen and Rozemarijn van Duursen

7.1 Setting the scene	167
7.2 Working with adults with personality disorder	167
7.3 The context in which we work	168
7.4 Working with your Patient	170
7.4.1 Example: Working with your Patient	171
7.5 Working with your Team	172
7.5.1 Example: Working with your Team	173
7.6 Working with your Network	175
7.6.1 Example: Working with your Network	175
7.7 Learning at Work	176
7.8 Concluding remarks	178
7.9 Implications	179

8. Enhancing multiprofessional cooperation in a child and youth social service institution: Vorarlberger Kinderdorf, Austria — **181**
Beate Huter and Michael Hollenstein

8.1 Setting the scene	181
8.2 Introduction	182
8.2.1 Who we are and what we did: the story in a nutshell	182
8.2.2 Initial contact with AMBIT	183
8.2.3 What were the problems we needed help with?	183
8.2.3.1 Staff well-being	183
8.2.3.2 The need to pay attention to the workers' state of mind	184
8.2.3.3 Pedagogy and the problem of help-seeking for workers	184
8.2.3.4 Increasing case complexity	185
8.2.3.5 The stress of working in networks	185
8.3 Implementation in practice	185
8.3.1 The 'bones': the implementation process	185
8.3.2 The 'flesh': implementation in practice	187
8.3.2.1 Working with your Client	187

8.3.2.2 Working with your Team: the role of mentalizing
in supporting collaboration   191
8.3.2.3 Working with your Network   200
8.3.2.4 Learning at Work   204
8.4 Evaluation   205
8.4.1 The clients' perspective: using the AIM outcome evaluation   205
8.4.2 The stakeholders' perspective: implementation process evaluation   206
8.4.3 What we learned about AMBIT implementation   208
8.4.3.1 Bumpy roads: what did not work so well   208
8.4.3.2 The little and big successes: what worked   209
8.5 Where are we now?   210
8.6 Looking back: the AMBIT implementation wheel   211
8.6.1 Core element: mentalizing   212
8.6.2 Working with the Implementation Team (local facilitators)   213
8.6.3 Working with the Teams (defining goals, Active Planning)   213
8.6.4 Working with the Network (cooperation across the organization)   213
8.6.5 Learning at Work (learning culture)   213
8.7 Implications   214

9. Creating and supporting a Team around the Worker   217
Laura Talbot
9.1 Setting the scene   217
9.2 Introduction   217
9.3 What is a Team around the Worker?   218
9.4 Learning from training about what supports a Team around the Worker   220
9.4.1 Mentalizing the worker: 'This Team around the Worker thing
seems like a good idea, so why don't I want to do it?'   220
9.4.2 Trying it out: the importance of helping processes for the Team
around the Worker   223
9.5 The Team around the Worker: a case example of AMASS in London   224
9.5.1 Building Team around the Worker into the service design   224
9.5.2 Requesting help versus making a referral   226
9.5.3 Seeking the family's perspective on whether working with AMASS
would be helpful   227
9.5.4 Supporting the development of helping processes between
the social worker and the team   229
9.5.5 Building relationships with the young person using the
Team around the Worker   232
9.5.6 Bridging other professionals into relationships where epistemic
trust already exists   233
9.5.7 Team processes that support the Team around the Worker   235
9.5.7.1 Having the right mix of people who can work flexibly
in the team   235
9.5.7.2 Establishing and sustaining help-seeking in the team:
make it part of the work   236
9.5.7.3 Applying 'Team around the Worker' to group supervision   237
9.6 Implications   238

10. **Working with networks: Implementing AMBIT in disrupted healthcare systems** — 241

Janne Walløe Vilmar and Stefan Lock Jensen

10.1 Setting the scene — 241
10.2 Introduction — 242
10.3 The value of values: AMBIT in the age of disruptive dynamics — 243
10.4 AMBIT as outpatient milieu therapy in the real world — 247
10.5 Nothing unites people like a common enemy … but an enemy could become a friend — 248
10.6 Can you establish mentalizing network meetings? The NET-Aim-Questionnaire — 249
   10.6.1 What will mentalizing network meetings improve? — 253
   10.6.2 Will using the NET-Aim-Q improve patient-related outcome measures? — 254
10.7 The mentalizing case manager: the new specialist-generalist — 255
10.8 The resonance of young people and their helping systems — 258
10.9 'The Case of the Teenager Behind a Closed Door' — 260
10.10 Implications — 265

11. **Applying AMBIT to teacher training: innovations in Germany** — 269

Andrea Dlugosch and Melanie Henter

11.1 Setting the scene — 269
11.2 Introduction — 269
11.3 The needs of young people in special education settings — 270
11.4 Introducing the pilot project: 'Mentalization-based support for teachers' — 270
11.5 Teacher training and stress levels in Germany — 271
11.6 Using Active Planning to design the seminars — 272
   11.6.1 Sensitive attunement—understanding the needs of the student teachers — 272
   11.6.2 Broadcasting intentions—sharing our own ideas about what might help — 273
   11.6.3 Setting the plan — 274
11.7 Reflections on the seminars — 276
   11.7.1 Using the mentalizing stance and AMBIT tools in team discussions about pupils — 276
      11.7.1.1 Vignette—helping a child who is persistently late — 277
      11.7.1.2 Conclusion to section — 278
   11.7.2 Developing mentalization-based collegial case counselling — 279
      11.7.2.1 Conclusion to section — 282
   11.7.3 Reviewing video logs using mentalizing techniques — 282
11.8 Overall reflections on the seminars — 283
   11.8.1 The student teachers' perspective — 283
   11.8.2 The facilitators' perspective — 283
   11.8.3 Creating epistemic trust within the group — 284
   11.8.4 Dealing with emotions in teaching–learning fields — 284

11.8.5	How to best capture learning	285
11.8.6	How to embed a mentalizing stance: what is good-enough mentalizing?	285
11.9	Implications	286

12. Applying AMBIT principles to the training process — **291**

Laura Talbot, Rebecca Smith, James Wheeler, and Peter Fuggle

12.1	Setting the scene	291
12.2	Introduction	291
12.3	An AMBIT-influenced approach to training and implementation support	293
	12.3.1 What do you need? Attending to the state of mind of the workers	293
	12.3.1.1 How do we help teams to work out what they need?	294
	12.3.1.2 Engagement call	294
	12.3.1.3 Consultation day	295
	12.3.2 Training as an AMBIT-influenced helping process	297
	12.3.2.1 Who's got your rope? Sustaining a mentalizing stance as a trainer	299
	12.3.2.2 Using 'Active Planning' to adapt the training process to the team	301
	12.3.3 Supporting implementation in complex multiagency systems	304
	12.3.3.1 Strengthening the well-connected team	304
	12.3.3.2 Using training to promote network integration	306
	12.3.3.3 Keeping a focus on implementation throughout the training	309
	12.3.3.4 Supporting teams to implement AMBIT after the training	309
12.4	Evaluating our training approach	310
	12.4.1 Is the training a positive experience?	311
12.5	Implications	313

13. Adopting a mentalizing approach to evaluating outcomes — **315**

Peter Fuggle, James Fairbairn, and Anna Oriol-Sanchez

13.1	Setting the scene	315
13.2	Introduction	316
13.3	Looking from the inside: outcomes work for the worker, manager, and client	317
	13.3.1 Mentalizing the worker's experience of outcomes work	318
	13.3.2 Creating a culture of curiosity about outcomes	319
	13.3.2.1 Sharing mental models about outcomes	321
	13.3.2.2 Connecting outcomes to interest in intentional states	322
	13.3.2.3 Using logic models to determine outcomes that matter	323
	13.3.2.4 Discussing and feeding back outcomes with the whole team	327
13.4	Looking from the outside: outcomes for AMBIT-trained teams	328

13.5 Creating a shared outcomes framework   332
    13.5.1 An example of a local evaluation using the AIM   334
    13.5.2 Establishing the international AMBIT Study Group   334
13.6 Implications   336

14. What are the future directions for AMBIT?   **339**
Liz Cracknell, Laura Talbot, Rebecca Smith, James Fairbairn,
Dickon Bevington, and Peter Fuggle
14.1 Setting the scene   339
14.2 Introduction   340
14.3 Developing the basic AMBIT approach   342
    14.3.1 Making AMBIT values explicit and improving our attention
        to EDI   342
        14.3.1.1 Articulate AMBIT values and ethics   342
        14.3.1.2 Uphold the values in our work   343
        14.3.1.3 Improve how the AMBIT approach promotes EDI   343
    14.3.2 A deployment-based approach to model development   344
    14.3.3 Improving our knowledge of routine client outcomes   345
    14.3.4 Developing a research programme on the core model   347
14.4 Increasing training capacity and widening diversity   348
    14.4.1 Setting up international AMBIT Training Centres   348
    14.4.2 Widening diversity within the AMBIT Programme Team and in
        the community of practice to improve learning and adaptation 348
    14.4.3 Widening methods of dissemination through training and
        consultation   349
14.5 Improving implementation   350
    14.5.1 Supporting implementation after training   350
    14.5.2 Improving the wiki manual   351
14.6 Conclusion   351

Index   **353**

Acknowledgements

AMBIT is built on the feedback of others; we are not being polite or modest or 'English' or any of these things, we are just describing what happens. And because of that we have a lot of people to thank! So, we would like to begin by thanking all the staff in teams that have taken part in AMBIT training, turning up for the first day with a coffee in their hand and wondering whether this was going to prove a good idea after all. We would like to show appreciation for those who question us strongly about the approach, who have challenged us about things that we should have known better, and for those who have shared their appreciation with us. To all of you, we hope this book reflects what you have shared with us. And to the wonderful contributors to this book, for demonstrating unambiguously that they have not implemented AMBIT, they have created it; they have taken the starting points and made it their own but also have added ideas that those of us who were here from the beginning would never have thought of. We very much hope this book gives you a sense of this evolving process.

Contributors

Dickon Bevington, University College London
Dickon Bevington, MA MBBS MRCPsych PGCert FRSA, is a child/adolescent psychiatrist with 30 years of experience in the NHS, initially in London and latterly in Cambridgeshire and Peterborough Foundation Trust, where he leads a team for multiply burdened youth with substance use disorders. In London he is Medical Director of the Anna Freud National Centre for Children and Families. With Peter Fuggle he is the co-founder of AMBIT and has published and taught widely on this, mentalizing theory and practice, and on evidence-based approaches to children and young people's mental health. Prior to medicine he studied anthropology and comparative religion.

Dr Chloe Campbell, University College London
Chloe is Deputy Director of the Psychoanalysis Unit, University College London, UK. Her research interests include mentalizing, epistemic trust, and attachment theory. She recently created and validated a new measure of epistemic trust, the Epistemic Trust, Mistrust and Credulity Questionnaire. She is series co-editor, with Dr Liz Allison, of the Anna Freud National Centre for Children and Families/Routledge Best Practice Series. She is particularly interested in pursuing the interdisciplinary implications of recent theoretical developments in the area of epistemic trust, culture, and psychopathology.

Liz Cracknell, Anna Freud National Centre for Children and Families
Liz is the AMBIT Joint Programme Director and a member of the adolescent therapy team at the Anna Freud National Centre for Children and Families, London, and honorary senior research fellow at University College London, UK. A registered mental health nurse and systemic practitioner, she has specialized in working with young people who have multiple needs in both outreach and secure in-reach settings. She has contributed to a number of key publications and the development of AMBIT and has trained and consulted with hundreds of workers in AMBIT in the UK and internationally.

Ernst Dahlquist, Psykolog Centrum
Ernst is a social worker, psychotherapist, and supervisor in psychotherapy and social work in Malmo, Sweden. His main theoretical orientation is psychodynamic, with an additional integration of other perspectives on psychotherapy and social work. Ernst has a background in child and adolescent psychiatric care, and since 2009 he has worked in private practice. During this period, he has also, together with a colleague, built a treatment team with a mentalization-based orientation. This is a private enterprise that receives referrals from the public social services. The team combines social work and psychotherapy and since 2016 it has been AMBIT influenced and supervised by Peter Fuggle.

Dr Mark Dangerfield, Ramon Llull University
Mark has a PhD in psychology and is a clinical psychologist and psychotherapist (European Federation of Psychologists' Associations and the Official College of Psychologists in Spain). He is a psychoanalyst and a member of the Spanish Psychoanalytical Society and the International

Psychoanalytical Association. He is now Director of the Vidal & Barraquer University Institute of Mental Health, Ramon Llull University in Barcelona and was formerly Clinical Manager of the ECID Project, a pioneering project in Spain, where AMBIT-influenced community outreach mental health teams work with non-help-seeking young people. He is also Lead AMBIT and mentalization-based treatment (MBT) for adults trainer and supervisor at the Anna Freud National Centre for Children and Families in London.

Professor Andrea Dlugosch, University of Koblenz-Landau
Andrea studied special education for teaching as well as a diploma in educational sciences and received her doctor's degree in 2002. Since 2013 she has been Professor of Pedagogy for Learning Disabilities and Behavioural Disorders at the University of Koblenz-Landau, Germany. She is an associated member of the MentEd network and completed further trainings in Theme-Centred Interaction (TCI) (diploma 2001, RCI International), AMBIT (Local Facilitator), and in mentalization-based therapy. Her main areas of work are professionalization research, inclusion as a multilevel constellation, mentalization-based pedagogy, and social network research.

James Fairbairn, Anna Freud National Centre for Children and Families
James is a clinical psychologist and AMBIT Lead Trainer based at the Anna Freud National Centre for Children and Families, London, UK. James also works in the NHS in child and adolescent mental health services where he has practised for a number of years in both inpatient and community settings. James is a systemic practitioner and has a particular interest in working with young people and families who have multiple needs, alongside a passion in learning how to support organizations to develop and provide effective help to clients who do not easily use conventional forms of treatment.

Dr Peter Fonagy, Anna Freud National Centre for Children and Families
Peter Fonagy, OBE, is Professor of Contemporary Psychoanalysis and Developmental Science, and Head of Division for Psychology and Language Sciences, University College London; Chief Executive of the Anna Freud National Centre for Children and Families, London; and Director, UCLPartners Mental Health and Wellbeing Programme, London, UK. His clinical and research interests lie in early attachment relationships, social cognition, borderline personality disorder, and violence. A central focus has been an innovative research-based psychodynamic therapeutic approach, MBT, which was developed in collaboration with a number of clinical sites in the UK and the USA. He has published over 630 scientific papers and 21 books.

Dr Peter Fuggle, Anna Freud National Centre for Children and Families
Peter Fuggle, PhD, is a clinical psychologist who has worked in child mental health services for over 30 years. He was clinical director of a community-based mental health service in London for 20 years and became concerned about young people with mental health needs who did not wish to attend mainstream services. His collaboration with Dickon Bevington at the Anna Freud National Centre for Children and Families, London, UK, was a turning point of his career and resulted in the start of the AMBIT programme. His focus now is on community approaches to mental health of which AMBIT plays the main part.

Melanie Henter, University of Koblenz-Landau
Melanie has a diploma in educational science for special educational needs. Since 2016 she has been a research associate at the University of Koblenz-Landau, Institute for Special Education and Pedagogy for Learning Disabilities and Behavioural Disorders, Landau, Germany. She is an associate member of the MentEd network and the AMBIT Study Group. She has trained in

AMBIT (Local Facilitator), MBT, MBT for adults (2017–2022, Anna Freud National Centre for Children and Families, London), as well as systemic counselling and is qualified in using the Reflective Functioning Scale. Her main areas of work are mentalization-based pedagogy and the implementation of AMBIT in youth welfare systems.

Michael Hollenstein, Sigmund Freud Private University
Michael studied psychology and political science in Innsbruck, Austria, and New Orleans, USA, and is a clinical, health and occupational psychologist, supervisor, coach, and organizational developer. He has a leading position at Paedakoop, Vorarlberger Kinderdorf, Bregenz, Austria. He and Beate Huter are joint leads of a team of psychologists, therapists, and social workers doing residential and outreach family work, assessment, and therapy of young people at high risk. He is a lecturer at Sigmund Freud University, Vienna, Austria, and has been trained in AMBIT and MBT for families. He develops and implements AMBIT in Austria together with Beate Huter. Michael is an active member of the AMBIT Study Group at the Anna Freud National Centre for Children and Families, London, UK.

Beate Huter, Sigmund Freud University
Bea is a paediatric nurse, clinical and health psychologist, supervisor, coach, and organizational developer. She is a lecturer at the Sigmund Freud University, Vienna, Austria, and works in private practice and at Vorarlberger Kinderdorf, Bregenz, Austria. She and Michael Hollenstein are joint leads of a team of psychologists, therapists, and social workers doing residential and outreach family work, assessment, and therapy of young people at high risk. Trained in AMBIT, MBT for families, and MBT for children, they implement AMBIT in Austria and try to shift a mentalizing culture across teams and organizations. She is responsible for national and international cooperation, and is a member of the AMBIT Study Group and the Welt der Kinder advisory board.

Stefan Lock Jensen, Roskilde Clinic of Child and Adolescent Psychiatry
Stefan is a clinical psychologist and a specialist in child and adolescent psychiatry. He is manager of an out-patient clinic working with Child and Adolescent Psychiatry in Roskilde, Region Zealand, Denmark. Together with Janne Walløe Vilmar he initiated the first AMBIT teams in Denmark and has been working for over two decades on trying to integrate the organizational and therapeutic aspects of complex psychosocial work. He completed his training in MBT and AMBIT at the Anna Freud National Centre for Children and Families, London, UK, and is a board member of the Danish Institute of Mentalization.

Saskia Knapen, Altrecht Mental Health Institution
Saskia is a psychiatrist and MBT therapist who specializes in severe and complex personality disorders at Altrecht Mental Health Institution, Utrecht, the Netherlands. She introduced the AMBIT method to the Netherlands and implemented five AMBIT-influenced teams who work with severe and complex personality disorders in 2017 as medical director at the Department for Personality Disorders at Altrecht. Together with Rozemarijn van Duursen they deliver a lot of AMBIT training throughout the country and are currently writing a Dutch book on AMBIT. Apart from this, she is a PhD candidate at Amsterdam University Medical Centre working on 'Epistemic trust as a psychomarker for psychosocial interventions'.

Anna Oriol-Sanchez, Vidal i Barraquer Foundation
Anna is a social worker based in Barcelona, Spain, who has worked in public mental health services for several years, focused on early psychosis and supporting educational and social

services in mental health prevention. She is currently leading the ECID in the Fundació Vidal i Barraquer, an outreach AMBIT-influenced team, working since 2017 with non-help-seeking adolescents and their families, with severe mental health problems, and providing consultation to other services helping in working with this cohort. She has been an AMBIT Trainer since 2019 and supervises teams which are using AMBIT local adaptations. She co-leads the international AMBIT Study Group.

Rebecca Smith, Anna Freud National Centre for Children and Families
Rebecca is a Lead Trainer in the AMBIT Team. Prior to this she worked for Wandsworth Local Authority, UK, for 18 years, as a team manager in the Evolve Team (who support young people and young adults impacted by gangs, youth violence, and exploitation), and as a youth offending team practitioner. She came to Wandsworth having trained as a probation officer, with experience of working with adults in the criminal justice system, particularly those convicted of violent offences.

Dr Laura Talbot, Anna Freud National Centre for Children and Families
Laura is the AMBIT Joint Programme Director and a clinical psychologist by background. She has specialized in working with adolescents and young adults in community outreach services across the health, social care, and voluntary sectors. Laura has held clinical lead roles in a number of AMBIT-influenced services, including teams working with young people on the edge of care, those affected by gang involvement, and those at risk of school exclusion.

Rozemarijn van Duursen, Altrecht Mental Health Institution
Rose is a psychiatrist in an AMBIT-influenced outpatient team for people with severe and complex personality disorders and is a member of the suicide evaluation committee. She is involved with the residential psychiatry training at Altrecht Mental Health Institution, Utrecht, the Netherlands. She is also an MBT therapist. Together with Saskia Knapen, she has been crucial to extending the AMBIT approach to working with adults and delivers AMBIT training throughout the Netherlands.

Dr Janne Walløe Vilmar, Roskilde Clinic of Child and Adolescent Psychiatry
Janne is a child and adolescent psychiatrist who works as the chief physician at the child and adolescent psychiatric clinic in Roskilde, Region Zealand, Denmark. She has had 15 years of clinical experience in child and adolescent psychiatric evaluation and treatment mainly with complex disease characterized by emotional and behavioural disorders, personality disorders, schizophrenia, and eating disorders. She is also an associate professor at the University of Copenhagen and is a specialist in psychodynamic therapy, a supervisor in MBT, and an AMBIT Trainer.

James Wheeler, Anna Freud National Centre for Children and Families
James was an outreach and substance misuse worker for many years working with young people in both youth and criminal justice settings. He then moved into leadership and commissioning roles in the local authority and successfully established AMBIT as a cross-agency approach in the London borough of Wandsworth, UK. He also became an AMBIT Lead Trainer, and supported the FCAMHS/Secure Stairs evaluation which led to the development and piloting of a peer mentoring programme with local youth charities. He is now in the process of completing his training in clinical psychology in Scotland.

Abbreviations

A&E	accident and emergency
ADHD	attention deficit hyperactivity disorder
AIM	AMBIT Integrative Measure
AMASS	Adolescent Multi-Agency Support Service
AMBIT	Adaptive Mentalization-Based Integrative Treatment
ARE	adverse relational experience
ASEQ	AMBIT Service Evaluation Questionnaire
BUP	Barn- och Ungdomspsykiatri (Child and Adolescent Psychiatry)
CAMHS	Child and Adolescent Mental Health Services
COVID-19	coronavirus disease 2019
CYSS	Child and Youth Social Services
ECID	Equipo Clínico de Intervención a Domicilio (Home Intervention Clinical Team)
EDI	equity, diversity, and inclusion
FACT	Functional Assertive Community Treatment
GP	general practitioner
MBT	mentalization-based treatment
MCM	mentalizing case manager
NET-Aim-Q	NET-Aim-Questionnaire
VBM	value-based management

1
Why has AMBIT come about?

Laura Talbot and Peter Fuggle

1.1 Introduction

Welcome to our second book about Adaptive Mentalization-Based Integrative Treatment, AMBIT for short. AMBIT is a mentalization-based approach designed to support teams who work with young people and adults with multiple needs who find help hard to trust. We use the term 'multiple needs' to describe clients who are simultaneously experiencing difficulties in a number of areas of life, including with their mental health, family relationships, peer relationships, educational or vocational experiences, exposure to criminality, exploitation or discrimination, their use of substances, and/or stressors connected to their socioeconomic status. The approach was first developed at the Anna Freud Centre in London. At the heart of AMBIT is the intention to help teams and workers design and deliver the best help that they can for a group of clients who are often in the greatest need, but, in our view, helped the least by our existing ways of practising. Over the past 15 years, the approach has attracted considerable interest from teams from a range of sectors both in the UK and across the world, in Europe, Australia, and the USA.

Why have we written this book? In 2017, we published the first AMBIT book (Bevington et al., 2017), which was a comprehensive guide to AMBIT, outlining all of the core principles, methods, and tools of the approach. In this second book, our main intention is to share what AMBIT looks like in practice. We are honoured to be able to include chapters written by members of several different AMBIT-influenced teams, who have shared accounts of their work that are very much grounded in the realities of doing this complex work. Other chapters are authored by members of the AMBIT team in London and focus on key aspects of the model that have developed further since 2017.

In this first chapter, we will set the scene as to why we think an approach like AMBIT is needed. We have developed and adapted our ideas over many years, by paying very close attention to the experiences of the hundreds of teams we have trained. This training and the subsequent supervision and ongoing relationships with these teams have radically shaped our approach. Before we undertake a training, we explicitly ask frontline workers, managers, and commissioners what makes their work hard, what it feels like, and what they need to do it better. We do this for a whole day and gain a powerful snapshot of their lived experience at work. From this process, we have learned a huge amount about the shared issues, preoccupations, and challenges that teams in this field face and are valiantly trying to overcome to do their work well.

The feedback from teams is surprisingly consistent, whether we are talking to a social care team, a mental health team, a youth justice team, a team supporting adults who are homeless, or a team at a residential children's home, and we have organized our learning from this feedback into four overarching themes. In some ways these themes are so familiar to those who do this work that we are reminded of the story of the fish who, when asked to describe what water is like, replied, 'What is water?' In the same way that the nature of water has determined why fish are the way they are, so it is with this work: unless we describe the themes that describe the conditions in which teams work, you, the reader, will not understand why AMBIT is the way it is. The four themes are:

1. Clients of these teams have *multiple needs* that interact with each other in complex and reciprocal ways, rather than being a series of separate problems. These needs are unlikely to fall within the skill set of any one practitioner, often have long-term roots, and, despite the interventions offered, may well endure for a long time into the future.

2. Our helping services are primarily organized into teams that each specialize in helping with a specific need (e.g. an eating disorder, domestic violence). Workers in such teams commonly provide relatively short-term forms of help, targeted at the specific problem they are trained (and commissioned) to help with. For clients with multiple, interconnected, long-term needs, this often results in having *multiple teams and 'helpers'* involved simultaneously but for relatively short periods of time. These different workers offer different interventions that often run in a parallel, rather than an integrated, way.

3. Having multiple needs and multiple helpers makes it more difficult to provide the client with a satisfactory experience of help. Being offered multiple forms of specialized help may be a confusing, contradictory, and overwhelming experience for the client because it does not necessarily take account of how their different needs fit together or their ideas about what would help. Having multiple needs and multiple helpers requires greater attention to be paid to the basic helping process (i.e. the way that the help is delivered). It is often the lack of an *individualized approach to the helping process* that results in clients experiencing the help they are offered as aversive.

4. Helping clients with multiple needs can be very rewarding but often takes place within an emotive and highly stressful context. Helping requires the worker to retain a balanced and reflective state of mind, but this is often undermined by both the complexity of the client's needs and the difficulties of interventions involving multiple helpers. The importance of the *helper's state of mind* to the helping process is not unique to working with clients with multiple needs, but, because of the significant emotional impact of the work in these contexts, it

requires significantly more attention. Effective help will be achieved only if the state of mind of both the client and the helper is properly attended to.

These themes present major challenges to frontline services and are usually, in our view, insufficiently addressed. They have a profound influence on why AMBIT is organized the way it is if it is to be helpful to workers and their clients.

1.2 Many clients have multiple needs

Let us begin with two case examples to clarify the important differences that we see as existing between clients with single difficulties and those with multiple needs. Erica, who is 14 years old, is developing eating problems (disruption of mealtimes and anxiety about weight loss) but has a generally good relationship with her parents and attends school. She lives with her mother and stepfather and, although her relationship with her parents is currently strained by her eating problems, the relationships in the family are caring and positive. Unknown to her parents, she has experimented with bulimic vomiting but did not like it. She believes her difficulties began at the time of her parents' separation 3 years ago. As with many eating problems, Erica's difficulties are multifaceted, involving her eating behaviour, relationships, and her emerging sense of identity. But the complexity is linked together in a way that is familiar and supported by research and practice, so the sort of help that she needs can be provided by a single team or service.

Compare this to a scenario with another 14-year-old young person. Ashley has emerging eating difficulties, is experimenting with bulimic vomiting, and has high anxiety about body image, but this problem is part of a wider set of more severe life difficulties. Although her eating difficulties are in some ways similar to Erica's, Ashley's overall distress is greatly exacerbated by how they interact with many other parts of her life. Ashley has never liked school and her attendance has been irregular for over a year, which is resulting in tensions and rows at home. Ashley increasingly finds it hard to keep up with her schoolwork and often loses her temper with teachers, especially when she has not eaten. She does not have a large friendship group but does have two good friends; however, they are not always in the same class and she becomes more anxious and self-conscious when she is alone at school. She spends a lot of time at home on social media, comparing herself to other girls her own age and talking to older boys. Her relationship with her parents is volatile and their rows are followed by silence rather than emotional repair. She has gone missing overnight from home on many occasions after family arguments and her parents are not sure where she goes, leading to some concerns that she is at risk of sexual exploitation. To address Ashley's needs, a range of different agencies, including social care, her school, the local youth work team, and Child and Adolescent Mental Health Services (CAMHS), have become involved. No one service can address this set of needs alone.

Rather than young people like Ashley being the exception, it turns out that young people with multiple problems are much more common than is often recognized. A large number of clients and families who use a combination of health, social care, voluntary sector, and educational systems fit into this category. For children and young people, the presence of multiple problems is particularly common. In a major study of 96,325 children and young people referred to CAMHS in the UK between 2011 and 2015, at least 51% presented with mental health problems that were related to life circumstances, particularly family relationship difficulties (52%) and peer relationship difficulties (48%) (Wolpert et al., 2016). The National Institute for Health and Care Excellence (2021) states that a significant proportion of looked-after children have mental health difficulties, and the Timpson Review of School Exclusion (2019) found that children with mental health needs and special educational needs were more likely to be excluded than children without such needs. These figures become even more compelling with respect to young people who are known to juvenile justice services. In one study, 70.4% of young people in such services met criteria for at least one mental health disorder (Shufelt & Cocozza, 2006). A similar picture of highly elevated rates of mental health problems (34%) emerges for non-heterosexual young people, young people who report being bullied (59%), and young people who are seen by substance use services, over half of which report very high levels of mental health needs in their clients (Cochran et al., 2007; Merikangas et al., 1998). It is likely that a large proportion of children and young people with mental health problems have other co-occurring needs (e.g. being bullied) that may require the involvement of other agencies and services.

Research reveals a similar picture for adults. A report by the charitable foundation Lankelly Chase estimated that there are around 5.3 million adults in the UK—approximately 11% of the adult population—with multiple needs (Bramley et al., 2015). Adults with multiple needs are distinguished from those with single problems by the presence of family difficulties (including a background of childhood trauma), social needs, mental health difficulties, poverty, and loneliness. The report concludes by questioning the usefulness of services focused on single problems (e.g. homelessness, offending, substance use). Even looking at health needs alone, in the UK, 25% of the population have two or more long-term conditions, which often require treatment from separate healthcare teams (Barnett et al., 2012; Taskforce on Multiple Conditions, 2019). We think the evidence is clear that clients with multiple needs are not a small minority but constitute a major proportion of the clients served by all health and social care agencies.

1.2.1 Problems are often highly interconnected

As we set out, Ashley can be described as having multiple problems: difficulties with eating, with going to school, with her family relationships, and potentially starting to be at risk in the community. Ashley does not experience these problems separately, but all together; she feels her life is a mess, she can't work things out, and at times the distress overwhelms her. Is it helpful for Ashley's problems to be seen as separate problems, or not? In one sense, they clearly are separate as they arise in different contexts of Ashley's life and what may be helpful in addressing these different needs may appear to be quite different. Making sense of her difficulties in school may focus on different parts of her life from trying to understand her eating difficulties. However, at the same time, the problems intersect with each other. The stress Ashley experiences when things go badly at school exacerbates her eating problems and, on days when she eats less, she is more irritable and struggles to concentrate in school. The connection between these problems rests in Ashley's lived experience and not in the nature of the problems per se. In her mind, she feels that her parents (particularly her father) are very critical of her. She thinks that she has disappointed them and they have never understood her. Feelings rapidly erupt in rows at home about her eating and her life at school. Because the family had moved around during her earlier life, Ashley changed schools frequently and never established a settled peer group at school. She feels that her parents have come to believe that *she* is the problem. In her mind, her difficulties are all of a piece. Life is too much, the demands are impossible; she moves between hating other people and desperately wanting to please them. She wishes all those helping people would just go away.

Some of the interrelations between these sorts of problems are well established in both research and practitioner experience. For example, the social determinants of mental health difficulties in children and young people (Alegria et al., 2018; Allen et al., 2014) are now clear, so it should not be a surprise that clients with a high frequency of social, economic, vocational, and forensic difficulties are experiencing mental health problems as well. For some mental health problems, such as eating disorders, these interconnections have been even more clearly specified. In the case of Erica and her family, her eating problems can be viewed through a well-researched understanding of how eating difficulties are often highly associated with family relationship difficulties. The interconnections between these different problems are well understood by eating disorder practitioners, and methods of help have been developed to address these interconnections. For Ashley, the situation is not so clear. Although in Ashley's experience her problems are all interlinked, there is no research and practice model that addresses her eating difficulties, possible family breakdown, and educational and school problems in the way that exists for Erica's type of difficulties. For Ashley, an understanding of the way her problems are linked together (and ideas about what might help) needs to be developed in conjunction with the workers in the helping system around her. Because of this, clients with multiple needs are usually offered multiple forms of help as a way of meeting their needs. Although this makes sense on one level, it can pose its own challenges, as we will discuss in the next section.

1.3 Multiple needs attract multiple helpers

Practitioners routinely convey to us that very often their clients have some needs that they are not trained to address. Whether the practitioners in question are therapists, social workers, or youth workers, many of these additional problems make it hard for them to do their job. Problems other than the one they are expected to focus on are often uppermost in the minds of their clients, which can leave workers feeling de-skilled, frustrated, or unsure how to best help. A common response to this situation can be for workers to enlist more help by making referrals to other services in an attempt to meet the client's full range of needs.

To explore how this looks in practice, let us return to the example of Ashley. The staff at Ashley's school first became worried about her eating and her weight, and made a referral to CAMHS. The therapist who undertook the initial assessment with Ashley's parents was concerned about some of the other issues that they spoke about, particularly the episodes of Ashley going missing, and made a referral to children's social care. The social worker suggested involving a youth worker to talk to Ashley about the risks of going missing (and possible sexual exploitation) as well as for the school staff to take on a more assertive role with Ashley in trying to help with her attendance, behaviour, and friendship problems. The school put in place regular meetings with the head of year and mentoring from the school's behaviour specialist. Although these workers and services were clearly relevant to Ashley's needs, Ashley and her parents felt overwhelmed by the involvement of social care, CAMHS, youth work, and school staff. Ashley found the demands of creating relationships with multiple workers too much and often avoided the multiple weekly meetings that were required, apart from those with Jason, her social worker, who she quite liked. Jason, however, was stressed about Ashley missing appointments with other professionals, as he did not feel equipped to help with issues like eating and school problems. Ideally, he would have liked help from CAMHS to address some of the family relationship difficulties, which he felt were beyond the limits of his usual parenting intervention skills. He was often contacted by the other workers with their worries and concerns about Ashley, which he found hard to keep up with.

Let us contrast this with the situation for Erica. Erica was prepared (albeit reluctantly) to attend her general practitioner (GP) with her mother to discuss her eating problems. Even though she went to the appointment, Erica did not really feel that she needed any help and believed the problem was exaggerated in the minds of other people. Nonetheless, she accepted a referral to the local eating disorder team, which managed to engage her in early prevention work to avoid her eating problems becoming more severe. The impact of the eating problems on other areas of her life was modest, and the eating disorder team was familiar with these issues and was set up to have the skills and experience to manage the interconnecting aspects of her problems. Because the team had a sense of competence around these matters, they did not require another team or agency to be involved in their work with her. For Erica, this specialist, well-targeted form of help worked well. It was reliant on the family having sufficient trust in the helping system to overcome their anxiety (and perhaps shame) about seeking help for the problems they were experiencing. Their relationship with Erica functioned sufficiently well for her to be positively influenced by this. Comparing these two scenarios, AMBIT has been developed to try to be helpful to young people like Ashley and has much less to say about how to be helpful to those like Erica, for whom we believe current services are often well designed.

These issues also affect adults and can become even more complex when the adult is a parent. Here, the needs of each family member have a reciprocal impact on each other, such that both the parent and the young person can be seen as having multiple and often interacting needs. These needs usually attract the attention of different types of helpers from both young people's and adult services, between which there is traditionally even less join-up. Let us introduce another example to explore this.

Alice (35 years old) is a single parent and is stressed about paying the rent, worried about her son Lucas (12 years old), who is being very challenging and uncooperative, and has recently discovered her own mother is having significant memory losses. Her ex-partner (Lucas's father), who was violent towards her, has recently been released from prison. There is now an order in place preventing him from having contact with Alice and Lucas, and a police officer has been assigned to Alice to oversee this. Lucas is angry with Alice, as he misses his father and blames Alice for not being able to see him. Every week, Alice has to deal with the housing office, Lucas's school, a family support worker, the police, and her mother's medical team. She has also been referred to a domestic violence worker, but has not been returning the worker's calls, as she feels that these issues were in the past and do not need to be thought about now. Alice is just about managing to continue working in her job as she has a sympathetic manager who has allowed some flexibility with her hours.

Alice, overwhelmed by the accumulating problems, went to her GP complaining of low mood, and was offered medication and psychological therapy for depression. However, she remains stressed by each of her problems, as the help for low mood did not (and of course could not) explicitly address them. Clearly, each of her problems requires different solutions but, for Alice (like Ashley), her capacity to receive (and give) help in relation to each of these problems was hugely affected by the impact of the other problems on her. So, for example, budgeting advice to help sort out the rent arrears might have been sensible in general but was unhelpful to Alice when she was faced with the additional costs of making sure that her mother was properly looked after. Advice from the family support worker to spend more time doing positive activities with Lucas to help repair their relationship made sense, but was hard to put into practice when Lucas generally refused to talk to her and Alice was feeling low. Alice's (and, we might imagine, Lucas's) problems were highly interconnected but each of the different teams and services involved with them focused on only one part of the problem, and this separation was increasingly not helpful to Alice.

The recognition that multiple needs can commonly lead to the involvement of multiple helpers is key, because we propose that some of the difficulties that arise when working with this client group are as much about the complexity in how the helping system is organized as the complexity arising from the multiple needs themselves. This view has been proposed by Malvaso et al. (2016, p. 129), who define complex needs among youth as 'situations where young people are burdened by multiple and co-occurring problems', problems that may be related to mental health issues, and/or social problems that often lead to multiple forms of assistance. Similarly, Ungar et al. (2014) use the categorization 'multiple service-using youth' interchangeably with 'youth with complex needs'. These themes have been recognized and highlighted in the UK by the prominence of the role of integrated care planning in 'The NHS Long Term Plan', which made this one of the central challenges for innovation and development of new healthcare models (NHS, 2019).

1.3.1 Collaboration between agencies is hard to achieve

Although workers in different services have the best intentions and know the benefits that collaboration between services would bring for clients like Ashley, Alice, and Lucas, we repeatedly hear from these workers how difficult it can be to achieve collaboration between the services in their locality, irrespective of the service to which they belong. When clients find it difficult to make use of the help offered to them, we believe that this should not be solely attributed to their personal history, but also seen as reflecting the less-than-ideal way in which help is offered when such *difficulties in professional collaboration* exist. Workers frequently voice their experience of feeling misunderstood or being blamed by workers from other teams, suggesting that trust between services is not easy to establish or maintain. This kind of behaviour between professionals has been termed 'finger pointing' by Pavkov et al. (2012), who attribute it to an understandable inclination for services to protect their own interests. We notice that workers can readily identify examples of this being done to them, but do not always show awareness or acknowledgement of their tendency to apportion blame to others or how they might contribute to perpetuating inaccurate beliefs about other services. In AMBIT we refer to this as 'dis-integration', a seemingly universal and inevitable experience, which simply recognizes that integrating help across agencies remains a perennial rather than unique challenge. This recognition is the first step in addressing the issue, as without a foundation of trust and respect between services, and sufficient time afforded to developing this, we know that these difficulties play out repeatedly to the detriment of clients.

So, how does this lack of collaboration play out for Alice and Lucas? For Alice, some of the solutions she is offered directly conflict with other solutions. For example, the school's suggestion for Alice to use a system of rewards and consequences to manage Lucas's behaviour is at odds with both the family support worker's plan (that Alice should first focus on rebuilding trust and connection with Lucas) and the police's advice (that Lucas is likely to be stirred up at this time of his father's release from prison, so Alice should just give him some space). As well as resulting in confusing or contradictory experiences for Alice and Lucas, the professionals find themselves becoming increasingly frustrated with each other because they experience their attempts to help as being undermined and thwarted by others in the network.

Of course, multiple forms of specialist help *can* work alongside each other well, but this requires the recognition that, in the same way that multiple problems interact with each other, so do multiple forms of help. The challenge for services is to ensure that they are supporting this to happen in a way that brings different forms of help together in a complementary and integrated way. As we frequently see, hear, and experience ourselves, achieving this is not always an easy process.

1.3.2 Involving multiple services does not necessarily mean better help

Having an array of helping services is not automatically of benefit to clients with multiple needs. Workers themselves often say that working where there are multiple services available can sometimes make it more complicated to work out how best to help clients, rather than making it easier. Workers describe feeling under pressure to make the best use of the different services on offer, resulting in multiple referrals to ensure that their clients' needs are met by the most specialist team possible, while being simultaneously aware that this can create duplication and become unmanageable for clients. Although such plans may look comprehensive on paper (and may be welcomed by clients who are able to manage multiple helping relationships), this is often not the experience for clients with multiple needs, especially those who may be more ambivalent about seeking help and less trusting of professionals.

Furthermore, having a number of different services in a particular locality can make it difficult for workers to keep up to date with what each service does. Workers frequently tell us that other teams don't know what they do, and they don't really know what other teams do, resulting in referrals between teams that are not always appropriate, which can be disappointing and frustrating for clients and workers alike. Even where the input of a particular service may be relevant, these services are often under pressure due to high demand, which exacerbates the tendency for clients to be passed back and forth between agencies. In these situations, it can be common for different services to frame different aspects of the client's problems as being the 'main problem', to try to get another service to take on responsibility for providing help, rather than their own. This often generates significant ill feeling, undermining not only the client's experience of help but also the relationships between teams themselves, which creates further barriers to collaboration.

For some readers, it may appear that we are being overly negative or pessimistic about the potential of joint agency collaboration to produce effective help. We understand this and are aware of many superb practitioners who do brilliantly coordinated multiagency work. We understand that people might be reading this and thinking 'Is it really as bad as this?' It does seem as though it *should* all work well in practice, because there are often a number of great individual parts (i.e. workers, teams), but these do not always work well together as a whole. Part of what may prevent us from attending to the 'whole' is that professional training in general focuses on equipping us to deliver our particular form of individual help to clients, not the *collective help* that we are proposing is needed for this group of clients. As a result, we just keep changing and improving the individual parts within the system and hoping for the best, rather than giving as much attention to how the system as a whole is working. The pervasiveness of these problems is powerfully conveyed to us by the teams we work with both in the UK and in other countries. One of the major arguments set out in this book is that these difficulties are intrinsic to our helping systems and often profoundly reduce the effectiveness of well-tested interventions to improve clients' life problems.

1.3.3 The limitations of service redesign in addressing these problems

One common response to the problems we have highlighted is for service planners to propose service redesigns that increase the likelihood of greater collaboration between workers. In our view, we do not believe that the problem of how to help clients like Ashley, Alice, and Lucas can be effectively addressed by service redesign alone, because multiple needs like theirs emerge in so many combinations, and collaboration between workers will still be needed. If we take Ashley and her helpers as an example, the challenge is how to enable the frontline practitioners to provide effective help for Ashley that addresses all of her needs in a way that feels manageable for her, while respecting and making best use of the important different perspectives and skills of the agencies involved in helping her. AMBIT is *not* advocating reorganizing the system so that there is only one team for young people with the sort of difficulties Ashley is having. We propose that Ashley's multiple problems are best addressed by strengthening the quality of the relationships between her and the practitioners, and the relationships between these practitioners and their respective colleagues both within their own teams and with colleagues in other agencies. This is what we mean by a 'relational approach', and the complexity and severity of the challenges that this presents are why it takes a whole book to show how this may work in practice!

1.4 The helping process is crucial

To explain what we mean by the 'helping process', let us again begin with an example. In one of the early projects before AMBIT was established, a team was created to work with young people with multiple problems with the explicit aim of reducing the number of professionals involved with a group of families with multiple needs. Each family had one main worker who visited them twice a week. One family was allocated to Paul, who was a social worker by training. He engaged well with Sam, a 12-year-old boy who was currently out of school and not attending the specialist education centre where he was on roll. Sam wanted to go back to school but wanted help from Paul with reading before he did, because he felt embarrassed by how far he had fallen behind.

Paul did not feel competent to do this and initially tried to persuade Sam to accept some help from a home tutor, but Sam refused. Rather than this becoming an impasse, Paul organized supervision for himself from the home tutor so that he could learn about how best to practise reading with Paul as part of his twice-weekly home visits. This lasted only a few weeks and Sam, with Paul's support, soon started going back to school a few days each week. We learned subsequently that it had meant a lot to Sam that Paul had changed his behaviour in response to Sam's request. The team reflected that this had probably increased Sam's trust in Paul and that it was this (perhaps more than the reading practice itself) that had enabled Sam to move forward with going to school. We see this as an example of how a practitioner attended more to the helping process (by responding to what the client asked for and how he wanted to be helped) than the specific problems he was having. It was easier for Sam to accept help for his reading from someone he trusted, rather than someone who was an expert in reading.

This small but crucial shift in practice has enormous implications for how we think about offering help. The system of services that is generally in place is based on the idea of connecting the person with the problem to the person with the greatest expertise about such a problem. The underlying belief is that expertise is the crucial component of effective help. This clearly makes sense in many areas of human life. If I am anxious about my tax returns, I seek out someone who knows about tax and then gauge whether I can trust that person's advice. The expertise is the primary criterion. However, for those who have a fragile relationship to help (or, by analogy, an anxious relationship to the tax authorities), the primary criterion may be that it is more important that the advice comes from someone they trust. In situations where the helping process is fragile, trust overrides expertise, and we have learned that this is the case for the population of clients AMBIT is designed to help. But expertise matters too. The challenge is how to funnel this expertise into relationships of trust. The practical implications (and potential disruption) of existing systems cannot be overestimated. In the example above, Paul adapted his approach to take account of Sam's preferences about how he wanted help with his reading, but this adaptation created anxiety for Paul ('I don't know how to do this'). Our suggestion is that the relevant knowledge ('how to do this') can be shared with Paul so that he can be *sufficiently* helpful to Sam, particularly in the early stages of help. We know how difficult it is to implement this in practice, as the context in which most teams work does not easily support this sort of practice.

1.4.1 The fragility of the helping process

Asking for help and offering help is a fragile process for all of us. This has been well described by Edgar Schein, who emphasized the vulnerabilities it evokes and how easy it is for things to go wrong (Schein, 2009). In Schein's approach, this fragility arises for many reasons but crucially from the failure to attend sufficiently to the vulnerability and loss of status of the 'helped' person. He proposes that effective help takes place when the helper and the helped achieve a degree of equitable status in their work together. He also suggests that anxiety is intrinsic to the process of help seeking, that this cannot be entirely eradicated by the skill of the helper, and that it is best addressed by enabling the anxiety to be jointly acknowledged by both parties. Schein's work also illustrates that too much help can be ineffective and aversive to the helped; the skill is in how the helper facilitates, rather than leads, the process, which he calls 'humble inquiry'. Interestingly, Schein also highlights that the capacity of the helper to demonstrate their own capacity to *accept* help is often highly significant in developing an effective helper–helped relationship. Creating conditions of safety for the helping process is particularly challenging for those in positions of power-lessness, disadvantage, or despair. Common vulnerabilities are easily exacerbated in such conditions and become major barriers to enabling others to provide support for change.

Going back to the example of Sam, Paul modelled the process of help-seeking by acknowledging to Sam his own need for support with the task of teaching reading and sourcing appropriate help with it, which he then used to help Sam. This prevented Paul from having to simply refer Sam on to home tuition; in all likelihood, Sam would have rejected tutoring, which in turn would have posed a major barrier to his return to education. We recognize that this approach took place as part of a highly experimental service that was explicitly set up to try out new methods of working, and that having such flexibility around roles may not always be commonplace. Providing help is not always the predictable, neat, and linear process that we might wish it to be; it is messy, uncertain, and easily undermined by a range of factors. In our view, services often are unable to sufficiently adapt the helping process in the way that we have illustrated here. Because of this, workers are at greater risk of being experienced by their clients as being unhelpful.

1.4.2   The role of attachment theory

Attachment theory provides a rich description of the helping process in early life where a fundamental developmental achievement for children is to learn and discover who they can—and who they cannot—seek help from. This profound process of learning provides the bedrock for helping patterns in later life, giving rise to ideas about the degree to which others can be helpful, comforting, and validating or whether they are humiliating, shaming, and hurtful. We also know from attachment research that help is successful when it is *contingent* to need (i.e. that the child experiences their carers as being responsive to their distress). In our experience, there is a group of clients and families who have profound sensitivities to engaging in a helping process because of their early relational experiences, out of which a stance of *adaptive mistrust* towards others has often developed. In this context, there is an even greater need for any help offered to be experienced as contingent, particularly in the early stages of relationship building. But this is easier said than done.

In the example with Ashley, her social worker Jason has arranged a meeting with Ashley's parents to think about how they can avoid the way rows with Ashley escalate out of control for all of them. This meeting has taken a long time to set up and both parents have taken time off work to be present. Ashley knows that this is happening as a first step and that this meeting will be followed by another meeting, which will include her. In the week of the meeting, the parents have received a letter from Ashley's school raising concerns about her attendance record. The parents believe that they may be vulnerable to being fined for her poor attendance and are angry and upset. Jason's careful efforts to provide a context for focusing on their relationship with Ashley has been disrupted by the letter. He cannot help feeling that it is not his job to deal with this, and feels frustrated and angry, but for different reasons from the parents. In our experience, this type of situation happens a lot. It is very difficult for Jason to know what to do. Does he change the focus of the meeting to the letter from the school, knowing that this is not his area of expertise; or does he continue with the original plan? For the parents, it is extremely easy for them to experience Jason as not being able to help them with what they are most worried about now, and that his interest is non-contingent with their current feelings and anxiety. This also results in Jason feeling a bit useless. Rather than the meeting developing a sense of engagement and trust, the parents feel frustrated and generalize their view of Jason to all social workers—that they are not helpful and do not know what they are doing. The meeting is characterized by high emotion and little focus. To offer contingent help, Jason needs to recognize the parents' state of mind and to demonstrate by his behaviour that he takes it seriously. Developing methods of addressing this kind of problem (without abandoning the plan of work entirely) is very much part of the AMBIT approach.

This perhaps familiar description of the problems of establishing an effective helping process arises out of the combination of the vulnerabilities that clients bring to the process alongside professional fragmentation in relation to providing help. As is the case with Jason, this may reduce the capacity of the worker to demonstrate helping behaviours consistent with evidence from attachment research. As in the example with Jason and Ashley's parents, the key is for the worker to attend to what the client sees as helpful *at that time* and not what the worker thinks they should be focusing on because of their expertise or preference. This is not easy in practice when there are multiple needs and multiple workers. As in this example, either the wrong worker is available for the wrong problem or the involvement of other services inhibits the worker from responding to what they see in front of them, as they believe that this is best dealt with by someone else with more expertise. These disruptions cannot be entirely avoided, but they highlight why trust is so central to effective help. If a client has had previous experience of being helped by a worker, or they feel that their frustrations are being recognized (mentalized) rather than defensively avoided, then this may enable the disruption to be repaired. In fact, as we shall see from many examples in this book, it may provide an opportunity for the client to feel understood about their experience of the fragmentation of help that clients like Ashley—and Alice and Lucas—commonly encounter.

1.5   The worker's state of mind is fundamental to help

One of the major themes that comes up in AMBIT training is the level of strong emotion that many practitioners experience in their work and the need for more attention to be paid to this. We routinely ask teams about the feelings the work brings up for them and they have no difficulty in generating a long list. Workers commonly report that they feel stressed, overwhelmed, frustrated, burdened, worried, misunderstood, doubtful of their own effectiveness, and hopeless at times. This enquiry has proved to have high resonance with the teams, as they are easily able to link these feelings to their experience of a range of different aspects of their work. Crucially, these feelings do not just arise in relation to their client work (as is sometimes too easily assumed) but are also felt in their interactions with their own team and members of their professional network. Teams and workers also tell us that they need a place within their work to share, reflect upon, and get help with the emotional impact of their work. They do not always feel that the culture and processes in their team support this. We have come to consider the absence of attention to the states of mind of frontline practitioners to be one of the key challenges faced by practitioners. The recognition of this is absolutely critical because it can very easily begin to negatively affect not just a worker's own emotional well-being but also their ability to help clients and collaborate effectively with colleagues.

In situations when these affect-laden states of mind are very prevalent, it is very easy for workers to fall into procedural methods of working that disregard or are insensitive to the beliefs, wishes, attitudes, and plans of others, including the client. In the AMBIT programme, we have become very interested in how processes of help (usually unintentionally) lose connection with the state of mind of the client or family. We see this as arising from a lack of attention being paid to the state of mind of the worker, for whom retaining a curious, open-minded, and flexible stance in their work becomes a tall order when they are repeatedly exposed to risk, uncertainty, pressure, and stress in a context of very limited support. We call this a *non-mentalizing* helping system. These systems tend to have several recognizable features.

1. *Lack of trust.* Clients and families may not trust that the worker is safe or reliable, or that the worker is motivated to be helpful. The worker may be distrustful about whether the client or family is committed to the intervention and wants to achieve change. Workers may not sufficiently trust their own team, which acts as a barrier to establishing mutual helping processes. Distrust between teams within the network may be high.
2. *A lack of making sense of behaviour.* The predominant focus is on action or plans and targeting behaviour, rather than exploring and addressing what might be underlying the behaviour (i.e. not making sense of behaviour by considering what is going in the minds and lives of those engaging in the behaviour). This applies equally to the behaviour of all players in the system, whether they are a client, team colleague, or member of the multiagency network.

3. *Loss of narrative continuity.* Problems are seen only in the current context and there is a lack of understanding of the chronology. There is a loss of understanding of the story of the client, which may have unhelpful consequences for interventions or decision-making, which could ultimately mean that help of a particular nature is not offered when it might be useful. Repeated attempts are made to help with the same issues despite lack of change, or the help is persisted with for too long without taking more definitive action (e.g. in situations of abuse/neglect).

4. *Not holding the balance between perspectives when designing help.* What is offered is driven by the workers'/system's ideas about what is helpful rather than ideas co-created with the client. There is a lack of attention to and curiosity about the client's state of mind. This can lead to plans being made on the basis of apparent certainties that have not been checked out with the client. Alternatively, there may be an insufficient balance in holding perspectives within a family, for example, being too focused on the adults' needs at the expense of the needs of the children in safeguarding contexts.

5. *Problems with planning.* The work is characterized by frequent changes of plans. Workers may not have confidence in the help they are offering and frequently change plans about how to help the client. This may be mirrored by the client, for example, by changing the focus of what they want help with at each appointment offered. The work may involve too little or no planning but lots of activity. Everyone is busy and often expresses that there is not enough time to think. Actual contacts with the client may be experienced as not being purposeful or collaborative.

These are not the only non-mentalizing patterns that may be experienced; they are presented as illustrations of the difficulties that commonly occur. AMBIT has been developed because these problems are due to complex systemic conditions that make it very difficult for workers and clients to hold a mentalizing and balanced position. It is, as described so meticulously in Chapter 3, the working context that easily overwhelms efforts to both hold a mentalizing stance and create conditions that facilitate trust between clients and colleagues. But, in our experience, it does not need to be like this. The whole purpose of AMBIT is to make sense of these difficulties and the behaviours they give rise to. This book will provide many methods and examples that enable a balanced, non-procedural approach to be retained that nurtures the possibility of trust between all those involved in the fragile process of helping.

1.6 Conclusion

At this point we appreciate that our summary of the difficulties of providing effective help for clients with multiple problems and with multiple helpers may not make for comfortable reading. As we have consistently emphasized, this is not a story that is critical of the individual workers who do this tremendously important and challenging work, but it reflects a problem of the whole system. One of the biggest benefits for us in the AMBIT programme has been the opportunity and honour of working with teams of workers who are inspiring in their determination to make things better for their clients.

In this first chapter, we have described that, although many clients and families are effectively helped through the current design and delivery of professional services, there is a significant group of clients and families with multiple needs, and who are involved with multiple helping agencies, for whom the current design of services works poorly. The size of this problem was highlighted in a UK NHS policy statement about integrated care, which stated that 'the patient's perspective should be at the heart of any discussion about their care. Achieving integrated care requires those involved with planning and providing services to impose the patient perspective as the organizing principle of service delivery' (Shaw et al., 2011, p. 7). This is a powerful call to arms that few would argue against, but many are unsure how to achieve.

To address these challenges, AMBIT sets out not to design a new therapy but to create an approach that has been designed to address the challenges presented here. The basic constituent of effective practice is a recognition that states of mind matter and influence behaviour. Supporting constructive states of mind cannot be achieved by individual practitioners on their own and can be achieved only by being part of a well-connected team. This team needs to have a strong multiagency approach to its work and to place the helping process at the heart of the endeavour. These are the building blocks of the approach. We are in no doubt about the scale of the challenge in doing this. It requires explicit team methods, values, and practices that effectively support practitioners in this difficult work. It advocates the need for a level of flexible practice that often places practitioners outside their usual area of expertise and competence. These are high requirements, but AMBIT sets out to support the ability of teams to work in this way. We are optimistic that the experience of help can be radically improved, and in the chapters that follow we will provide many examples of how this is being done by teams using the AMBIT approach.

1.7 The plan for the book

Our aim in this book is to go beyond a basic description of the AMBIT approach, to bring the work to life; to enable you, the reader, to see what it looks like in practice; to understand the systemic problems it is trying to address; to see how it is has been adapted in different service settings; to share what we have learned about what has worked, and what has not; and to introduce you to some of the remarkable AMBIT practitioners and their clients along the way.

The authors who have come together to produce this book bring a range of unique perspectives. In keeping with the many possibilities of mentalizing, the chapters will move between emphasizing feelings and thinking, between considering the perspective of the client and that of the worker, between the abstract and the concrete, and between the managerial and the relational. Some authors will bring a philosophical perspective, and others will focus on the science of what AMBIT is about. There will be perspectives from educationalists, service leaders, therapists, social workers, youth workers, parents, and young people. As one of our authors helpfully reminds us, we cannot entirely tidy up the mess because the unpredictable intersectionality of people's lives is what AMBIT aims to embrace. But we will do our best and tidy up where we can. Throughout, we will call those who do the work 'workers' or 'practitioners' to emphasize that much of the challenges of this work are shared rather than unique to one profession, discipline, or level of experience. Each chapter will begin with a section called 'Setting the scene', written by the editors, in which the content of the chapter will be linked to other parts of the book, and will finish with a section called 'Implications', where we will try to draw out some key learning points that apply to AMBIT in general. We hope that, despite the diversity and lack of uniformity across the chapters, the coherence of the AMBIT approach will appear.

Chapter 2 provides a summary of the AMBIT approach. Chapters 3 and 4 elaborate recent developments in AMBIT, namely around the role of trust and mistrust, and then describe ways of opening up communication with clients using specifically designed playing cards to explore their perspective on their problems. Chapters 5–10 describe the implementation of AMBIT in a range of centres in Europe, each of which focuses on different parts of the AMBIT approach, whether clients, teams, or networks. Chapters 11–13 are more future focused, considering mentalizing approaches to training and to the evaluation of outcomes. We finish, in Chapter 14, by sharing our ambitions for the development of the AMBIT community of practice over the next few years. We very much hope that you will enjoy reading about them.

References

Alegria, M., NeMoyer, A., Falgas Bague, I., Wang, Y., & Alvarez, K. (2018). Social determinants of mental health: Where we are and where we need to go. *Current Psychiatry Reports, 20*(11), 95. https://doi.org/10.1007/s11920-018-0969-9

Allen, J., Balfour, R., Bell, R., & Marmot, M. (2014). Social determinants of mental health. *International Review of Psychiatry, 26*(4), 392–407. https://doi.org/10.3109/09540261.2014.928270

Barnett, K., Mercer, S. W., Norbury, M., Watt, G., Wyke, S., & Guthrie, B. (2012). Epidemiology of multimorbidity and implications for health care, research, and medical education: A cross-sectional study. *Lancet, 380*(9836), 37–43. https://doi.org/10.1016/S0140-6736(12)60240-2

Bevington, D., Fuggle, P., Cracknell, L., & Fonagy, P. (2017). *Adaptive mentalization-based integrative treatment: A guide for teams to develop systems of care.* Oxford University Press.

Bramley, G., Fizpatrick, S., Edwards, J., Ford, D., Johnsen, S., Sosenko, F., & Watkins, D. (2015). *Hard edges: Mapping severe and multiple disadvantage.* Lankelly Chase Foundation. https://lankellychase.org.uk/wp-content/uploads/2015/07/Hard-Edges-Mapping-SMD-2015.pdf

Cochran, S. D., Mays, V. M., Alegria, M., Ortega, A. N., & Takeuchi, D. (2007). Mental health and substance use disorders among Latino and Asian American lesbian, gay, and bisexual adults. *Journal of Consulting and Clinical Psychology, 75*(5), 785–794. https://doi.org/10.1037/0022-006X.75.5.785

Malvaso, C., Delfabbro, P., Hackett, L., & Mills, H. (2016). Service approaches to young people with complex needs leaving out-of-home care. *Child Care in Practice, 22*(2), 128–147. https://doi.org/10.1080/13575279.2015.1118016

Merikangas, K. R., Mehta, R. L., Molnar, B. E., Walters, E. E., Swendsen, J. D., Aguilar-Gaziola, S., Bijl, R., Borges, G., Caraveo-Anduaga, J. J., Dewit, D. J., Kolody, B., Vega, W. A., Wittchen, H., & Kessler, R. C. (1998). Comorbidity of substance use disorders with mood and anxiety disorders: Results of the International Consortium in Psychiatric Epidemiology. *Addictive Behaviors, 23*(6), 893–907. https://doi.org/10.1016/S0306-4603(98)00076-8

National Institute for Health and Care Excellence. (2021). *Looked-after children and young people.* NICE guideline [NG205]. National Institute for Health and Care Excellence. https://www.nice.org.uk/guidance/ng205

NHS. (2019). *The NHS long term plan.* https://www.longtermplan.nhs.uk

Pavkov, T. W., Soloski, K. L., & Deliberty, R. (2012). The social construction of reality in the realm of children's mental health services. *Journal of Social Service Research, 38*(5), 672–687. https://doi.org/10.1080/01488376.2012.717864

Schein, E. H. (2009). *Helping: How to offer, give, and receive help.* Berrett-Koehler Publishers, Inc.

Shaw, S., Rosen, R., & Rumbold, B. (2011). *What is integrated care?* Nuffield Trust. https://www.nuffieldtrust.org.uk/research/what-is-integrated-care

Shufelt, J. L., & Cocozza, J. J. (2006). *Youth with mental health disorders in the juvenile justice system: Results from a multi-state prevalence study.* National Center for Mental Health and Juvenile Justice. https://sites.unicef.org/tdad/usmentalhealthprevalence06.pdf

Taskforce on Multiple Conditions. (2019). *The multiple conditions guidebook.* The Richmond Group of Charities. https://richmondgroupofcharities.org.uk/sites/default/files/multiple_conditions_report_a4_digital_spreads_noembargo_1.pdf

Timpson, E. (2019). *Timpson review of school exclusion.* Department for Education. https://assets.publishing.service.gov.uk/government/uploads/system/uploads/attachment_data/file/807862/Timpson_review.pdf

Ungar, M., Liebenberg, L., & Ikeda, J. (2014). Young people with complex needs: Designing coordinated interventions to promote resilience across child welfare, juvenile corrections, mental health and education services. *British Journal of Social Work, 44*(3), 675–693. https://doi.org/10.1093/bjsw/bcs147

Wolpert, M., Jacob, J., Napoleone, E., Whale, A., Calderon, A., & Edbrooke-Childs, J. (2016). *Child- and parent-reported outcomes and experience from child and young people's mental health services 2011–2015.* CAMHS Press. https://www.corc.uk.net/media/1544/0505207_corc-report_for-web.pdf

2
An introduction to AMBIT

Liz Cracknell and Dickon Bevington

2.1 Setting the scene

This chapter will provide an overview of the AMBIT approach, including a kind of glossary of common AMBIT phrases and terms that will be referred to in the other chapters of this book. More details about specific aspects of AMBIT described in this chapter can be found in Bevington et al. (2017) and on the open-source AMBIT wiki (https://manuals.annafreud.org/ambit), which has a wide range of download-able resources about AMBIT, including teaching videos, which are freely available to everyone. We will also include other key references where these are helpful.

The authors of this chapter could not be more qualified to provide this introduction. Both have been central to the development of AMBIT over the past 10 years and have day-to-day roles operating both as trainers and as practitioners. Liz Cracknell works as a mental health nurse and Dickon Bevington as a child and adolescent psychiatrist, but their intention is to write from a more general professional position that would be relevant to, for instance, a youth worker, a probation officer, a social worker, a ther-apist, a youth participation worker, a teacher, a drugs worker, a gangs and violence worker, a police officer, a prison officer, a support worker, or a psychologist—all of whom have both received training in AMBIT and, as we will describe later, have con-tributed so much to the development of AMBIT.

One key aspect of the AMBIT approach concerns the role of trust and mistrust in helping systems. This is common to all mentalization-based approaches and has been the focus of much interest in recent years. Because of its importance to AMBIT, this aspect of the mentalizing approach will be covered in more detail in Chapter 3, once the reader has gained an oversight of mentalizing and the basic AMBIT framework and approach.

2.2 Introduction

In this chapter, we will begin by introducing the overall AMBIT approach and the core construct of mentalizing that is at its heart. We will then outline the four core areas of practice, referred to as the *quadrants* of the AMBIT wheel, which need to be held in balance if work is to be safe, effective, and sustainable. The four quadrants are:

1. Working with your Client
2. Working with your Team
3. Working with your Network
4. Learning at Work.

For each quadrant we will describe the role of mentalizing in this area of work, the features of the stance, basic practice, and specific tools and techniques found to be helpful by workers who have applied them in a wide range of work settings and tasks.

AMBIT is best thought of as a foundational approach or framework for supporting a wide range of helping practices to be more effective. As we have highlighted, it is practised by a range of different kinds of helpers, in teams working in a range of different settings, serving different groups of people. As described in Chapter 1, what these teams have in common are an experience of working with clients with a multiplicity of needs, difficulties collaborating with other professionals to design and co-ordinate a helping offer that the clients trust, and the significant impact of this work on the practitioners.

Over the years we have trained and consulted with hundreds of teams around the world and have been struck by the apparent universality of these problems, despite the wide variations in how helping systems are financed and organized. AMBIT seeks to equip teams to tackle these problems. Whether underlying or overarching, in the foreground or the background, AMBIT works to make a team's existing practices more helpful in the context of multiple needs and helpers. This is why, as you will read in Chapter 11, the training process for AMBIT begins with AMBIT trainers seeking first to understand the nature of a team's work, the areas that are already working well (which need scaffolding), and the areas where the team needs help (for which change is sought). We aim to influence practice by adapting the AMBIT training to meet these needs. Our curiosity about these needs (and how to address them) means that AMBIT continues to develop in order to make it relevant to these real-world difficulties. In a very real way, AMBIT has been built on the feedback and contributions that we have gained from the many teams we have worked with.

AMBIT is not a therapy or a treatment but is intended to support and strengthen the approach and interventions that a team already uses. An analogy that is sometimes used to capture the nature of AMBIT is that, if helping interventions were some kind of digital device, AMBIT would be the operating system (e.g. Windows or Android) and any specific interventions that a team or worker might deliver (e.g. cognitive behavioural therapy, safeguarding work, or housing support) are the apps that run on the system. AMBIT, the operating system, works in the background to make the apps accessible to the intended users of the device and to ensure that the apps work effectively in the ways they were designed to. Just as apps sitting on a memory chip with no operating system are, no matter how brilliantly designed, quite useless, high-quality helping interventions offered in the absence of certain necessary conditions (e.g. a trusting relationship, a well-supported helper, and flexibility to arrange the help around the needs of the client) will be ineffective.

Where the problems outlined in detail in Chapter 1 do not exist (as in the example of Erica, who had fewer needs and a relatively trusting relationship to help), a standard operating system will most likely be sufficient, and a foregrounded 'AMBIT-influenced practice' may not be required: the team's usual methods work well to address the client's presenting needs, and any barriers encountered along the way can be relatively easily resolved. AMBIT is, in the context of this analogy, an 'upgrade' or 'patch' to be installed when the existing operating system is not working as it should. In this way, although AMBIT is not a therapy in itself, it aspires to be therapeutic in the sense that it enables a helping process to take place that is both experienced as and measurably more helpful. While this analogy might be quite neat, and gets us close to what AMBIT is, it is deceptive. The framing of AMBIT as simply creating the necessary conditions for helping interventions or therapy to take place, or as a 'foundation', perhaps rather misleadingly minimizes the complexity of this type of work and the degree of skill, understanding, adaptability, and emotional labour it requires from workers. If anything, AMBIT seeks to do the opposite. It attempts to articulate (intentionally moving from implicit to explicit) the art and science (it offers some science behind effective relational practices that some helpers will realize they have developed somewhat instinctually) of some of the most intricate and carefully balanced practices that are required to offer effective help, especially in the many contexts where this is not straightforward.

By offering an evidence-based and theoretically grounded shared language to explain the types of practices that get referred to (sometimes, perhaps, dismissively) as 'engagement work', 'relationship building', 'outreach', 'teamwork', and 'multiagency working', AMBIT not only recognizes that these skills are often absent from core professional trainings but also seeks to elevate such work from 'basic' to advanced practice. This represents a rebalancing of the value that we ascribe to different aspects of helping work. In this line of work, should we not value equally the 'textbook' delivery of a clever therapeutic manoeuvre and a thoughtfully composed email to workers in other agencies that tries to make sense of (or, in our language, to mentalize) the different perspectives held across the network about what should be done, and, in so doing, creates coherence and conditions for collaboration? Or the patience, compassion, and resolve required to slowly build trust with a person whose mind has quite understandably adapted to multiple experiences of trauma and marginalization by taking a position of automatic distrust of others (even where on paper this looks like lots of missed appointments and trips to cafés)?

2.3 Mentalizing: AMBIT as a mentalization-based approach

Mentalizing is at the heart of AMBIT. It has been previously described in detail (Bateman & Fonagy, 2016a; Fonagy et al., 2002), and active research continues to enrich and expand our definition of mentalizing. Mentalizing refers to one very specific example of the many and varied types of activity that minds engage in. This specific activity involves making sense of behaviours through the work of imaginatively creating more or less coherent narratives—stories that 'make sense' (a kind of 'folk psychology') of why behaviours happen. The stories that mentalizing concerns itself with are those about the mind behind the behaviour—its beliefs, feelings, memories, hopes, fears, and intentions. We will say more about why mentalizing is so important to the work that AMBIT teams do after exploring more about what mentalizing looks like when it is happening.

When someone is actively mentalizing:

- They exhibit *authentic curiosity* (an application of imagination in the service of 'working out', not just a mechanical asking of 'I'm curious about ...' questions) instead of a confident state of already knowing about a mind. This might apply to another person's mind or equally to their own mind. We all find ourselves doing things that we are not necessarily immediately able to explain; there are non-conscious biases, prejudices, and processes that are active, or easily become activated, in all of us. Mentalizing can be directed either *outwards* towards other minds or *inwards* towards the self; we can be as curious about better understanding our own mind as someone else's.
- They demonstrate a tolerance of *not-knowing*, alongside an implicit valuing of the progress of coming to know. Mentalizing is thus not a lazy, laissez-faire surrender to the impossibility of 'mind-reading'; it is an acknowledgement that while mind-reading is impossible, improved 'mind-estimating' is always desirable.
- They cannot help but communicate a *belief that their own mind will be enriched* by better understanding, as well (if the person being mentalized is someone other than themself) as the likely *benefit to the other person* if they come to experience themself as being more accurately understood. This helps explain why empathy is a sub-component of mentalizing.
- They demonstrate an awareness that *different emotional states (what we sometimes call 'affects') will have different impacts* on the mind's capacity to do this kind of sense-making. Someone who is furious might just be able to pause, mid-tirade, to say 'Look, I can't think straight as I'm so angry right now, but this is definitely something we need to talk about when I'm calmer ...'.
- They are more likely to be able to grasp or introduce *humour*: shared laughter is a biological signal that just at this moment our minds 'overlap', and most humour revolves around understanding misunderstandings ('getting' the joke). Shakespeare refers to the 'Comedy of Errors', which is a catchy summary for all human relationships, and a clue to the last, most important fact about mentalizing...
- They *recognize the fragility of this 'capacity to make sense of behaviours'*, and can predict the inevitability of their own misunderstandings, which manifests as a

kind of humility. A study by Tronick and Cohn (1989), which examined in minute detail the micro-communications between securely attached mothers and their own infants, calculated that only 30% of the mothers' reciprocal communications showed a close fit with their infants' behaviours: so, even in our most intimate closest relationships we are all beginners at making sense of each other. Recognizing that misunderstandings between humans are inevitable helps us to expect them, look out for them, and repair them as part of keeping our relationships working well.

This process of mentalizing is at the centre of the AMBIT approach, which is summarized in the diagram of the AMBIT wheel shown in Figure 2.1.

This adaptive positioning of mentalizing at the centre of AMBIT occurred for a variety of reasons—perhaps not least because at its heart (and in contrast to some of the science that underpins it), mentalizing is an easy idea to grasp that can nonetheless transform practice. As Bateman and Fonagy (2016b) have put it, this involves turning from the therapist-centric question of what the therapist needs to change in

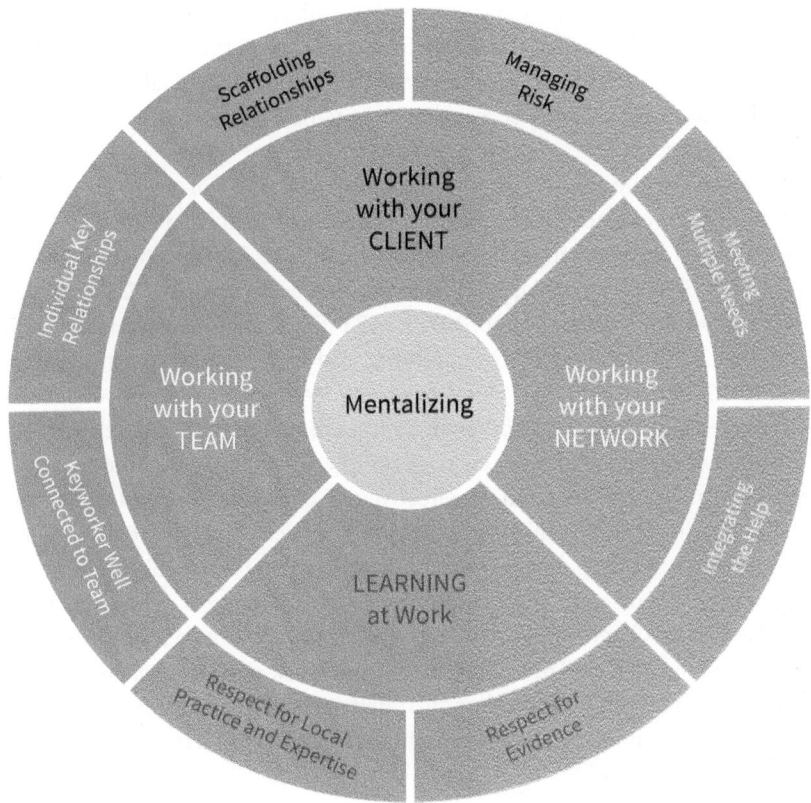

Figure 2.1 The AMBIT wheel.

the mind of the client to make things better, to the client-centred question of what the *client* needs to see change in the mind of the *therapist* in order to feel understood, enabling a trusting relationship to develop in which the client's own mentalizing capacity is 'regenerated'.

AMBIT trainees also repeatedly referred to the fact that this frame of reference for thinking about human communication offered them the promise of a 'common language' that appeared to speak respectfully in relation to and across a wide range of existing models and frameworks, coming alongside and enriching existing practices and experiences, rather than invalidating them. This was particularly important to us in trying to design an approach that would be inclusive of professionals from different backgrounds, all of whom have a valuable role in supporting clients with multiple needs. Mentalizing addresses what can perhaps be seen as a universal drive (notwithstanding cultural variations in how it is expressed): the drive to understand and be understood.

Another reason for the centrality of mentalizing in the AMBIT framework is that it offers something of a transdiagnostic approach, describing and manualizing some elements of what research into the common factors of effective therapy has uncovered. It has been argued (Fonagy & Allison, 2014) that effective mentalizing is the final common pathway achieved by most, perhaps all, of the many and varied effective psychotherapies, regardless of the theoretical model underpinning them. Although the various therapeutic modalities have very different intellectual frameworks and practices, research consistently shows that they achieve surprisingly similar levels of positive outcomes.

AMBIT can be thought of as a member of a 'family' of mentalization-based interventions—for example, mentalization-based treatment (MBT) for adults with a diagnosis of borderline personality disorder (Bateman & Fonagy, 2016a); MBT-F for families (Asen & Fonagy, 2021); MBT-A for adolescents (Rossouw & Fonagy, 2012); MBT-C for children (Midgley et al., 2017); MBT-ED for eating disorders (Robinson & Skårderud, 2019); and reflective parenting and reflective foster care (Cooper & Redfern, 2016; Redfern, 2019)—and it has some features in common with each. All have developed alongside one another and, rather like siblings, have been shaped over time by some of the same influences. For example, our developing understanding of the centrality of *epistemic trust* to the effectiveness of any helping endeavour and the role of mentalizing in the establishment of that trust (see Chapter 3) can be seen in all of these therapies. AMBIT differs from the others in that it is not best thought of as a therapy, or even as a discrete intervention for a particular type of need or client group, as it can be, and has been, applied by different types of teams in a range of contexts. The exact position that AMBIT takes within the work of a team or helping system varies quite significantly, which is demonstrated markedly—and wonderfully—in the later chapters of this book written by practitioners working in a range of very different settings around the world.

2.3.1 The fragility of mentalizing: a great power leveller

One of the most important things to understand about mentalizing is its fragility and the implications that this has for our work as helpers of those with multiple needs. When mentalizing collapses, it is replaced by other, *non-mentalizing*, mental states that are in most cases much less likely to promote safety, learning, adaptation, and satisfying relationships. This fragility is something that is shared and experienced by clients and workers alike. Once mentalizing is lost, it is most effectively repaired when one experiences another mentalizing mind. There is no space for individual heroism in the work of an AMBIT team; all workers, no matter how experienced or skilled, are vulnerable to losing their capacity to mentalize, on account of being human.

When we lose our capacity to mentalize, our thinking becomes characterized by a non-mentalizing state of mind. The most common non-mentalizing states are in fact (developmentally speaking) the building blocks of mature mentalizing; they are certainly not to be seen as intrinsically pathological. In their right place, when required—and just like any good tool—nothing else will do! Evolution sees to it, however, that these non-mentalizing states of mind are very easily and rapidly triggered because our survival has depended on our brain being able to respond rapidly to environmental (including social) threats. The common perceived threats that arise nowadays are perhaps different from earlier millennia (there are fewer man-eating tigers around!) but nevertheless trigger the same responses. In the wrong context, these non-mentalizing states of mind are frequently at the root of, or at least exacerbate, relational difficulties (towards the self and others). It is important to recognize that even quite moderate levels of arousal will derail the brain from the slower, imaginative, musing qualities that it displays when mentalizing.

In neurological terms, mentalizing is mainly located in the most recently evolved (and the most uniquely human) part of the brain, the prefrontal cortex. When we feel threatened or fearful, the sympathetic ('Stay alive!') nervous system is activated, resulting in the release of adrenaline and other factors that rapidly reroute blood from the skin to more survival-critical machinery such as the large muscles and the heart (this explains why we go pale when frightened). Similarly, in the brain, the outer folds of the prefrontal cortex are rapidly abandoned by the precious blood (that powers 'thinking energy' as well as muscles); it is sucked deep inside to the ancient core of the brain—to the centres dealing with threat appraisal and action, such as the amygdala. Within seconds, even a moderate rise in stress and arousal, which may, for many reasons, be frequently experienced by clients or helpers in the context of AMBIT work, can activate one or other of these three non-mentalizing states of mind:

- *Certainty* (or 'psychic equivalence'), in which the mind's ideas about something (especially about the intentions of another mind) are seen in that moment as directly equivalent to the *reality* of that thing, not just as a theory about it. In survival situations this can be very useful: I don't get curious about why you are approaching me with a knife, I simply know in an instant that you mean to do me harm. By contrast, sacrificing the capacity to wonder about alternative explanations and perspectives is very often deeply damaging to relationships ('You saunter in half an hour late because you just want to belittle me!')—and these kinds of encounters are much more common than people coming at us with knives.

- *Action* ('quick-fix' or 'teleology') often flows directly on from psychic equivalence; it is the mind's attempt to relieve arousal or distress through some physically observable action that results in physical/observable change ('I won't feel this sense of revulsion about myself once I feel the blade cutting my arm or see the blood'). Of course, there are many examples of where teleology is exactly what is required ('We're hungry, let's eat!') because these are based on an accurately mentalized connection, but workers in health and social care or education will recognize many responses to the inevitable stresses that work contexts can create that are unhelpfully teleological (e.g. managing anxiety by making multiple referrals, which may not be wanted and do not change the immediate situation).

- *Pretend mode* ('waffle', or the 'veil of words') is the state of mind that offers self-soothing via the comfort of words and often a sense of 'cleverness': the words might be strictly true, or not, but they are used in ways that comfort the speaker rather than to establish or sustain an authentic reciprocal relationship and connection with the person in front of them. An example might be the doctor droning on to a parent (who is sobbing and feeling horrified) about the 'complex interplay of aetiological factors that have led inexorably to this challenging situation' where their son is now under arrest for arson. Or professionals engaging in a highly theoretical exchange of hypotheses in a review meeting, which masks the absence of progress and a workable plan of action. Or the parent justifying their binge drinking to a social worker, saying 'My drinking isn't really an issue. I know people around here who drink more than me, and it doesn't affect the children as I only drink in the evening', as the worker anxiously remembers the bruising on their child's cheek and surveys the empty kitchen. On the other hand, this sense of interiority, the 'play of ideas' or of getting into a 'dialogue with oneself', is often precisely where new ideas and creative inspiration can spring from. For example, trying to imagine the impact for a young person of moving from living with her mother in a rural part of Nigeria to living with her father in London. Really trying to imagine what this may be like for a 14-year-old young person without constraining this to just the presenting problem itself. Different food, different TV programmes, thinking about her friends back home, the grandmother she has had to leave behind … just trying to imagine what it's like to be her, as an actor might do when preparing to play a part. So, the pretend mode—just like psychic equivalence and teleology—is not without value when used in its proper context.

So, for all humans, mentalizing is an ephemeral, fluctuating, minute-by-minute state of mind rather than a skill that once learned is there to stay like a degree certificate on the wall. Lacking awareness of the fragility of our mentalizing can lead to us engaging in patterns of thinking and behaving that have unhelpful consequences for our work. In this sense, our *shared* experience of the fragility of mentalizing can make for a great 'power leveller' between worker and client. Having the confidence to expect one's own mentalizing errors, and so to get quickly into the work of repairing these 'in the open air' when they inevitably occur, or referring to the help that is given by teammates with this task, allows workers to model mentalizing and its repair, but without creating (or at least emphasizing) an unhelpful power differential. This is especially relevant when we consider the belated focus on systematic discrimination, the impact of microaggressions or misinterpretations relating to race, gender, sexuality, or other characteristics of difference that so easily create additional barriers to help. Following the lead of systemic practitioners, mentalizing in the context of an explicit acknowledgement of how power is manifested and experienced in the here and now of any working relationship should be a standard part of practice.

In concluding this introduction to mentalizing, we acknowledge it may be easy to regard mentalizing as a professional skill, one that we must learn, practise, and hone until, eventually, we achieve the level of a 'mentalizing ninja'. Perhaps mentalizing is a skill, in the sense that anything that we do could be considered a skill, but, unlike other skills we might develop in our professional lives, we do not begin professional training in mentalizing as novices. Instead, we have been in training for this skill since infancy, when our caregivers paid attention to our minds—when they mentalized us—gradually teaching us that we have minds, and that others have minds that are separate from our own. Our basic capacity to mentalize continued to develop well into our late adolescent years, and, with it, our increasing ability both to make sense of our own minds (and, in turn, to regulate our emotions) and to make sense of the minds of others, helping us to navigate relationships and the social world. In AMBIT, we emphasize that mentalizing is a *basic human function* that fluctuates according to our affective states that we each experience and have been doing, day in and day out, for years before we ever heard the word 'mentalizing' for the first time. Whether professionals or clients, we share this common heritage.

2.3.2 Mentalizing in four directions: balancing the wheel

In AMBIT training, we often talk about applying mentalizing in four directions, which can sound like an overwhelming task. By this we mean that the theory and practice of mentalizing can assist us not only in our work with our clients, but also in how we approach team working, multiprofessional network collaboration, and learning together as a team about how to do our work well. In order to best serve our clients, we must pay equal attention to our own minds and those of our teammates, to the minds of the various members of the wider networks around our clients, and—somewhat more figuratively—to our 'collective organizational minds', in terms of their capacity for continual organizational learning ('Who are we?' 'How do we work?' 'Why do we do things like this, and not like that?').

To those who would say in response to AMBIT 'But we do this already!' (which we sometimes hear from the groups we are training), we would perhaps half-agree. There is much about AMBIT that people might find familiar, or at least intuitive, and yet our experience is that teams tend not to practise in these ways consistently. Just as it is inevitable that at times our minds fall out of balance (into non-mentalizing), so too is it inevitable that we, as helpers, will fall out of balance in terms of attention to the four broad areas of the work laid out in the quadrants of the AMBIT wheel. AMBIT seeks to help workers to notice when they are off-balance and to get back on track faster when they are. A comment from a participant in a recent AMBIT training put it like this:

> We're good at x and y therapy, but it's the secret sauce around it that makes it work or not work, and that's what we need some help to think about because we're not quite sure what that secret sauce is—sometimes we have it, sometimes we don't!

In the following sections, we lay out the key principles and practices of AMBIT, one quadrant at a time: 'Working with your Team', 'Working with your Client', 'Working with your Network', and 'Learning at Work'. For each quadrant we will describe the following:

- How mentalizing and non-mentalizing can manifest in that quadrant's area of the work.
- The pair of 'stance features' associated with the quadrant. Each pair of stance features (situated around the edges of the AMBIT wheel shown in Figure 2.1) highlight two important aspects of the work relating to the quadrant they are associated with, but are often in tension with one another, pulling us in opposite directions—risking imbalance not just between the quadrants of practice but within each quadrant, too.
- The basic practice of how the stance features are enacted.
- An overview of tools and techniques. Links are provided to pages within the on-line AMBIT manual (https://manuals.annafreud.org/ambit) where detailed descriptions of the tools and techniques are provided.

2.4 Working with your Team

2.4.1 Mentalizing and non-mentalizing in teams and workers

Two core assumptions organize the principles and practices in AMBIT's Working with your Team quadrant (Figure 2.2) and create the paradox we describe above:

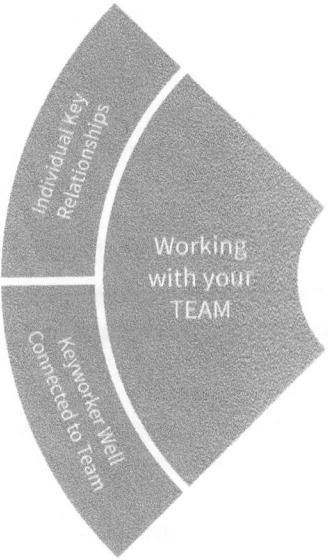

Figure 2.2 Working with your Team.

1. Whatever form of help a worker is offering, the capacity of that worker to mentalize themselves, the client, and others in the client's network (both informal and professional) is central to the effectiveness of the help.
2. Working alongside people who are experiencing problems and distress of any kind, and within the associated helping systems, will inevitably cause the worker stress at times, and that stress will interfere with a worker's capacity to mentalize, probably just when they need it the most.

Worker stress—and the accompanying loss of mentalizing—is seen not as an indication of worker weakness or some other failing, but as a normal feature of the work and entirely in keeping with the ways our brains work. In some ways, stress is even a necessary feature of the work, because to experience emotion is part of engaging with the realities of what is happening in front of, around, and within us. Completely uncontained expressions of strong emotions or prolonged non-mentalizing on the part of the worker in front of the client may not be helpful, but, if the client feeling understood by their worker is a necessary condition for epistemic trust (see Chapter 3) and supports the client to mentalize better, then some impact on the worker of the client's circumstances surely needs to be evident to the client. A client facing a worker who appears to be completely unaffected by the client's story may feel invalidated and misunderstood, feelings that may in turn reduce the client's ability to mentalize. Just as an infant learns about their own mind in what they see reflected back from a caregiver, the client's experience and ability to mentalize is influenced by what they see in their worker. In situations where the client is uncertain about the nature of what has happened to them, as is seen in clients who have experienced gaslighting by an abuser, exploitation, or chronic marginalization, the emotional response (or lack of one) of the worker may have a particularly painful significance.

The aim of AMBIT is not to entirely prevent worker stress, but to attend to it. We want to reduce the negative impact of stress on workers' mentalizing by ensuring that there is an explicit culture in teams of acknowledging worker stress, encouraging workers to seek help at times of stress, and ensuring that there are clear team methods and routines for supporting workers' mentalizing when the inevitable collapses occur. The intention of this focus is primarily to improve client outcomes through supporting workers' well-being, as these are inextricably linked; we want workers to be able to work to their full potential and for systems to be able to retain their staff, as we know that high staff turnover can significantly undermine the continuity of help that clients receive. Workers whose minds are attended to by colleagues are better able to mentalize. When workers mentalize, they can, for example:

- Become more curious about behaviour: they attempt to make sense of both their own and others' behaviour in terms of mental states and understand misunderstandings better because of this
- Be self-reflective: they notice and reflect upon their emotional responses to situations and the influence of their own previous experiences, prejudices, and biases; they notice and make sense of ways in which they may be behaving differently from usual
- Take multiple perspectives: they remember that their understanding of a situation is just their perspective and are genuinely curious about, and open to, the perspectives of others.

Non-mentalizing in workers can take many forms, but examples, following the three main types of non-mentalizing, include:

- *Pretend mode*: workers may protect their minds from overwhelming stress by not connecting fully with certain aspects of reality. This could include not connecting with the client's emotional state (which could lead to the worker being perceived as uncaring), avoiding a particular area of the client's needs, or ignoring a problem in the client–worker relationship
- *Certainty*: workers under stress can become very fixed in their view of a situation or person and lose the ability to take different perspectives, even when new information arises. This could lead them to behave in ways that are unhelpful because their actions are based on inaccurate understandings of people or situations
- *Quick-fix*: workers can be strongly organized by the wish to *do something* in response to stress, resulting in reactive, rather than thoughtful, responses to crises. Clients can be unhelpfully impacted by workers who move too quickly into doing without first taking the time to adequately understand or collaboratively plan with the client.

Although these examples illustrate some of the impacts of worker non-mentalizing on clients, these states of mind can also be triggered and play out unhelpfully in our relationships with teammates and network colleagues. High-pressure service contexts for teams may easily support aspects of non-mentalizing, encouraging quick-fix solutions, certainties about the roles of other agencies, and pretend-mode formulations apparently disconnected from the immediate needs of the client. Some teams develop a culture of self-protective pretend mode; for example, as workers from a crisis team told us: 'You develop a tolerance for risk—we deal with suicide attempts all the time and you can't let it affect you or you'd become too ill to do the job'. The same team described the side effects of this approach: workers felt scared to acknowledge when things did affect them, for fear of being judged, and their strategy meant they could lose the ability to connect with clients: 'I got really annoyed with this patient's mum because she wasn't being reasonable. Looking back, I realize I deal with this [suicidality] every day and it's become weirdly normal to me, but it was her child who had tried to kill himself. It was probably the worst day of her whole life and I just completely lost sight of what that must be like'. In such a context, the matter of supporting the workers' mentalizing is a major task.

2.4.2 Working with your Team: stance features

This courageously shared story was a powerful example of how challenging it can be to keep in balance the two stance features associated with the Working with your Team quadrant:

- Individual keyworker relationship
- Keyworker well connected to the team.

2.4.2.1 Individual keyworker relationship

This stance feature emphasizes the importance of the relationship between the worker and client when delivering help. Help occurs most meaningfully and effectively when it happens within a relationship where trust has developed. In general, in an AMBIT-trained team, one member of the team will be allocated to each client and will take a lead in trying to build a relationship with the client. This often takes time, patience, persistence, and creativity on the part of the worker, particularly when client mistrust is high (see Section 2.5). We have encountered many teams whose workers possess these skills and qualities in abundance and who are excellent at building trusting relationships as a result. We emphasize this stance feature not because it is a new idea, but because it is not enough for this adaptation to take place at the practitioner level only; workers need to be embedded in teams and organizations that have adequately adapted their expectations about what this work requires to accommodate this focus on engagement and relationship building as part of routine practice with this client group, rather than placing workers under additional pressure to achieve concrete outcomes within short time frames. What may also be a little different about the framing of this work within AMBIT is the explicit recognition of the high risk of worker stress and isolation in such roles.

The AMBIT-trained team may be aware that the client they are trying to engage already has a trusting relationship with another worker from another team. Indeed, we encourage workers to actively check out whether this is the case before automatically assuming that a new relationship of help needs to be established. These ideas will be discussed further in relation to the Working with your Network quadrant (see Section 2.6), where we will discuss 'Team around the Worker', but we want to acknowledge here that it is not a necessity for workers in an AMBIT team to be the ones who have the key relationship with the client in the first instance. This does not negate the need for workers to be well connected to the team (as we describe below), since it is likely that they will be taking on a more direct keyworking role with some of their clients, even if not for all of them.

2.4.2.2 Keyworker well connected to the team

As we have described above, worker stress and consequent losses of mentalizing capacity are a frequent and an expected part of the work, meaning that we must take seriously the need to create relationships within teams in which mentalizing can be restored. The most effective way of supporting any person's mentalizing capacity is relational, through a safe, trusting relationship of the type that has the best chance of being developed with a relatively small group of people with whom we have the most regular contact—such as our team colleagues. This may seem like common sense and something that all teams should have, but even though teams can often describe some of the ways in which they already support each other, the presence of these conditions within a team should not be taken for granted because they tend not to flourish without conscious collective effort. Sometimes, it is in teams that encounter the most severe stresses and risks (e.g. prison, police, child protection, and crisis teams) that we hear of cultures in which shame is attached to worker stress. Some systems rely on a hierarchical 'command and control' style of leadership to create safety, in which a reluctance to share worker stress is modelled from the top down. We will explore the helping processes that we see as being important in teams in more depth in the following sections.

Balancing our efforts to establish and maintain team connectedness with the need to establish strong keyworker relationships can be challenging. For example, in the simplest of terms, it can be hard for teams to schedule and protect time to meet together alongside remaining responsive to their clients and their changing circumstances. Just as leaning too far towards connectedness to the team would have a potentially negative impact on helping relationships with clients, the opposite can also be true. In some ways, the more effective the worker has been in attuning to the client, the more they are at risk of losses of mentalizing, because they are in closer proximity to the distress of the client and more likely to experience powerful emotions themselves. At these times, the need for connection to the team is paramount in order for the worker to restore and optimize their effectiveness as a helper, but may also feel most difficult to prioritize.

Even though our team is best positioned to help us sustain and regain a mentalizing stance in our work, this is not without its complexities. In teams, we are all moving in and out of being able to mentalize in relation to our own work and can be as easily dysregulated by our own work as by that of others. For this reason, we emphasize the need for teams to have methods to support a culture of mentalizing within the team (which will be explored further in the sections below), as captured in the following vignette:

> An example from a recent AMBIT supervision involved a worker, Ajay, and his client, John. Ajay had a good relationship with John and was working hard to build his trust, after learning of John's previous negative experiences of help. Ajay's team thought that he was doing too much for John and told him to turn down some of John's requests, fearing that he was being 'manipulated'. Ajay felt stuck, as whatever he did felt as if it might alienate him from either John or the team. What was missing from the team's response was any mentalizing of Ajay and John and including consideration of their perspectives in the subsequent plan.

2.4.3 Working with your Team: basic practice

2.4.3.1 Helping processes in teams

For each individual worker in a team, there are two sides to the basic practice of Working with your Team. First, there is practice relating to one's own workload (whether this is direct client work, leadership responsibilities, or administrative duties) and how one remains connected to one's team while carrying out that work. This involves both seeking and accepting help from colleagues, which requires an ability to acknowledge and recognize our inevitable need for help at times. We share a model of help-seeking in training that was developed to conceptualize client help-seeking (Rickwood et al., 2005), but for us this can apply equally to make sense of worker help-seeking. The model proposes that in order to receive help, we need to have awareness of our need and a way to express it, for there to be an available source of help, and for us to be willing to use it. Our ability to be aware of and express our need for help involves us being able to mentalize ourselves just well enough to be aware that we are working under conditions that are making it hard to mentalize. We may not be able to express perfectly what we need, but we are in a position to be able to signal our need for help. At other times, we may not recognize our need for help, but someone else makes us aware of this—not an uncommon scenario given that working under stress makes it hard to mentalize oneself and others. Whether we seek out or take up an offer of help will depend on whether we perceive that other people are available enough for this task and that we feel willing to use them. As we have framed it before, there is no role for 'lone rangers' in this kind of work (Bevington et al., 2017); AMBIT is explicitly a team approach, even when only one member of the team might have contact with each client. AMBIT encourages workers to share with clients the ways in which they have sought help from their colleagues and why, thus modelling effective help-seeking and educating clients about how mentalizing can be supported by reaching out to other minds.

Second, and of equal importance, is one's role in being a member of a well-connected team and taking on one's share of the responsibility for offering and providing help to colleagues by attending to the minds of one's colleagues and supporting them to restore their mentalizing when it is lost. Adopting this shared responsibility across a team can represent a considerable change for many teams, and we see this as being an addition to, rather than a replacement for, a team's existing hierarchical structures in which some workers will be accountable for the work of others. Put simply, a worker in an AMBIT-influenced team sees it as part of their job to look out for their colleagues and play a part in creating a team culture that supports mentalizing. While sometimes the help a worker needs is that of someone with greater knowledge or expertise (i.e. a supervisor or senior colleague), very often the help that is required is something that can be offered by someone whose own mind is better able to mentalize because they are a step removed from the strong emotions around the circumstances that are affecting the worker. For this reason, the most junior member of staff can be in a position to provide effective, contingent help to the leader of the team. In fact, we have found that a key factor in creating a culture of help-seeking and help-offering in teams is the willingness of those in leadership positions to ask their colleagues for help.

All of these aspects link to what we mean by being a 'well-connected' team: the extent to which there are shared values about how we will help each other with our work and sufficient trust in the team to make it feel safe to do so. A few key metaphors have developed in AMBIT to convey some of these central aspects of practice. These metaphors have become commonly used by AMBIT teams to reflect and communicate together on cases. These metaphors are referred to in some of the subsequent chapters, so it is helpful to clarify them now.

2.4.3.2 'Ripples in the pond'

One metaphor is about the sense of being overwhelmed by a particular case. This is represented by the image of turbulence in a pond created by a stone being dropped into it (Figure 2.3). The worker is at the point where the stone has dropped into the water, surrounded by chaotic movements of water that gradually resolve into orderly circular waves. These waves can more easily be seen from the bank of the pond than from the chaos and enactment at the point of contact. In the same way, those outside the immediate situation may be more able to see the 'bigger picture' than the worker in the middle of the pond. The function of the well-connected team is to bring together perspectives from the bank with the perspective of the worker in the pond. Often AMBIT teams talk about workers 'falling in the pond' and the value of others 'staying on the bank' rather than jumping in and splashing around too.

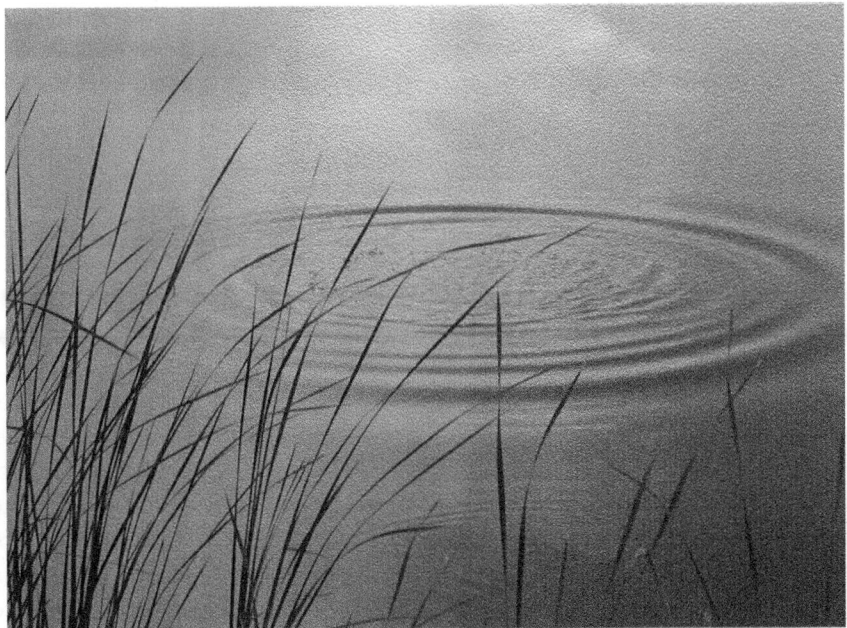

Figure 2.3 Ripples in the pond.

2.4.3.3 'Who's got your rope?'

A second key metaphor is based on mountaineering and the importance of climbers being connected by a rope so that the lead climber is held by the rest of the team. This 'rope' involves a sense of feeling connected to others, as well as a set of disciplines to sustain that connection. It may reveal itself in the practical realities of encouraging telephone contact between workers during client contacts or of team members using text messages to monitor each other. The metaphor represents the fact that mentalizing takes place through a connection between people, and this sense of connection needs to have some concrete reality and social rituals and disciplines to sustain it. Our experience is that teams adapt their practice using this metaphor as an organizing idea.

2.4.4 Tools and techniques for Working with your Team

The tools and techniques in this quadrant include strengthening a culture of helping within the team, as well as a structured tool ('Thinking Together') for supporting a mentalization-based approach to helping conversations (Box 2.1). Helping conversations may take place within formal structures (e.g. team meetings or supervision) as well as in more informal exchanges between team members (e.g. peer to peer throughout the day). Thinking Together can be used in a one-to-one conversation or in a group format.

2.5 Working with your Client

2.5.1 Mentalizing and non-mentalizing in working with clients

AMBIT-trained teams work with a wide range of client groups. Despite the differences between these contexts, we have learned from workers that the mentalizing challenges that occur in relation to their client work have a number of similar themes.

First, the personal histories of clients have often not prepared them well to deploy their mentalizing capacities in ways that help them negotiate their paths through challenging territories. They have often grown up (and sometimes continue to live) within extremely hostile or 'non-contingent' contexts, to which they have had to adapt. These contexts include not just their family, but also their interactions with wider professional and societal systems. For example, consider the past experiences of 'help' that many of our clients will bring: of people with power (parents, professionals, etc.) who might have offered 'help' that ended not in an experience of being helped, but in something quite the opposite—such as exploitation, abuse, racism, humiliation, neglect, or broken promises. Against this backdrop of negative relational experiences, the emotions that may be triggered in our clients when faced with a new professional may be significant and make it very difficult for them to engage in the curious, open-minded thinking that might assist them in accurately mentalizing the worker in front of them. Instead, it is far more likely that these high emotions will give rise to non-mentalizing states of mind, which might be expressed as certainty about this worker's harmful intentions or inability to be helpful, or by them moving into a more pretend state, where they minimize their needs. For some clients, these states of mind can lead to a purposeful rejection of help even before there is an opportunity for the helping relationship to begin. For others, these states may be more fluctuating but continue to be a significant feature of the relationship that they are slowly able to form with a new worker. This has been termed *epistemic hypervigilance*—a state of being in which the 'door' through which any kind of learning or transfer of help might pass is locked shut, for the adaptive reasons that we have described. Sometimes, however, this reaction is labelled by helpers as 'non-engagement' or as 'refusing help'. It is crucial that workers take a mentalizing stance in relation to these behaviours and use this understanding to adapt their own behaviour towards the client, rather than labelling these clients as 'hard to reach' (a term we now reject as pejorative) and simply closing the case.

As we have suggested above, the fragility of the client's mentalizing and its associated impacts are to be an expected part of the ongoing work. Because of their multiple needs and the hostility of the environments in which they live, our clients' presentations may fluctuate not only because of changing internal states (of mind or of body; consider the impact of food poverty or addiction) but also external challenges. Repeated crises of various kinds may form a key backdrop to their presentations, so that a worker may experience the best of their helping intentions as being constantly knocked off course. Despite the abundance of evidence for the regular

Box 2.1 Tools and techniques for Working with your Team

Help-seeking, help-offering, and the well-connected team
Teams are encouraged to have explicit conversations about help-seeking and help-offering, and to agree upon rituals and routines to support mentalizing:

- What are our attitudes towards help-seeking, both positive and negative?
- Do we know what it looks like when each of us needs help?
- Can we agree on some shared language to offer one another help without it being experienced as shaming?
- How can we increase opportunities for connectedness and help-seeking in our team?

Thinking Together
Thinking Together is a four-step process for improving the helpfulness of conversations between a worker and their team. The emphasis is on attending to the mind of the *worker* and supporting the worker's own mentalizing, rather than leaping in to offer ideas about the *client*.

1. *Mark the task*:
   - What does the worker need from the conversation?
   - Kick-start the worker's mentalizing ('What do I need?').
   - How long have we got?
2. *State the case*:
   - Worker provides only the information relevant to the task.
   - No problem-solving or long storytelling.
3. *Mentalize the moment*:
   - First, mentalize the worker: how is the worker feeling and thinking?
   - How might the client (and others) be feeling and thinking? How can we make sense of this situation?
4. *Return to purpose*:
   - Return to the task set at the beginning to ensure this is met.
   - Does the worker have any new thoughts or ideas?
   - What ideas do colleagues have?

For more information on these tools and techniques, visit the online AMBIT manual: https://manuals.annafreud.org/ambit

collapse of a client's mentalizing, it is important to remember that those same clients will certainly also have capacities in this domain, which may easily be overlooked by workers. For example, a team that engaged young people involved in serious youth violence described how their clients were able to co-create advice for how the group should respond if a client was ever found to have brought a firearm on-site. Their advice was emphatic, easily agreed upon, and showed excellent mentalizing skills: in such an event, everyone in the building should sit on the floor, and place both of their hands flat and visible on the floor, before the weapon holder is reminded calmly that they cannot have a firearm here and should leave immediately. Their rationale for this plan was that 'If you are carrying a firearm, you are always afraid ...' (either that's why you are carrying it in the first place, or you are afraid of getting caught with it) '... and people who are sitting down in that way are the least frightening'.

We now consider some of the mentalizing challenges that might be present for workers in relation to the Working with your Client quadrant (Figure 2.4). There are features of supporting clients with multiple needs in particular that may make it more likely that workers' mentalizing capacity is vulnerable to collapse. As we have noted, our clients are often embedded in contexts that make them vulnerable to a number of risks that are often linked to their relationships with others (e.g. abuse, neglect, exploitation, social isolation, being out of education or employment, estrangement from family, or marginalization).

The challenges of supporting clients who face multiple risks will be all too familiar to workers in the field. Our responsibility as helpers to promote safety for our clients, while operating in contexts over which we have limited control, is significant and often daunting. Expecting that we will be able to sustain our mentalizing when immersed in such emotive work is unrealistic, and we must recognize the impact that this can have on our practice. We may find ourselves regularly tipped into non-mentalizing states, which can significantly undermine the process of forming and sustaining a trusting relationship with our clients, as well as our ability to develop and follow collaborative plans for our work.

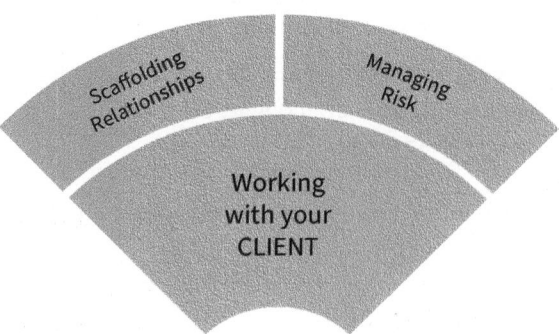

Figure 2.4 Working with your Client.

2.5.2 Working with your Client: stance features

The two (often mutually contradictory) elements of the AMBIT stance that are most often relevant to this quadrant are:

- Scaffolding relationships
- Managing risk.

2.5.2.1 Scaffolding relationships

'Scaffolding relationships' (previously named 'Scaffolding existing relationships') refers to strengthening the network of relationships around a client in order to promote their well-being and safety. We originally wanted to emphasize the significance of the existing relationships around a client to remind workers that we never create a helping network around a client—we only join existing networks, however precarious these may sometimes be. Scaffolding means paying attention to what needs to be strengthened and repaired in the relationships that already exist around clients, in terms of their informal network of family and friends. For those clients who experience more extreme isolation, creating new relationships may also be a focus of the work (e.g. Jensen et al., 2021). As epistemic trust (see Chapter 3) develops in the client–worker relationship, it forms a critical part of enabling these new relationships to eventually develop. If a client has developed epistemic trust in their worker, they are (a) more likely to try out the worker's suggestions for what might help in the context of their other relationships (this is sometimes referred to as 'generalization of learning') and (b) more likely at least to 'open the door' to a helping relationship with another person if they witness the worker's positive relationship with that person.

Scaffolding is, of course, by its nature temporary. The goal of encouraging workers to build around what is already there is key to ensuring that a client has an informal network around them that is more long-lived than any professional relationship, which is important for sustainability. Focusing on the network of helping relationships around a client also acts as a helpful signal that the worker's own professional role in their life will be only temporary. This mitigates the risk of creating a temporary dependency without considering sustainability once the worker's role has come to an end.

2.5.2.2 Managing risk

As with all quadrants in the AMBIT wheel, there is a tension between the two stance features. We cannot afford to overlook the significant risks that are present in the relational contexts of our clients' lives and simply busy ourselves with scaffolding relationships, even though this might feel like a more comfortable task. An over-focus on scaffolding relationships can overlook the fact that some 'helping' relationships (as far as our clients may see them) are far from safe (as we would see them).

In engaging with and managing risk, we almost inevitably tend to be drawn into more assertive (and in terms of power, more asymmetrical) relationships. The worker who can use their connectedness to a supportive team to help them hold the right balance between relational engagement and safe intervention, and who in so doing can model transparently to their client the universality (and universal challenges) of help-seeking and help-receiving, is working in an AMBIT-influenced way. If this uncertain balancing of two vital but often mutually incompatible intentional stances conjures in the reader a feeling of familiar discomfort, then it is hoped that in doing so it validates the difficulty of this kind of work.

2.5.3 Working with your Client: basic practice

Within this quadrant, as well as basic practices that support us to attend to the stance features, we share some of the practices that help us to build relationships with our clients in the context of mistrust.

2.5.3.1 Epistemic trust

The critical task—especially in the early stages of face-to-face work—is to create conditions in which the client not only experiences themself as having been adequately understood by their worker but also feels that their existing capacities and personal agency are acknowledged. It is this experience of 'being seen' (i.e. being accurately mentalized) that our theory predicts can help facilitate the development of epistemic trust (see Chapter 3) towards that helper—that is, trust in the social value of what the helper might know, and the possibility of it being helpful. In turn, this improves the likelihood of learning from the helper, and in particular the generalization of this learning via behavioural experiments conducted away from the helper in the real world of the client's life (e.g. something as 'simple' as walking away to cool off when an argument is erupting). If the world is then just benign enough to give positive feedback in response to the client's attempts at changing patterned behaviours, lasting change might take root.

2.5.3.2 The mentalizing stance

Given the mentalizing vulnerabilities that both client and worker are likely to have, it is important for workers to work within a stance that attends to mentalizing. The worker's connections to their team will be critical in ensuring that they are emotionally regulated enough to be able to enact and model a mentalizing stance when interacting with their clients. The 'therapist's mentalizing stance' has been written about extensively elsewhere (Sharp & Bevington, 2022). It includes efforts to (a) maintain an open, authentically and respectfully curious, 'not-knowing' stance; (b) hold a flexible balance between the various dimensional 'poles' of mentalizing (affective and cognitive, self and other, internal and external, automatic and controlled); (c) intervene actively to punctuate obvious non-mentalizing with manoeuvres that offer the possibility of kick-starting the client's own mentalizing again ('Did you notice the temperature between us change just now? I am sorry, I think I may have said something unhelpful—I want to fix that, but first, can I just check if I'm right to say things feel a bit more awkward than they did a few minutes ago?'); and (d) intervene in positive, affirmative ways to mark, describe, and label any instances of effective mentalizing that the client demonstrates.

2.5.3.3 Scaffolding relationships

Scaffolding relationships encourages us to do what we can to strengthen, rebuild, and repair the relationships around the client. We may do this through exploring some of the following questions (or similar ones) with the client:

- Who is already in the client's life that they experience as helpful?
- What is the quality of their relationship towards their own self, and how might that relationship be improved?
- What do these relationships tell us about the client's existing 'relationship to help' in general?
- Are there existing sources of help that, with some focused work, could function better for the client? Might such relationships be strengthened or repaired?
- Are there potential new relationships whose establishment we could support that might supply longer-lasting or very specific temporary forms of help that our own contribution cannot provide?

2.5.3.4 'Active Planning'

AMBIT promotes an approach called Active Planning, which helps workers to deploy mentalizing in relation to planning. We know that without a plan (long-term goals and objectives, with steps and processes, and perhaps even timelines and measures for progress) achieving significant change in highly complex cases is unlikely. On the other hand, simply making and carrying out plans can easily become highly teleological and counterproductive (e.g. if a young person has not eaten for 24 hours and is hungry, he is unlikely to want to think about why he gets so stressed at college). If we do not attune to what is on our clients' minds, our clients—as we have already seen—may find it extremely difficult to mentalize us as workers, requiring us to 'go the extra mile' in broadcasting what our intentions are. For this reason, Active Planning promotes attention to workers balancing three kinds of effort: (a) making and carrying out plans, (b) broadcasting intentions, and (c) sensitive attunement.

Keeping these three elements in balance can support us with developing shared goals (which include attending to risk areas), working towards these goals purposefully, and managing any crises or new risks that may continue to come up in the course of the work. There are some specific tools, namely the AMBIT Integrative Measure (AIM) cards and the 'Egg and Triangle', that can support us to take an Active Planning approach within our work, and these are detailed in Box 2.2.

2.5.4 Tools and techniques for Working with your Client

See Box 2.2.

Box 2.2 Tools and techniques for Working with your Client

AMBIT has developed a 43-item, multidomain clinician-rated assessment and measure called the *AIM* based on a larger research instrument. Services that use the AIM report its helpfulness in framing a broad, contextually rich narrative of a client's strengths and challenges that can also be used to measure progress. In addition to this, there is a pack of *AIM cards* (or digital equivalents for online use) that can be used as a client-rated version of the same questions, and which enable workers and clients to explore the connections between problems, and to cluster and rank them in terms of what areas of difficulty should be prioritized for attention and help. Working with the AIM cards is described in detail in Chapter 4.

Active Planning can also be helped with an *Active Planning Map*, more commonly referred to as the 'Egg and Triangle' (Figure 2.5).

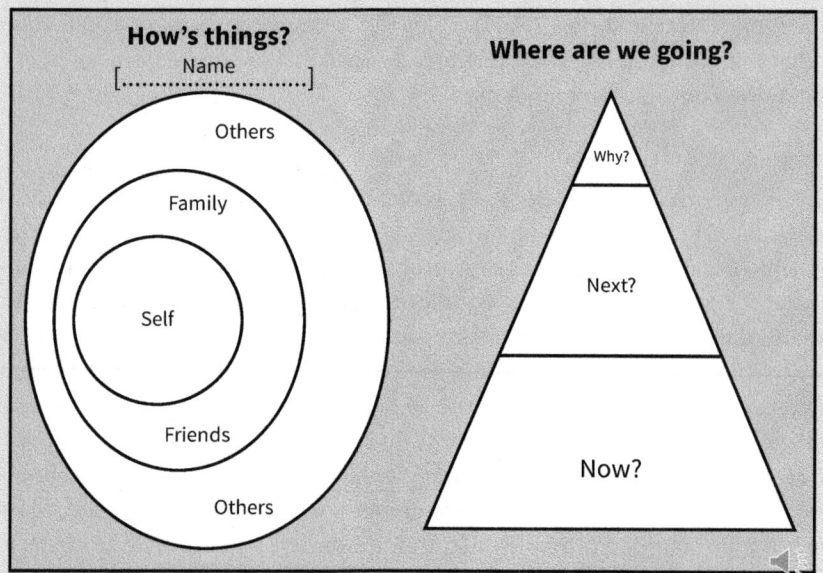

Suggestion: worker fills this in after initial discussion, *then asks young person to help correct it*

Figure 2.5 The Egg and Triangle.

The point of this tool is to facilitate co-created plans, and (if the recording of the client's dilemmas is accurate enough) to begin the process of developing epistemic trust. First, the worker can 'broadcast' their own intentions by filling in the 'egg', which is a visual representation of how they have currently understood the client's struggles. This might be done ahead of or during a meeting with the client and should represent the client's words and thoughts as a 'best estimate' (mentalizing) of their predicament. The client is invited to write their own adaptations and additions, which offers an opportunity for the worker to sensitively attune to the client's ideas. The 'triangle' can be seen as a grossly simplified adaptation of Maslow's Hierarchy of Need, focused on helping actions. It is used to share ideas about work or help that makes sense in the light of what is recorded in the 'egg'. The top slice ('Why?') offers a place to record more aspirational goals (which are often easier for a client and worker to agree upon—things like 'living independently' or 'feeling happier'), while the lower two slices enable discussion about priorities (e.g. activities to address significant safety/risk issues will come under 'Now?' rather than 'Next?').

For more information on these tools and techniques visit the online AMBIT manual: https://manuals.annafreud.org/ambit

2.6 Working with your Network

2.6.1 Mentalizing and non-mentalizing in networks

Many workers in teams attending AMBIT training tell us how difficult they find it to coordinate their work with that of the other agencies that are also involved in helping their clients. Recently, for example, we delivered training for workers in child and young person mental health crisis teams in England and carried out a pretraining consultation to understand some of the challenges faced by this workforce. The workers felt confident overall in managing presentations that they perceived to be un-ambiguous crises of mental health (e.g. self-harm and suicidality in the context of a mental disorder), even though these were of a severe and highly distressing nature. They were less confident in dealing with the significant number of clients whose problems were less easy to define and therefore did not easily fit with the help provided by one particular service. A common scenario was one in which they perceived a young person's distress to be related to their family environment and therefore deemed a 'social care issue', while social care teams viewed the young person's distress primarily as a 'mental health issue' that required treatment from Child and Adolescent Mental Health Services, resulting in a heated debate between the services. This is one of hundreds of similar stories we have heard that demonstrate the challenges of multiprofessional collaboration.

This, combined with the inevitable stress of this work, creates conditions in which it is difficult for members of a multiprofessional network to effectively mentalize. This impacts their ability to make adequate sense not only of the client and their circumstances, but also of each other and how they might best collaborate around the task of helping the client collectively. In AMBIT, we use the term 'dis-integration' to describe these commonly occurring features in networks around clients with multiple needs. We have come to see that there are predictable ways in which networks are poorly integrated around these clients, in that they lack and struggle to reach shared understanding and ideas about several important matters. These are:

- What the problem is
- What to do about the problem
- Who is responsible for doing what.

This is not intended to be critical of workers; dis-integration is inevitable in networks, despite the assumed best intentions of all involved. If we apply mentalizing to such dis-integration it starts to make sense that it should so commonly arise in these ways. Reasons for dis-integration include:

- Different training backgrounds, theories, and models
- Different—or contradictory—priorities of different services
- Access to different information about the client
- Competitive commissioning environments
- Misunderstandings about what each team does, particularly when services are reorganized frequently.

We have also noticed that as workers we can sometimes be a little less inclined to apply our mentalizing ability to trying to make sense of the minds and behaviour of other workers than we are towards mentalizing our clients, particularly if we feel that this will not be reciprocated. All of these factors combine to mean that we can quite often become stuck in non-mentalizing states, which can play out in the following ways within networks:

- *Certainty*: workers can become fixed in their own perspective of the client and what help the client needs, which can leave them closed to new information and thus *certain* that others' ideas are wrong. Workers can also become fixed in their view of other workers/teams because of inaccurate stories that often develop over time within teams as a result of repeated unsuccessful attempts to get into collaboration with each other (e.g. 'Housing workers don't care about our clients').
- *Quick-fix*: in a crisis, when there is an increase in risk and, with it, an increase in worker anxiety, there can be a desire for action. This can result in referrals being made to more services, perhaps more specialist services, even when a large professional network is already in place. This might reduce anxiety in the worker, who feels they have at least done something (and perhaps some relief that accountability has been transferred on to another team), but the addition of more workers may achieve little for the client or, worse, be detrimental, adding yet more complexity and dis-integration.

- *Pretend mode*: such scenarios ('quick-fix' by referral on) sometimes also contain an element of pretend mode—the idea that there exists somewhere a worker of sufficient expertise who can make things better where all others have failed. Workers or teams who find themselves positioned as this 'expert' may feel unable to do anything other than play along, using their expertise to profess certainties when the reality of the situation is that certainties are not currently possible to grasp. (This is not to say that referral out and expert input are never helpful—clearly, sometimes they may be exactly what is required—but the point is that they are often unhelpful when they are the result of non-mentalizing states of mind in workers, rather than a well-thought-out, co-constructed plan.)

By contrast, a mentalizing network contains members who:

- Remain curious about what is behind the different perspectives held by others
- Take alternative perspectives by trying to put themselves in the shoes of others (e.g. 'If I were my client's teacher, it would make sense that I would be most concerned about x, y, z ...')
- Help others to understand their own perspective while avoiding certainty that their perspective is correct and being willing to change their own mind
- Notice any unhelpful assumptions they are forming in their own mind about others
- Pursue shared understanding by recognizing that a richer understanding will be reached by combining multiple perspectives, rather than seeking to impose a single perspective.

2.6.2 Working with your Network: stance features

The two stance features relating to Working with your Network (Figure 2.6) are:

- Meeting multiple needs
- Integrating the help.

We have recently changed the names of these stance features. The adapted stance features, 'Meeting multiple needs' (formerly 'Working in multiple domains') and 'Integrating the help' (formerly 'Keyworker responsible for integration'), simplify the language while broadening the scope of the stance. It is the responsibility of all involved to step outside of traditional siloed working and consider how their own role fits within the client's wider system of care and to make explicit, proactive efforts, within one's ambit (sphere of influence), to ensure that there is a plan for meeting all of a client's needs in an integrated way.

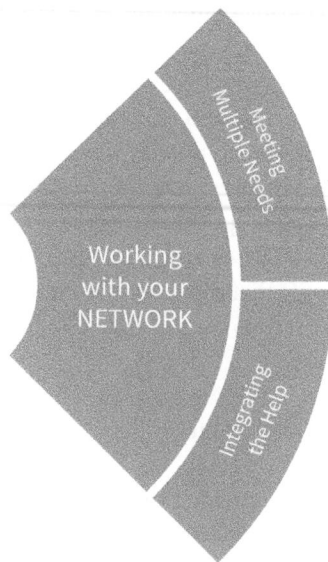

Figure 2.6 Working with your Network.

2.6.2.1 Meeting multiple needs

This stance feature simply reminds us that when we are working with a client with multiple needs, we need to ensure that the help they are offered takes account of and tries to address their various needs. As we have emphasized, these needs are not separate from each other but are often highly interconnected. It is important that any help offered is based on an understanding of how these different needs fit together. Because the needs are not separate, a client does not necessarily need a separate intervention for each one, which is what can commonly happen in our landscape of specialized services, as we described in Chapter 1. The interconnection between their needs means that help in one area may impact positively on another, if we plan and sequence our interventions well.

2.6.2.2 Integrating the help

Help needs to make sense and feel manageable to the client as well as responding to all of their needs. This stance feature reminds us to focus on the client's experience of how the help is organized. The inherent tension between the two network stance features remains unchanged; they can be viewed as two ends on a continuum. At one extreme, a helping system could seek to meet a client's multiple needs by allocating an expert worker for each need. Each expert worker would attempt to build a relationship with the client directly and deliver their particular intervention within their own timescales. The client would be seen not as a whole person but as a constellation of separate needs, and the result would almost certainly be a highly dis-integrated and unhelpful experience for the client. At the other extreme, a high level of integration could be achieved by allocating a single worker to the client and entirely excluding any other services and perspectives. The worker and client might develop a trusting relationship—a prerequisite of effective help—but the worker is likely to be unable to effectively meet the client's multiple needs alone. The best balance on this continuum will vary for each client and will most likely change over time, but usually requires the involvement of several different specialist workers who are prepared to adapt the way that they would work with a client with a single problem (see Section 2.6.3.1). If there is a call to commissioners and service designers, it is to balance the need for clear service specifications with the need for flexibility (so that systems can shape-shift to arrange help around the needs of clients) and adaptability (to allow the shape to change as the client's needs and capacity to trust change).

2.6.3 Working with your Network: basic practice

2.6.3.1 Team around the Worker

Team around the Worker (Figure 2.7) is a principle that encourages us to think about a different way of organizing a network of help around a client. We explore the Team around the Worker more in Chapter 9. To summarize here, it is an alternative to the more usual practice of Team around the Client/Family, whereby a client accesses help by forming individual relationships with a number of different workers whose specialisms are relevant to meeting their needs. These arrangements tend to work well for clients who are trusting of and seeking out help, so we do not seek to replace them in these contexts. However, they usually work less well for clients with multiple needs, due to their adaptive mistrust and the number of relationships that they would have to form in relation to needs that they may not currently acknowledge or wish to seek help for.

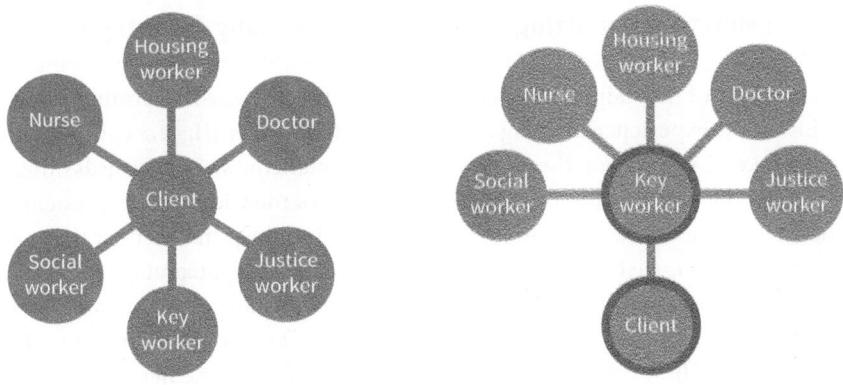

Team around the CLIENT   Team around the WORKER

Figure 2.7 The traditional Team around the Client model compared with the Team around the Worker approach.

Team around the Worker encourages us to mentalize the experience of the client at the centre of the network, to identify who the client trusts most in the current network, or to think about who might be in the best position to develop a trusting relationship with the client if no such relationship already exists. This worker then becomes the bridge between the client and other people in the network. This relationship of trust is centralized, and the network assembles around this relationship to work out how the worker might be best supported to meet the client's multiple needs—which is something they are not going to be able to do on their own (both because it would be an overwhelming task and because the worker is unlikely to have all the knowledge and skills required across different specialisms). The worker will help to broker relationships between the client and other workers, or they may be supported (e.g. through consultation) to deliver interventions that are needed by the client but outside their usual specialism (e.g. a youth worker delivering an intervention to support low mood; a psychologist working through some careers guidance). The number of workers with whom the client has a relationship may grow over time as trust develops, and this is important. We want the worker who the client trusts to support them to develop trusting relationships with others, not to remain or become the only person the client trusts.

This principle does not always sit comfortably with helping systems that are often designed around the expertise of the worker, with workers delivering only the interventions they have been directly trained in or being able to hold cases open only if they are directly seeing the client. As will be discussed in Chapter 9, Team around the Worker is an attempt to design help in a way that adapts to the client's current capacity for trust and help-seeking. Importantly, the idea of the Team around the Worker should not be seen as an inflexible structural prescription for how services should be arranged or commissioned, and certainly not as a map for how accountability should be distributed.

2.6.3.2 Taking a mentalizing approach to addressing dis-integration

For any worker, the practice of Working with your Network involves applying one's understanding of mentalizing and epistemic trust to the networks around one's clients. Just as the experience of being mentalized by the worker triggers epistemic trust in that worker for the client, the application of a mentalizing stance towards others in the network increases epistemic trust between parts of the wider helping system, enabling knowledge and learning to flow in ways that best help the client at the centre. The worker's task is first to recognize the inevitability of dis-integration in networks when clients have multiple needs and then to understand the contribution that non-mentalizing states of mind (one's own and others') make to the creation of that dis-integration. The worker can apply mentalizing to reduce the negative impact of dis-integration within networks by:

- Maintaining curiosity about the client's experience of the network (which is easy to lose sight of amid our own confusion and frustration as a player in that network)

- Helping the client to mentalize the different behaviours and perspectives of the different workers involved in their care (avoiding the temptation to bolster one's own relationship with the client by joining in with non-mentalized criticism of other workers)
- Mentalizing others in the network and seeking help from one's team when one is aware that one is working under conditions that make it difficult to maintain a mentalizing stance towards others in the network
- Noticing when one's teammates enter into non-mentalizing states in relation to others in the network, and offering them help to regain their mentalizing when this occurs
- Making explicit efforts to help others in the network to mentalize oneself, re-membering that if a worker is finding others difficult to understand then it is very possible that others are finding that worker difficult to understand, too.

2.6.4 Tools and techniques for Working with your Network

See Box 2.3.

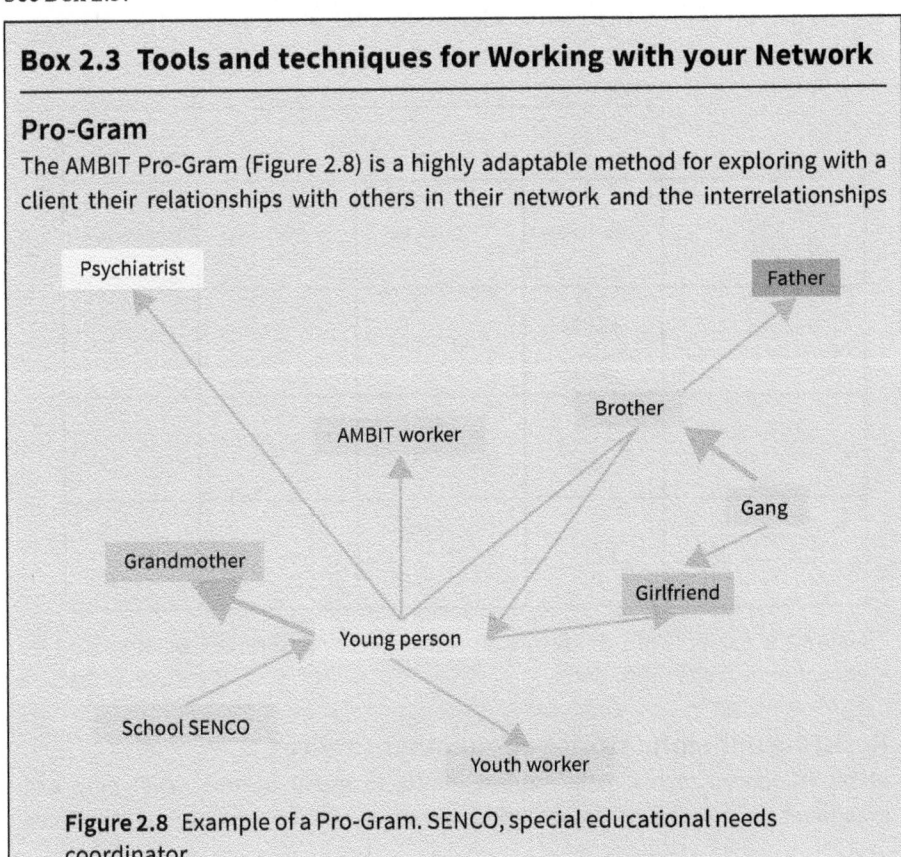

Box 2.3 Tools and techniques for Working with your Network

Pro-Gram

The AMBIT Pro-Gram (Figure 2.8) is a highly adaptable method for exploring with a client their relationships with others in their network and the interrelationships

Figure 2.8 Example of a Pro-Gram. SENCO, special educational needs coordinator.

between those others. In mapping out the network with the client—either on paper, or by 'sculpting' the network with objects—the AMBIT-influenced worker is particularly interested in matters of trust, helpfulness, and understanding, and encourages the client to position people according to their own point of view. Those people who the client trusts or finds helpful are positioned closer to the client at the centre, and levels of understanding or coordination between people are indicated by their proximity to one another.

Dis-integration grid

The dis-integration grid (Figure 2.9) is another tool for mapping out networks and making sense of dis-integration. Most often, dis-integration grids are used by workers in case discussion or supervision, but some teams have successfully used the grids with clients too. The first task is to mentalize each person in the network—to think about what is in the mind of each person in relation to each of the three main levels of dis-integration. The dis-integration grid is a tool to support mentalizing that can open up new perspectives and help one to discover how the current dis-integration makes sense. Often, it reveals gaps in one's understanding of others' perspectives ('Actually, I don't have a clue what the school thinks needs to happen!'). The second step is to use the new ideas to make a plan to address dis-integration, by identifying the 'connecting conversations' that need to take place.

DOMAINS				
LEVELS OF INTEGRATION	Grandmother	Youth worker	School SENCO	Young person
Explanation What's the problem?	Peer relationships —links to gangs	Use of drugs	Lack of family authority to support school attendance	No money
Intervention What to do?	Send him to a boarding school	Engage him with drugs team Alter friendship group	Needs to go into foster care	Have money to stop offending
Responsibility Who can help?	Education authority	Drug and alcohol team Youth club team	Social care	My Dad

Figure 2.9 Example of a completed dis-integration grid. SENCO, special educational needs coordinator.

Resisting unhelpful stories about other services

AMBIT-influenced teams make explicit efforts to guard against developing and maintaining unhelpful, non-mentalizing narratives about other services. A training exercise called 'Wearing Different Hats' explores the stories that teams hold about other teams in the network and those that are held about them. Reflection is encouraged on how these stories develop, their accuracy, and actions that can be taken to promote more mentalized understandings between teams. The aim is to promote integration between teams at a general level, with the hope that this reduces mistrust and improves their capacity to collaborate around shared clients.

For more information on these tools and techniques visit the online AMBIT manual: https://manuals.annafreud.org/ambit

2.7 Learning at Work

2.7.1 Mentalizing and non-mentalizing in relation to learning

AMBIT sets itself up as an open system that is continually receptive to development and improvement and by necessity needs to be adapted to local service contexts. We use the analogy of considering AMBIT to be like open-source software, being refined by users and needing to adapt to new problems and challenges. Teams and practitioners are invited to adopt a stance of always being open to discovering that there may be different and better ways of working—which is a big undertaking. In short, we invite them to become curious about their own methods of practice. In our experience it is a major challenge for both teams and workers to hold a position of serious commitment to the well-being of their clients while at the same time being open to questioning whether what they are offering is the best way of supporting their needs. A mentalizing position in relation to learning involves the capacity to adopt a position of curiosity about one's own work, about 'why we do things in the way that we do'. In many ways, adopting a mentalizing stance with respect to one's own learning represents a bigger challenge than those raised in the other three quadrants of AMBIT. It requires holding a balance between working with conviction around the needs of the client while at the same time holding a position of curiosity about one's work (Figure 2.10). A fuller exploration of this dilemma is described in Chapter 13, where we explore a mentalizing approach to evaluating outcomes.

A mentalizing approach to learning involves creating a team culture in which there is curiosity about the work, skills, and practices of a team and an interest in coming to shared understandings of 'how we do things around here'. When this occurs, it can be very creative and validating for the team and enables workers to move from positions of isolation to a position in which there is shared recognition of the challenges and triumphs of the work itself. The paradox is that we have seen teams develop a greater sense of confidence in their own work as a result of being able to question whether the way they do things is already the best or could be changed. Sometimes this works

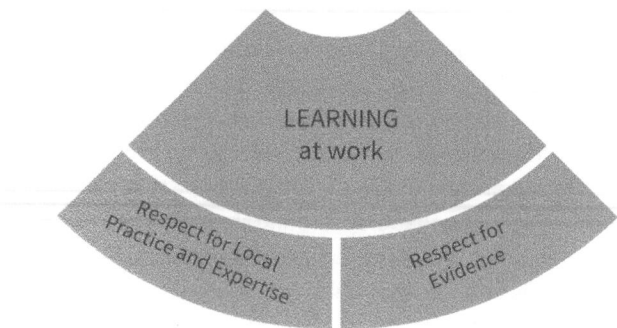

Figure 2.10 Learning at Work.

by teams being able to share common practitioner anxieties. For example, the discovery that everybody in the team privately believes that they each have the worst therapeutic skills in the team may enable the team to find a position of warmth and humour about their uncertainties and, with it, the potential to learn from each other in an authentic and mentalized way. As is the case with clients, the feeling of being understood is likely to lead to a sense of epistemic trust between members of the team, enabling team members to learn from each other.

In relation to Learning at Work, non-mentalizing states of mind are easily generated in work environments in which a perceived lack of effectiveness may trigger feelings of professional shame or represent a threat to the viability of a team. This modern-day 'tiger' that stimulates non-mentalizing may take the form of service reviews, reorganizations, or evaluations, and may represent a threat to survival that is (on one level) experienced as no less significant than a real-life tiger. Such threats easily create non-mentalizing states of mind characterized by certainty ('We know what to do and just need to prove it works'), pretend mode ('Nobody believes all that research, it's got nothing to do with the real world'), or quick-fix ('Just use a standardized outcome measure for every case and we'll be fine'). All of these states are understandable adaptations to service settings but, as is obvious enough, they lack a sense of curiosity about what sort of things have worked for which clients.

For learning to happen, various things need to be in place:

- First, at an individual (or group) learner level, there needs to be awareness and acceptance of the need for learning; in the preceding paragraphs we addressed some of the common ways blind spots arise in this respect.
- Second, again at the individual or group learner level, there needs to be a degree of epistemic trust in the source of potential new learning so that new ideas or learning can be taken in and tested out. For instance, acceptance of evidence from trials requires a certain amount of confidence that the trial has been set up, conducted, and analysed accurately, and that its findings are relevant for the challenges and contexts experienced by the client (or the team). Training models

(such as AMBIT), too, should at least speak in an authentic way to the condition of prospective trainees ('Does this model appear to recognize the particular challenges of my work, or not?'). Epistemic trust is also a necessary condition for team-based learning, where team members need to see each other as trustworthy sources of knowledge to create the openness to learning from each other.

- Third, at a team, organizational, or cultural level, there needs to be what Senge (2006) has described as a shift from an atmosphere of control ('doing as we are told', or, in our language, top-down teleology) to one of learning, in which a group of people experience themselves as permitted—or even encouraged—to explore each other's mental models, to seek out and define their shared intentions and understandings about what help works for which type of client. One of the key points of an AMBIT training is to help teams to mark their shared experience and shared intentions in this regard, and the need for appropriate senior management 'buy-in' to such trainings is therefore critical.

- Finally, at a pragmatic level, there needs to be a sustainable structure that consistently and persistently holds open the space and offers tools for both engaging in and (we would argue strongly) recording the fruits of this process.

2.7.2 Learning at Work: stance features

For AMBIT, the balance to be achieved in learning is between respecting what has been shown to be effective in research and clinical trials and recognizing the practice expertise of workers. The two elements of the stance are summarized as:

- Respect for evidence
- Respect for local practice and expertise.

2.7.2.1 Respect for evidence

Helping clients with multiple needs is difficult work because these different needs interact with each other, making standard interventions or treatments less easy to apply. This can lead to practitioners feeling that conclusions drawn from research are not relevant to the needs of their clients. AMBIT adopts a stance in which what is known from evidence-based practice should be properly considered in relation to the needs of the client. AMBIT does not replace these areas of well-researched practice, so, for example, the use of motivational interviewing for clients with substance use problems would be strongly supported. Similarly, clients experiencing high levels of anxiety (including social anxiety) should be offered help that is consistent with understanding of the role of graded exposure in enabling clients to function well. It is unlikely that any one worker will be versed in all the evidence-based approaches that might be required to support a client with multiple needs. A worker in an AMBIT-influenced team may be able to provide some evidence-based interventions, according to the team's expertise, but will probably also need to look for help for the client outside their team too. This might mean the AMBIT worker being supported by a worker from another team (via a Team around the Worker arrangement) or through the client accessing this help independently.

2.7.2.2 Respect for local practice and expertise

Respect for local practice and expertise is needed on the grounds that 'pure' academic research-based evidence, developed in settings and with populations that are likely to differ (often substantially) from your client's, will always lack the situated and relational knowledge that a practitioner on the ground—with a connection to the client (and understanding of their individual choices) and knowledge of local culture and the local service ecology—can bring. Respecting local practice and expertise alone, of course, risks inviting people to 'make it up as they go along', so again it is the uncertain balancing point between the two principles of respect for evidence and respect for local practice and expertise that the AMBIT-influenced team seeks to find and hold on to. This is much in keeping with the original definition of 'evidence-based medicine' outlined by Sackett et al. (1996, p. 72):

> Because it requires a bottom-up approach that integrates the best external evidence with individual clinical expertise and patients' choice, it cannot result in slavish, cookbook approaches to individual patient care.

As well as relating to the domain of learning and the power relationships that systems of learning and training implicitly carry, we should also add that the stance of respecting local practice and expertise is equally applicable to how team members stand in relation to each other's expertise, and collectively towards their wider local multiagency network colleagues. This may support a more 'whole-systems approach' to the team's internal culture: increased awareness of this stance element allows team members to challenge each other (albeit with humour and compassion) when they notice instances of non-mentalizing (and non-respectful certainty) about the qualities or intentions of other workers or agencies.

Clients with multiple needs require help that is adapted to the details of their particular needs, as highlighted by the case of Ashley in Chapter 1. Workers in AMBIT-influenced teams will have developed many approaches to practice that work well through their experience of doing the work in their local context. The expertise of practitioners is often about how we enable something to happen with this specific family, in this specific school, working alongside this specific social care team. Without this local expertise, evidence-based practice would not have a proverbial leg to stand on. However, the introduction of a training such as AMBIT may inadvertently risk evoking experiences of invalidation in those whose hard-won existing practices and expertise may be implicitly construed as 'replaceable' or 'outmoded'. AMBIT explicitly sets out a model in which both types of expertise are respected, and begins the training process by making the current strengths of the local teams and service a point of interest (this is explained in more detail in Chapter 12).

2.7.3 Learning at Work: basic practice

Holding a team's attentional focus on Learning at Work is challenging because, while few would argue explicitly against it, it can also be hard to know where to start. Consideration of the other three quadrants of the AMBIT wheel is helpful here:

- In the *Client* quadrant, what client outcome measures does the team use, and what evidence is there that they are feeding back into helpful adaptations of individual casework and of the team's shared practices in relation to commonly recurring scenarios?
- In the *Team* quadrant, what forum is available for the kind of shared exploration of mental models and measures that we have described, and what measures of team satisfaction, coherence, and shared practice are available?
- In the *Network* quadrant, what feedback from multiagency stakeholders and partners is available for the team to assess their impact on the coherence of the whole system around clients and their role as 'helpful collaborators'? What feedback is available from clients to enable the team to assess their role as an advocate/broker/interpreter in addressing the multiplicity of the clients' needs across different domains?

In our view, there is a risk both in rigidly following evidence-based protocols for families with multiple problems and in uncritically supporting any type of practice enthusiastically advocated by a local team. How can a balance between these two risks be struck? AMBIT has proposed several tools to mitigate these risks. The first tool is that AMBIT teams are invited to explicitly describe their practice using locally adapted online manuals, which are accessible to all. This creates transparency and also proposes a discipline of making implicit team procedures and ways of working explicit. How does a team working with a client who is subject to a safeguarding plan ensure that their treatment plan is coherent with the social worker's understanding of the family's needs? How does that happen in practice—not just because a practitioner has been prepared to go the extra mile, but what is the general approach of the whole team? When a client is admitted to hospital following attendance at the emergency department, how does the team link up with the hospital team to improve the overall coherence of the client's care? Such knowledge may exist in experienced practitioners' heads, but AMBIT would try to ensure that this knowledge is shared and agreed by the team and becomes an example of 'how we do things in this team'. This process is called *manualizing* and AMBIT places great store in this process as providing a way of balancing what is generally known with local expertise. Transparency of practice is what is needed, with clear shared descriptions of good practice that have been drawn from the collective knowledge and training of the whole team.

AMBIT also promotes a second balancing tool to this dilemma, namely the use of outcome measures that focus on clients' overall functioning rather than their symptoms. This enables teams to track the proportion of cases that show progress that relates to clients' multiple problems rather than only specific mental health matters. We have developed a measure called the AIM, which monitors functioning such as school attendance, relationships in the family, and individual well-being. The ambition is to enable teams to learn more about which of their clients they have successfully helped and those who have made little progress despite the skilled and persistent efforts of the team. Similarly, clarifying what problems the team is more effective in addressing may also be crucial information for the team to come to understand.

We appreciate that lack of time and resources may make some aspects of this work difficult for teams. We have listened carefully to many teams discussing the challenges they face in the 'Learning' quadrant of the AMBIT wheel and have aimed to design methods of learning that are as embedded in team processes as possible. The aim has been to extract learning from events that already happen, such as team meetings, supervision, and informal discussions, rather than allocate large-scale meetings to this task. Our belief is that many opportunities for learning are easily lost, and that valuable learning and discussion are not adequately respected and recorded. This may result in repetitive processes in which familiar issues repeatedly come up and are discussed, taking up a lot of team members' time; these issues may be more effectively addressed by manualizing them. A full description of manualizing can be found in the first AMBIT book (Bevington et al., 2017) and the online AMBIT manual (https://manuals.annafreud.org/ambit).

2.7.4 Tools and techniques for Learning at Work

See Box 2.4.

Box 2.4 Tools and techniques for Learning at Work

AMBIT has developed a range of measures that teams can use, some of which are listed below, but its most unique contribution to the practice of Learning at Work is its wiki manual, the core shared content of which is available at https://manuals.annafreud.org/ambit. Each team that is trained is given their own local version of this wiki, in which their own local edits (new pages, or locally 'attuned' or adapted versions of the core content pages) can be saved and shared online. The key features of the local wiki manual are as follows:

- It is the *process or practice* of a team's (regular and, to a degree, 'ritualized') coming together and collectively sharing learning around a topic, the key outcomes of which are then recorded, that is most important—not the 'technical' aspects of publishing their work in a public-facing wiki.
- Nonetheless, when a team examines a specific element of their practice (looking for the 'marginal gains' that might be won by improving practice in this area),

and *then puts a summary of its learning and intentions into the public domain* on the wiki, this process has an enlivening impact on the team members—who are implicitly invited to find ways to express their shared intentions. A team, as it consists of multiple minds, cannot, strictly speaking, 'mentalize', but a team that is involved in manualizing is probably closest to a group expression of mentalizing: working out 'why we do things like *this*, and not like *that*'.

- There is by design an implicit generosity in the sharing of best practice, and the wiki is an attempt to build this into the model, but AMBIT is also literally built (and continues to be developed) in the wiki, and this transparency of practice at the level of the team and the whole AMBIT community of practice mirrors something of the mentalizing practitioner's radical transparency, where ideas are enriched through exchange and the addition of feedback and new perspectives.

Other key learning tools that AMBIT has developed include the following measures and instruments:

- The *AIM* Version 2 is a 43-item, Likert-scaled, clinician-rated questionnaire with pegged scoring descriptions to help inter-rater reliability. Version 2 added three new items to the original 40 items in Version 1. It probes a wide range of functional domains and is sensitive to clinically relevant change.
  - There is a *client-rated version* of the same questions that can be deployed as a set of *playing cards* (or remotely, using online playing cards) to help in building a client-centred narrative, care planning, and identifying goals-based outcomes.
  - There is also an *online interactive version* (in the AMBIT wiki manual) that easily and safely exports data for collection.
- The *AMBIT Service Evaluation Questionnaire* (ASEQ) is a brief survey using non-technical language that probes team practices across all four quadrants of the AMBIT wheel and enables a team to get a measure of where future training or learning efforts might best be directed to maintain an AMBIT influence in their ongoing practice.
- The *AMBIT Practice Audit Tool* (APrAT) is a simple case audit tool that probes the extent to which there is balanced activity in all four quadrants.
- There is an active *AMBIT community of practice* that seeks to connect workers around the world whose work is influenced by AMBIT so that expertise can be shared more effectively. The community uses online forums, as well as conferences and workshops, and has a mailing list and newsletters to help maintain connections.

For more information on these tools and techniques visit the online AMBIT manual: https://manuals.annafreud.org/ambit

2.8 Implications

This chapter has outlined how AMBIT is a multifaceted, multimodal approach, or, in ordinary language, it is an approach that has many interlocking parts. As with clients, not all services have the same needs; some may have very well-established team processes that would be unhelpfully disrupted by imposing new techniques on to the team, and others may have very well-established and trusting cross-agency arrangements so that some aspects of AMBIT may seem superfluous to this context. This means that AMBIT should be adapted to specific service contexts so that some parts of the approach are prominent in local implementations and other parts may be less so. To realize its adaptive capacity, we see AMBIT as an approach that is half formed as an overall model, in which the gaps are filled by local provision. There is no particular virtue in services aiming to 'do AMBIT' in its entirety. More important is the degree to which AMBIT can be adapted to local service provision in an effective way. In Chapters 5–11, we will illustrate some of the range of settings in which AMBIT has been implemented and the differences that they demonstrate, with each bringing its own area of expertise and existing practice. Beyond the differences, what unites them is the experience—and recognition—of the difficulty of mentalizing under conditions of stress and the difficulty of keeping in balance all of the different aspects of work required to offer effective help to clients. Each of these teams tells a story that is inspirational and valuable in its own right; together they demonstrate AMBIT's adaptability to the context and provide examples of how the four areas of basic practice and eight features of the AMBIT stance we have outlined in this chapter can be applied in different settings.

Before coming to their stories, we will now turn to considering in more detail the theory and role of epistemic trust in the AMBIT approach. Epistemic trust is a component of all mentalization-based interventions, but in AMBIT we apply this creative and highly productive idea to both clients and workers in order to explore how trust and mistrust operate not just between clients and workers but between teams and networks too. We will explore this in Chapter 3.

References

Asen, E., & Fonagy, P. (2021). *Mentalization-based treatment with families*. Guilford Press.

Bateman, A., & Fonagy, P. (2016a). *Mentalization-based treatment for personality disorders: A practical guide*. Oxford University Press.

Bateman, A., & Fonagy, P. (2016b). What is mentalizing? In *Mentalization-based treatment for personality disorders: A practical guide* (pp. 3–38). Oxford University Press.

Bevington, D., Fuggle, P., Cracknell, L., & Fonagy, P. (2017). *Adaptive mentalization-based integrative treatment: A guide for teams to develop systems of care*. Oxford University Press.

Cooper, A., & Redfern, S. (2016). *Reflective parenting: A guide to understanding what's going on in your child's mind*. Routledge.

Fonagy, P., & Allison, E. (2014). The role of mentalizing and epistemic trust in the therapeutic relationship. *Psychotherapy, 51*(3), 372–380. https://doi.org/10.1037/a0036505

Fonagy, P., Gergely, G., Jurist, E., & Target, M. (2002). *Affect regulation, mentalization, and the development of the self.* Other Press.

Jensen, S. L., Bo, S., & Vilmar, J. W. (2021). What is behind the closed door? A case illustration of working with social isolation in adolescents using Adaptive Mentalization-Based Integrative Treatment (AMBIT). *Journal of Clinical Psychology, 77*(5), 1189–1204. https://doi.org/10.1002/jclp.23145

Midgley, N., Ensink, K., Lindqvist, K., Malberg, N., & Muller, N. (2017). *Mentalization-Based Treatment for Children (MBT-C): A time-limited approach.* American Psychological Association.

Redfern, S. (2019). Parenting and foster care. In A. Bateman & P. Fonagy (Eds.), *Handbook of mentalizing in mental health practice* (2nd ed., pp. 265–279). American Psychiatric Publishing.

Rickwood, D., Deane, F. P., Wilson, C. J., & Ciarrochi, J. (2005). Young people's help-seeking for mental health problems. *Australian e-Journal for the Advancement of Mental Health, 4*(3), 218–251. https://doi.org/10.5172/jamh.4.3.218

Robinson, P., & Skårderud, F. (2019). Eating disorders. In A. Bateman & P. Fonagy (Eds.), *Handbook of mentalizing in mental health practice* (2nd ed., pp. 369–386). American Psychiatric Publishing.

Rossouw, T. I., & Fonagy, P. (2012). Mentalization-based treatment for self-harm in adolescents: A randomized controlled trial. *Journal of the American Academy of Child and Adolescent Psychiatry, 51*(12), 1304–1313. https://doi.org/10.1016/j.jaac.2012.09.018

Sackett, D. L., Rosenberg, W. M. C., Gray, J. A. M., Haynes, R. B., & Richardson, W. S. (1996). Evidence based medicine: What it is and what it isn't. *BMJ, 312*(7023), 71–72. https://doi.org/10.1136/bmj.312.7023.71

Senge, P. (2006). *The fifth discipline: The art and practice of the learning organization* (Rev. ed.). Doubleday.

Sharp, C., & Bevington, D. (2022). *Mentalizing in psychotherapy: A guide for practitioners.* Guilford Press.

Tronick, E. Z., & Cohn, J. F. (1989). Infant-mother face-to-face interaction: Age and gender differences in coordination and the occurrence of miscoordination. *Child Development, 60*(1), 85–92. http://www.ncbi.nlm.nih.gov/pubmed/2702877

3
Epistemic trust and mistrust in helping systems

Peter Fonagy and Chloe Campbell

3.1 Setting the scene

Distrust of those who offer help is an insufficiently recognized difficulty in the work that is covered in this book. In this chapter, distrust is not framed as a negative attribute of a client but is considered, from the perspective of mentalizing theory, as an adaptive response to living in threatening and unsupportive social contexts and environments—and one that can be generated in both clients and workers. For many of our clients, mistrust makes sense. The task for the practitioner is to develop a creative, non-defensive response to this aspect of the state of mind of their clients. To this end, the chapter will provide a theoretical framework for approaching this challenging problem by outlining the theory of *epistemic trust* and *epistemic vigilance*. In doing so, this chapter will be more theoretical than any of the others in this book. We are aware that for some readers establishing practice on a strong theoretical foundation makes a lot of sense, whereas others are more comfortable relying on their implicit understanding of these things and can find theory a bit like a forest in which they can easily get lost. So, we have provided a number of worked examples throughout the chapter, like the breadcrumbs in the story of Hansel and Gretel, to help readers find their way back through the forest if they need to. In this journey, we ask you to trust us!

3.2 Mentalizing in real-world settings

One of the authors recently visited a prison where a mentalizing group was implemented highly successfully by a number of prison officers for prisoners serving sentences for violent crimes. The meetings were also attended by interested prison officers. The young men in the prison on the whole enjoyed the group meetings, which took place in a special rehabilitation unit. They claimed to have benefited in terms of improved well-being and having a better appreciation of their past experiences. They evidently valued the feeling that the officers were careful to express curiosity about the thoughts and feelings of the prisoners and were mindful about making unwarranted assumptions before offering alternative perspectives. They uniformly echoed the sense that the mentalizing group was the first experience they had had of any institution (including school, the youth justice service, and, in most cases, social care) appearing to have what felt to them like a meaningful interest in their understanding and experience of events. 'They care what things make us feel', one of them said. However, just before the author, who was introduced as one of the originators of the mentalizing approach, was about to immerse himself in a self-satisfied bubble of contentment, one young man—let's call him Kevin—who had been referred to the group because of repeated violent incidents with fellow prisoners, asked whether he could ask him a question. He said: 'This group and mentalizing is really good and I like it a lot. But when I get back on the wing, it's ****ing useless'. Kevin's insight into the limits of psychological intervention captures one of the main ambitions of AMBIT: how can you support mentalizing in someone when the world around them is often resolutely non-mentalizing?

Kevin's recognition of how difficult it is to generalize skills gained in therapeutic environments to real-world settings is not unique to mentalizing approaches. Kazdin (2013) noted that the generalization of therapeutic gains was perhaps the biggest single challenge shared by all psychological therapies. This is not necessarily surprising: it mirrors the challenges faced by children (and adults) as they acquire new understandings and try to apply these skills to new situations. Vygotsky (1978) highlighted this issue for children and famously suggested that a 'zone of proximal development' was what was needed—that is, space for a child to practise new skills and understandings while scaffolded by the attention and interest of a concerned other. This need for scaffolding applies to psychotherapeutic change, and we have increasingly emphasized that the conditions in which the client is able to apply their 'learnings' (we mean this term in its broadest sense, to refer to new knowledge and understanding acquired about the self or about the social world) in their lived world, outside the confines of the clinical environment, are one of the central and essential components of any effective form of intervention (Bateman et al., 2018). The challenge for the client is to not only understand and take in new ways of thinking about the self and others, and how they interact, but also to use and adapt this social learning in their own environment. This can be hard, and it is made far harder if the environment does not support these changes, especially given that the environment may well also be the one in which the client's original suboptimal (albeit often understandable in the context of that environment) ways of operating had developed. This point was eloquently made by Kevin, and it is supported by research.

In 2019, the Task Force of the Division of Psychotherapy of the American Psychological Association produced its third report, summarizing in a comprehensive way research and clinical practice on most elements of the therapeutic relationship (Norcross & Lambert, 2019). We know that clients do not benefit equally from psychological interventions, and this research focused on understanding the factors that contribute to the variation in client outcomes that we commonly see. Some of the differences were due to the specific therapeutic model used (15%), others to the quality of the relationship formed between the worker and client (30%), but the largest factor influencing outcomes was what happened in the client's life outside the therapeutic relationship (40%). This includes aspects of the client's lived environment, such as a change in their circumstances or their social support. The idea of focusing on the aspects of the helping process that are most likely to impact on the client's day-to-day life, outside of therapy, is at the heart of the AMBIT approach.

The radical aspect of AMBIT is that this observation is not uniquely applied to the experiences of clients in treatment; we believe that the same social learning challenges apply equally to practitioners, and that this challenge must be considered if we expect any real form of openness to learning at work to emerge. The findings of Norcross and Lambert (2019) indicate that providing good outcomes for clients depends on helping systems working together to scaffold the help that might be provided by any one individual worker. This makes a particular demand on helping systems: it means that a single practitioner, no matter how talented and committed they may be, is simply not going to cut it, because one person does not make a social environment. The AMBIT approach is focused on helping teams work together and create networks to build this scaffolding. AMBIT training is less about teaching content, techniques, or clinical skills; rather, it more broadly seeks to develop the social environment of the workplace or network into one that is characterized by openness to social learning, allowing individuals to develop and show their mentalizing processes and express curiosity and interest in the minds and contributions of clients and colleagues alike. To put it in Vygotskian terms, the AMBIT approach is designed to create zones of proximal development in relation to mentalizing within care and support networks: AMBIT seeks to set up the psychological scaffolding that enables new learning to be safely practised.

To illustrate this, let us return to the scenario in the prison outlined at the start of this chapter and come to Barry, a prison officer, who also found the mentalizing group stimulating. He found that it opened up his interest in taking a psychological approach to making sense of the lives of the young prisoners whom he worked with. Not in the sense of Sondheim's quip 'finding deprivation behind depravation' and not resting until sufficient neglect and abuse has been unearthed to 'explain' the young person's behaviour (which remains socially unacceptable in any case). Rather, he found that trying to see the world with the distorted perspectives of the young person, regardless of how they came to be the way they are, made for the possibility of a conversation that was more satisfying for both than the fruitless attempts at persuasion he had previously been inclined to indulge in. We imagine that Barry, as someone trained to immediately apply 'consequences' when he observed unruly behaviour in young people, was initially quite sceptical about this application of the mentalizing approach to the young people he considered to be perhaps the least deserving of sympathy on his wing in the prison. However, Barry reported that he had been surprised to find that he came away from the mentalizing group thinking more seriously about what it might be like to be living the lives of those he was charged with protecting. But Barry, like Kevin, also reported that using his capacity to mentalize out on the wing was often challenging. He described how he had been quite successful at times in applying this type of thinking to situations outside the group when he had been reasonably calm (e.g.

sorting out minor disputes between prisoners) but that it was much harder to think in this way on the more stressful days, 'and those are the times when you really need it'. When these moments of strain happened during the mentalizing group itself, he and the group co-facilitator were able to help each other out, but they worked in separate parts of the prison for their regular shifts and the rest of Barry's colleagues were not able to support him in the same way. So Barry would go back to a world of shifts and unpredictable changes in his work routines; he would be tasked with implementing procedures that are essential to the functioning of the prison but this would rarely take account of the individual experiences of the prisoners themselves. At times he thinks he has 'gone soft' and, more crucially, finds it very hard to see how mentalizing relates to most aspects of his job. We hope that these examples illustrate how Kevin and Barry share the problem of how to make use of the mentalizing approach in their everyday, real-world setting.

In this chapter, we are going to explore how recent developments in academic research have changed our understanding of what supports mentalizing for clients and practitioners. We have rehearsed some of the ideas we touch on here elsewhere (Fonagy et al., 2015, 2022)—however, in relation to AMBIT, we use these ideas from a different perspective. Our previous accounts have focused on problems associated with mental ill health, written from a clinical perspective; we have theorized on conceptualizations of mental disorder and wrestled with notions about what might make therapeutic interventions effective. Here, we will focus on mentalizing difficulties and the disruption in *epistemic trust* among practitioners and within services, rather than in their clients. Epistemic trust is defined as *trust in the communication of knowledge*: it is a concept that has traditionally mostly preoccupied sociologists and philosophers. Epistemic trust involves social judgements about the reliability, relevance, and value of information provided by other people, including those working in helping systems; it is a social-cognitive adaptation that enables us to fast-track social learning (Csibra & Gergely, 2011). Crucially, the great advantage of having epistemic trust in someone is that it enables us to be able to learn from them, which builds our cultural and social understanding of the world and how best to navigate it, and strengthens social bonds. Developmental psychopathologists have proposed that entrenched disruptions in the capacity for epistemic trust, which may be rooted at least partially in adverse childhood experiences, are a key factor in the emergence of mental disorders (Fonagy et al., 2015, 2017a, 2017b), We will explain epistemic trust further later in this chapter, in Section 3.5.1.

Thinking about epistemic mistrust within professional networks is not an attempt to pathologize our often already rather put-upon colleagues, fellow mental health practitioners, and other service providers. Rather, our perspective here is to articulate one of the central points of mentalizing theory: that we are all subject to breakdowns in mentalizing, and these are more likely to happen when we are operating in a non-mentalizing social environment. All of us, when we find ourselves working in non-mentalizing conditions, will find it difficult to work effectively: this is probably true of almost any work environment, but when the work is in a helping profession, in which interacting with others in complex networks and being highly aware of mental states and how they affect behaviour are critically important tasks, these issues are particularly significant.

Before going further, let us describe another example of what we mean. Claire is an outreach worker going to visit Saffron, a 15-year-old who is currently not attending school. Claire is building a relationship with Saffron, and she is planning to introduce Saffron to the head of the local boxing club. Often at these visits, Saffron's mother, Denise, shouts at Claire about how useless she is and how she doesn't understand that Saffron is just bad and needs someone to tell her how to behave. Claire finds these meetings very hard to manage, and often goes silent in response to these attacks and feels incompetent. In this state, she (quite understandably) finds it hard to think clearly, and it becomes difficult for her to mentalize Denise and imagine what must be going on for her. Ahead of this particular visit, Claire has discussed this problem with her supervisor, and they have rehearsed some ideas about how to respond if something similar happens again. Having had this thinking space, Claire is able to stay calm and to share with Denise that she imagines that Denise is increasingly worried that something awful might happen to Saffron. This effort to mentalize Denise changes the dialogue, which now focuses on Denise's worries about Saffron rather than her criticism of Claire. This small step produces a small change in an otherwise repetitive pattern of non-mentalized interactions that had been happening previously. It also creates the potential for Denise and Claire to start working together to protect Saffron.

3.3 Mentalizing: a strength and a vulnerability

Mentalizing is by its very nature an act of imagination—the contents of our mind are never entirely visible to us, and any attempt to think about the thoughts, feelings, or ideas that underpin our behaviour can only be reconstructed in our own minds through an act of imagination. However, our capacity for imagination also creates a significant Achilles' heel: an unmoored imagination, fuelled by either excessively elaborate mentalizing (hypermentalizing) or inadequate mentalizing, can cause significant distress and maladaptive social functioning. This kind of distress is a very common human experience: we know that only one in five people are thought *not* to experience a diagnosable mental health condition during their lifetime (Schaefer et al., 2017). The near universality of psychological distress severe enough to be diagnosed as a disorder suggests that there may be something about human experience, and being in possession of a mind, that leaves us with an intrinsic vulnerability. We have suggested that the risk of mental disorder may arise out of our social-cognitive complexity, in particular our capacity for imaginative thought, which is also the vital ingredient in the process of mentalizing (Fonagy et al., 2022).

We have proposed that our tendency to get caught up in unhelpful ways of imagining what is going on both for ourselves and for other people is the price human beings pay for the immense benefits of our imagination. The advantages of being able to think about mental states in this way are substantial; mentalizing enables us to think together with other people, to cooperate with them, empathize, align perspectives, teach, learn, and create (Fonagy et al., 2022). Mentalizing is a complex and difficult skill, and, as with all such skills, it is easy to get wrong, particularly when we are stressed out and emotionally overloaded. The problem is that being overwhelmed and stressed out and then making mentalizing mistakes, especially when we do this consistently and significantly, is liable to cause further difficulties in our relationships and social functioning, in turn increasing the risk of more stress and distress. We can illustrate how our capacity for imaginative thought can negatively affect our social functioning by returning to our earlier example. Denise imagines that Claire is being duped by Saffron to not understand Saffron's malign intentions and to be on her side against the rest of her family. This makes it impossible for Denise to develop a relationship with Claire that would benefit Saffron.

Some particular modes of thinking emerge when mentalizing goes offline. Previously, we have often described them in relation to clinical work and assessment, but they apply equally to the mentalizing system of a workplace, and we would like to consider them in relation to professional functioning here. These modes of functioning all create situations in which there is a risk in terms of the capacity of a team's ability to make reasoned decisions together on the basis of the shared but different perspectives that should be considered to give a richer and broader view of the needs of a client.

The first of these, already mentioned above, is the *pretend mode*; this describes a form of functioning in which mentalizing appears to be present, but it is superficial and not thought through or deeply meant. Its hallmark is a failure to provide examples, and to elaborate hypotheses and provide speculations in excess of the information that is available. For example, the problems of a young client may be talked about, often with great detail and even greater complexity (including details of their history and the intricacies of their current problems and their motives in relation to their family and friends), but in the end, the general experience is that there is little grounding in reality. A network meeting characterized by pretend mode (which may not be unfamiliar to many readers) is a meeting in which matters are discussed in great detail and with great apparent gravity, but no real progress is made, no meaningful contributions arise that can move the situation forward; there is just a semblance of busyness and concern. The risk in such a situation is that the really important, and perhaps more difficult to consider, issues and needs of the client are subsumed by process and detail. It is often an 'Emperor's New Clothes' scenario. Everyone who is present feels that their understanding of what is being discussed is incomplete but feels unable to speak up about this in case their lack of understanding reveals them to be 'inadequate' or 'incompetent' as a professional. Mentalizing theory refers to this phenomenon of the unsaid thought as 'the elephant in the room'. Sometimes, the one person who can call out the challenge is as gratefully welcomed as the child in the Hans Christian Andersen story.

In the *teleological mode* (also described in Chapter 2 as the 'action' or 'quick-fix' mode), those in the meeting might become concerned with the urgency of doing something in a manner that is reactive to a situation but closes off the possibility of understanding it more deeply. There may be a sense that an action has to be performed, and a visible outcome achieved, for any of the professional activity to be taken seriously. There is a threat or a risk that must be addressed, and often it is the background of intense but justifiable anxiety that understandably compromises mentalizing. The risk, in this mode, is that simply doing something becomes the priority, without adequate reflection or consultation. The joint action that comes out of the meeting achieves a kind of 'we-mode' (a form of co-mentalizing discussed in more detail below in Section 3.5) and trust, but this is based not on shared understanding but on shared fear and shared relief that something has been done. Thus, while there is trust and even a 'we-mode', its value is limited, and the exchange of knowledge between the professionals about the case does not follow. There is also a we-mode in everyone running to the same fire exit when someone shouts 'Fire!' We may be doing something together but, if we cannot get through the exit because of the crowd then, on reflection, it may not have been the best thing to do.

The third mode of functioning is *psychic equivalence*: this is a state in which the capacity to separate inside worlds from outside worlds (we believe that we know *exactly* what is going on), and others' mental states from our own (we *know* what is happening in someone else's mind), is lost. In this state, if we feel something, then it must simply be the case; it is how it is, and it is impossible to entertain another way of looking at things. In psychic equivalence the internal is insufficiently distinguished from the external. This adds an excessive certainty to impressions: 'how I see it is how it is'. It may lead to lengthy discussions in which points of view do not shift. If my perception is reflecting reality, what room can there be for alternative perspectives? As there are no alternative views, the potential for joint intentionality is limited. In a state of psychic equivalence, it is hard to achieve a state of 'we-ness' predicated on the assumption—and tolerance—of different perspectives within the group that come together in a shared understanding, moving to a joint resolution. In fact, when psychic equivalence dominates a group, the potential for different states of mind and ways of thinking to become aligned is usually negligible.

3.4 Mentalizing and collaboration within helping systems

Collaboration is key within helping systems. In AMBIT terms, helpers need to be able to collaborate with their clients, their teammates, and, particularly, with other helpers in their network to promote the best outcomes for their clients. As helpers, we also want to enhance our clients' capacity to relate to and collaborate with others in their own personal networks. In the following section we will share some theoretical ideas that help us make sense of some of the processes that underpin and undermine successful collaboration.

3.4.1   Joint attention and the 'we-mode'

Thinking and working together in complex collaboration is made possible by the ability we have to 'think together' with others. We have suggested that this is why mentalizing, despite the disadvantages and difficulties that go along with being able to think about mental states, is something that evolution has protected. The developmental and evolutionary psychologist Michael Tomasello has written extensively about what is unique about human cooperation. He has pointed out that human cooperative thinking involves the coordination of perspectives (O'Madagain & Tomasello, 2019). Coordination draws on quite a complicated triangle of understanding: it is dependent on drawing a distinction between what one is thinking oneself and what the other person is thinking, and viewing both of these perspectives in relation to the reality of what is 'out there'—the issue that each party is actually focused on. At around 9 months of age, infants, having already learned to track where other people are focusing their attention, develop the additional skill of holding attention jointly with other people. Joint attention is what makes this coordinated perspective possible—it is what happens when two or more people who are interacting notice that they are focused on the same thing at the same time, but perhaps see that object (or person or event) from different perspectives. The two minds are joined but are also, critically (unlike in the blind panic of the teleological state), aware of being separate. Implicit in this process is the awareness of having potentially different perspectives on the shared experience: joint attention depends on a robust and coherent sense of one's own perspective and the recognition of the other person as a separate intentional agent. We will come back to the benefits and risks of this fundamental facet of human cognition in relation to helping us understand and support individuals with multiple needs later in this chapter.

This joint attention and coordination of perspectives generates a particular subjective experience of social cognition that has been labelled the 'we-mode'. The we-mode, or, as we have also termed it, co-mentalizing or relational mentalizing, is an interpersonal experience where intentional mental states are shared and joined together with a common purpose. In the we-mode, Claire and Denise do not have to agree about everything, but they share their intention to help Saffron and recognize each other's intentions as benign and that there may be more than one way to help her. The we-mode broadens awareness of the options available for action and generates new solutions (Gallotti & Frith, 2013). When she is in a calmer state, Denise can see that Claire is trying to help Saffron engage in positive activity and not spend all day in her room playing computer games. She still thinks that Saffron should not be rewarded for avoiding school and thinks that Claire is naïve about what Saffron is really like, but she agrees to support Saffron doing boxing if she wants to do this.

Considerable benefits arise from being able to form this kind of we-mode when we are facing complex and demanding issues in our work: different knowledge and perspectives can be drawn on to resolve a problem that one person alone does not have the capability to deal with. It is not surprising that we are motivated to share our inner states (beliefs, thoughts) and understanding of the social world (Hardin & Higgins, 1996), because this convergence of mentalizing gives us greater confidence when it comes to communicating with other people and understanding where they are coming from. Perhaps most significantly, it changes the character of the relationship and subsequent interactions between the people operating in the we-mode: it contributes to the formation and the maintaining of social bonds.

3.4.2 The we-mode and epistemic trust

Along these lines, we have suggested that the we-mode, or relational mentalizing, may serve as a trigger for epistemic trust. If we hold a position of epistemic trust towards someone, we regard information they communicate as relevant and of shared value and interest: a useful piece of cultural currency. The transmission of knowledge through the channel of epistemic trust allows us to take in and pass on cultural knowledge: information can be passed on to the next generation without infants and children needing to work out the way the world works on their own or by simply watching and imitating others. But this openness to information relies on us being able to quickly recognize communicators that we can rely on, their trustworthiness, and their accuracy (Wilson & Sperber, 2012). While being able to trust is highly beneficial, it is essential to also retain the capacity for *epistemic vigilance* (Sperber et al., 2010). We need to be able to identify when an informant is untrustworthy, or whether what we are being told does not add up. Experimental research suggests that young humans seem to look for certain characteristic features in a communication that encourage us to switch off this vigilance and to accept what is being communicated as something known and appropriately shared by everyone belonging to the group (Gergely & Jacob, 2012). These communicational features, or *ostensive cues* (Sperber & Wilson, 1995), are the signals to alert the recipient that what is being communicated is something beneficial and that a relaxation of epistemic vigilance is safe (Csibra & Gergely, 2009). Infants have been found to be sensitive to ostensive cues such as eye contact, turn-taking, and the use of a special vocal tone (so-called motherese) (Csibra & Gergely, 2006, 2009, 2011); these cues appear to trigger an openness to learning new information from the communicator.

Let us go back to Denise, Saffron, and Claire for a moment. It is incredibly easy for Denise to be positioned as a 'difficult client' and for Saffron to be seen as 'hard to reach'. But their epistemic vigilance may be highly adaptive to both past and present circumstances. Saffron has had difficulties attending school ever since she started in secondary school. Claire is the last of many workers who have offered her help. Saffron got on particularly well with one education support officer, who then left her post without any warning for Saffron. So Claire may be nice, but will she stick around? Denise, meanwhile, hated school. She discovered she was dyslexic when she was an adult so, although she wants Saffron not to have the same bad experience as her, she has no lived experience that school is a safe place for her daughter. The challenge for Claire is to understand the epistemic vigilance as adaptive rather than simply unco-operative. Saffron and Denise *shouldn't* trust her, at least not immediately. How they might come to trust her is what we will now turn to.

Everybody seeks social knowledge to help them navigate the interpersonal world, and we are all sometimes uncertain in relation to our own beliefs and intuitions and seek input and reassurance from others. There is one particular form of ostensive cue that is particularly salient when it comes to activating or deactivating epistemic trust: the experience of being mentalized. As such, mentalizing should not be re-garded as an end in itself: a key aspect of its importance is the role it plays in enabling us to overcome our natural vigilance and benefit from the learning opportunities that social interaction offers.

3.4.3 Co-mentalizing and an epistemic match

Co-mentalizing, or relating to each other via mentalizing each other, is the key to establishing epistemic trust. We will now describe how we understand that learning via interpersonal communication is supported by particular social processes. At its most simple, we have described this thus:

> If I feel that I am understood, I will be disposed to learn from the person who understood me, who I feel is a trustworthy potential collaborator. This will include learning about myself but also learning about others and about the world I live in. (Fonagy et al., 2022, p. 1211)

Let us unpack this, because feeling understood can be quite a complex process, which involves feeling a recognition of one's personal narratives or self-perspectives. Narrative approaches are frequently applied to understand the complexity of identity development (McAdams, 2008; McAdams et al., 2004). The ability to reflect on events and use personal narratives to consolidate something about oneself, to create a social knowledge of the self, is one of the major processes by which one's identity is con-structed during adolescence and adulthood (McLean & Breen, 2009). Personal narra-tives are multilevel structures. We are more aware of some narratives (the dominant ones, which we would bring forward to give an account of our behaviour in terms of our thoughts and feelings); underneath these, and less in our consciousness, are a number of other constructions that we will call subdominant personal narratives. A client may present with a dominant personal narrative focused on, for example, feeling exhausted by having to comply with the multiple demands of carers, man-agers at work, friends, and the social worker who is involved with the family. As she relays this to her social worker, the social worker becomes aware that a subdominant narrative may be resentment or even rage at the impossibility of fulfilling all these expectations. The practitioner recognizes the subdominant personal narrative and empathizes not just with the client's reported sense of fatigue. She also expresses the client's sense of exasperation in relation to the complexity of the demands, suggests that she might feel quite angry and frustrated in similar circumstances, and supports the client in relation to her level of self-restraint. The client perceives the practitioner's recognition of the subdominant personal narrative; there is an epistemic match and an experience of 'we-ness'. The challenge for the practitioner is to gain the client's epistemic trust, which is readily achieved if she can not only perceive the client's subdominant personal narrative but also re-present it to the client in such a way that the practitioner's appreciation is evident to the client. This shared recognition is the we-mode that presents an opening for genuine communication (meaningful listening). The feeling of 'we-ness' is hard to describe; it is almost a bodily state of feeling together with the other person. It is a qualitatively different state where we have voluntarily and consciously subsumed our 'I-mode' to something where our purpose is shared and success no longer means 'I am right' but instead 'We got it right'. There is an essential feeling of collaboration characterized by a sense of mutual presence without any diminution of the importance of the 'I'. The 'I' becomes more important and feels validated by having joined in the 'we'. Going back to our example, Claire feels better about herself as a professional because she and Denise can now work together to support Saffron, while recognizing that her professional ambitions may need moderating—as well as developing a touch of generosity about Denise as a mother. An analogous change occurs in Denise's 'I-mode' as she now feels that her protective maternal instincts, which motivated her suspiciousness towards Claire, have been recognized and she can now listen to (rather than just hear) Claire.

We can break down the mentalizing process involved in creating an epistemic match as follows. It requires the listener to (a) have a coherent enough sense of self to be able to create a self-narrative and recognize the 'match' in the first place, (b) recognize the image of themselves that the communicator is describing to them, and (c) judge the similarity or difference between their self-perception and how the communicator is describing them. The mentalizing demands on the communicator are also considerable. The process requires the communicator to have mentalized the listener well enough to have a good understanding of them—that is, the communicator needs to have recognized the subdominant personal narrative. Mentalizing skills are also required so the communicator is able to convey their understanding of the listener in a clear and empathic way. Thus, epistemic trust as a social process depends on mentalizing on the part of both the listener and the communicator. A major reason for encouraging mentalizing in social environments (e.g. families, schools) is to enable epistemic trust within the system, which in turn enables social learning. This is essential for the system to achieve its primary social function of creating a learning environment—which, in the social context of the psychotherapy clinic, we might describe as 'therapeutic change'.

When there is a disruption in epistemic trust, the process described above also becomes disrupted, as a number of patterns may play out:

- Unease in relation to mentalizing and worry about what others might think or feel, leading to a general avoidance of discourse in mental-state terms and lack of interest in a social knowledge of self, which is likely to compromise a large proportion of social communication.
- Inadequate mentalizing that disrupts the representation of how an individual is perceived by their conversational partner. The individual misrepresents how others represent them, leaving the individual to feel persistently misunderstood and open to experiencing an intense and consistent sense of epistemic injustice, which ruptures communication. In our example, at various times both Claire and Denise experienced difficulties because they felt that their reasons for doing what they were doing were not understood, at least as reflected by the other's actions.
- A deeply inaccurate view of the self can lead the listener to feel misunderstood, and so even if the communicator's representation of their personal narrative is accurate, it is not experienced as a match, creating a rupture in communication. So, if Denise had (inaccurately) felt herself to be the perfect mother, Claire's accurate empathic recognition of her concern about Saffron would have got nowhere.

The disruption of epistemic trust generates a subjective sense of epistemic injustice (being misunderstood) and the person feels stuck in 'epistemic isolation'. To others, such a person appears to be rigid, 'hard to reach', brittle, and not open to communication or influence. However, this perception reflects as much the communicator's failure of mentalizing as anything about the listener.

So how does all of this help Denise, Saffron, and Claire? First, it takes an enormous effort for Claire's mental state not to be dominated by her experience of Denise's and Saffron's negative behaviour towards her, which can very easily dominate and undermine the interactions between them. Claire is able to hold to a mentalizing stance by communicating that her own behaviour may trigger strong reactions for Denise and Saffron. She verbalizes some of what she imagines to be in the minds of Denise and Saffron: 'I'm sure you've experienced workers who come and go'; 'Schools are not always supportive or safe for pupils'. She expresses interest in Denise's point of view and asks about her experience of school, and then she is able to recognize that Denise wants things to be different for Saffron compared with what happened to Denise at school. Denise experiences Claire as trying to see things beyond her own immediate experience and to see Denise's subdominant personal narrative of worry for Saffron that drives her fear of Saffron being overindulged. They can both experience and see similarities and differences between their own experiences. But the process is fragile, as Saffron experiences the growing alliance between Claire and Denise as a threat to her, which risks undermining the sense of parent–professional collaboration. Saffron focuses on creating conflict be-tween Claire and Denise by giving selective accounts to Denise about Claire and vice versa. Cooperative work is re-established by ostensive recognition that the key intention of the shared attention on Saffron is for Claire to work with Saffron with Denise's support.

3.5 What do we mean by non-mentalizing helping systems?

Non-mentalizing social systems have been characterized as ones that create fear and hyperactivate attachment, which undermines mentalizing and precipitates the use of non-mentalizing modes. Such social systems can be self-reinforcing and therefore highly stable in their instability, as they undermine the capacity to negotiate and col-laborate as well as openness to the mutual epistemic trust that would normally allow the social learning and adjustment to take place that might restore more adaptive functioning (Bateman & Fonagy, 2016). An effectively mentalizing social system, by contrast, has been described as flexible and relaxed, that is, not 'stuck' in one point of view. It can allow for give and take and playful problem-solving, without seeking to define others' experiences or perspectives. Individuals within such a system have a sense of agency, that is, that they 'own' their behaviour rather than being passive (Bateman & Fonagy, 2016).

At the start of this chapter, we suggested that non-mentalizing social systems are not the exclusive experience of the history of AMBIT clients. Given specific team his-tories and high levels of background emotion, workers are likely to find themselves operating within—and indeed (although usually not deliberately) contributing to—equally non-mentalizing environments. In fact, there are many aspects of 'helping' workplace cultures that lend themselves to a breakdown in mentalizing. These issues have been discussed before (Bevington et al., 2017), but here we will briefly sum-marize some of the highly legitimate causes of an ineffectively mentalizing culture. First, the pressures involved and the anxieties that arise when working with vulner-able client groups can easily lead to non-mentalizing modes of thinking. Second, substantial external pressures—heavy workloads, funding constraints, lack of organ-izational support, and absence of supervision and collegiality—inevitably take their toll on workers' capacity for reflection and shared thinking. This is an entirely natural response to the 'emergency functioning' that we switch into in pressurized circum-stances: no matter how capable we may be, individually, as mentalizers, the simple fact of the matter is that mentalizing is an interpersonal process, and it can realistic-ally be sustained only with recalibrating contact with other minds. Third, the history of a team may contain within it sensitive points that trigger high emotion and impair effective mentalizing—for example, memories of situations where there has been a sense of competition or of being undermined, unfairly criticized, or blamed within the workplace. Fourth, system-wide epistemic mistrust when repeated communication failures (hearing but *not* listening) occur can lead teams to fragment and individuals to withdraw.

3.6 Why focus on mentalizing in systems?

As a result of a breakdown in the capacity to mentalize others, team members are likely to feel that their perspective is not being understood, or even countenanced, and epistemic vigilance starts to dominate the discourse. We have all been part of teams where suspicion about team members' 'real' motives undermine the potential for collaboration. More commonly, the failure of trust in a system just leads to a reluctance to listen, manifesting as network members tuning out, opening their laptops 'to take notes' but really going through their emails, and listening at best partially. What they are hearing is felt to be from someone who does not really understand their perspective; if they did, they would not be speaking in the way they are. They understand what they are hearing and can make a pretence of responding, but the kind of detailed listening that would imply using the information to inform their subsequent actions is not accessible to them. Why should they listen? They know that what they are hearing is not relevant to them; their mind is firmly made up and their views are locked in a mode of psychic equivalence. Without epistemic trust, the team/network is not working productively in the interest of the client.

An effective team (or network) is one in which colleagues are open to learning from one another and develop new perspectives and ideas about the most appropriate possible courses of action for each client. A mentalizing environment that facilitates the opening of epistemic trust can generate *salutogenesis* (a term we use to mean the factors that support health and well-being) in socio-emotional functioning. In brief, we suggest that a generally mentalizing social environment engenders epistemic trust, which facilitates learning. Thus, AMBIT, if it is successful in creating a working environment imbued with mentalizing, potentially opens *all* participants within a social system (both clients and workers) to alternative ways of seeing things and also increases the likelihood of this new knowledge being internalized and becoming not just information to be recited, but knowledge laid down and embedded into the structures that govern behaviour.

Epistemic trust can colour the potential for social learning of an entire social system. We have recently published a self-report measure of epistemic trust that distinguishes three dimensions on which individuals vary: epistemic trust, mistrust, and indiscriminate trust, or *credulity* (Campbell et al., 2021). We found that mistrust and heightened credulity characterize individuals with a history of childhood adversity. We suggest that a history of trauma, particularly following neglect, generates a general background expectation of an imminent rupture of communication for individuals acting as either listeners or communicators in any social exchange. When an individual has a history of being repeatedly exposed to the communication of unreliable or malintentioned information, they may learn to reject such communications

(Fonagy et al., 2015; Mascaro & Sperber, 2009). Epistemic mistrust reflects persistent scepticism regarding the trustworthiness of a communicator and the information they communicate (Fonagy et al., 2017b). This results in a compromised capacity for social communication and a vulnerability to experiences of ruptured communications. We have described elsewhere (Fonagy et al., 2022; Luyten et al., 2020) the significance of these processes in terms of their developmental impact, and also in terms of understanding personality pathology and the process of change in psychopathology. However, the truth is that everyone experiences these types of disruptions in communication and co-mentalizing in certain situations and, in the face of such disruptions, becomes more vigilant. Certain prolonged experiences of a breakdown in co-mentalizing will cause individuals to become quite firmly epistemically mistrusting—in this state, the possibility of any new communication being meaningful, sincere, or accurate will be entirely disregarded. We maintain that, although severely traumatized individuals are likely to be more mistrustful than others, the non-mentalizing communication systems (which AMBIT aims to address) have the capacity to make all of us behave mistrustfully and be part of dysfunctional communication structures characterized by 'pathological' levels of epistemic mistrust, without individual histories of personal trauma playing a major part.

The potential for disruptions in trust within a system (or team) will reflect that system's own history. The trustworthiness of key actors within a team, as experienced by others in the team, will reflect the history of past interactions as well as the structure of the team. When individuals within the team do not feel adequately recognized or understood by others (see Section 3.4.3), a rupture in communication will follow; if the pattern is repeated or occurs in particularly traumatic ways, it will leave the individual concerned feeling isolated and shamed. For a typical worker, the common subjective experience of not having one's perspective recognized is that it generates ill-feeling, frustration, hopelessness, helplessness, and anxiety—especially if it feels as if something important is being overlooked. The disruption of learning and adaptation within the system can become just as difficult to shift as if it had been caused by the betrayal of trust by an abusive parental figure.

Regardless of its cause, damaged epistemic trust closes the mind to processing socially presented new information, and the 'epistemic superhighway' for the transfer of knowledge within the system is ruptured. There may be a destruction of trust in social knowledge of all kinds. The ability to explore new ways of behaving and responding becomes highly restricted. We are highly attuned to breakdowns in mentalizing in our colleagues and peers, and once a significant breakdown occurs, there is a toll on the ability of the group as a whole to 'think together'. Fresh information that is presented cannot be internalized and knowledge (including social knowledge about the self) is not updated, as it is not trusted.

There is a complication here that will inevitably be encountered in trying to manage epistemic mistrust in social systems such as teams. Failure of communication can, and often does, increase emotional arousal. Not feeling recognized is not a passive experience or even a feeling of emptiness. It is a painful sense of feeling unjustly treated, a sense of threat to the self, which understandably needs to protect itself by raising a shield of high emotion. Similarly, epistemic isolation—feeling excluded from the community of those who are engaged in learning social networks—can generate strong emotion. Rejection hurts, via pathways similar to those involved in physical pain (Eisenberger, 2012). Feeling rejected also interacts with mentalizing. If we know, for example, that someone who appears to be deliberately ignoring us is unusually shy, we rethink why they are avoiding eye contact with us and feel less rejected, because rejection normally has something to do with how we think someone might be thinking and feeling about us. Misinterpreting a neutral reaction as distant, cold, or uninterested may lead us to ask a question such as 'Why don't they like me?' Clearly, many instances of rejection are linked to how another's thoughts or feelings are seen, that is, how we perceive their intentions.

As mentalizing is the key to creating epistemic trust and optimal arousal is the key to effective mentalizing (Arnsten, 1998; Schulreich et al., 2022), it will be challenging to establish epistemic trust against a background of high emotion, which may be the result of feeling excluded or resentful about feeling neglected. As stress (and consequent emotion) increases, individuals tend to switch from relatively slow, controlled, and nuanced mentalizing to more rapid, automatic, and typically biased mentalizing (Luyten & Fonagy, 2015). This means (as most of us know from experience) that when we are stressed, we tend to think a different way. This can be useful—it enables us to make snap decisions and work on the spot—but it also involves a change in our epistemic stance: we are less able to take things in or to make thought-through judgements about the reliability of what we are being told. In a clinical setting, this can create therapeutic ruptures that can be understood as part of a vicious circle in which increased anxiety, or heightened arousal motivated by intense attachment, short-circuits controlled mentalizing and fills the client with further anxiety driven by mistrust, with the result that the emotion becomes even less manageable and can be handled only if it is thrown back at the therapist. As we seek to continually emphasize, workers, too, can experience lapses in mentalizing—particularly in highly stressful contexts—which inevitably leads to a further deterioration in proceedings.

We will use a clinical anecdote to illustrate this. A well-known senior therapist working in a unit specializing in treating individuals with borderline personality disorder supported a severely suicidal patient, who phoned the unit in a crisis. A member of the unit returned the call within the contracted time of 30 minutes but was unable to settle the patient's anxiety. Following the clinic's protocol, a 20-minute appointment was offered for the next day, 4 days before the patient's next scheduled meeting. With great effort, and as an exception to the rule, the patient's senior therapist is made available for this appointment. Unfortunately, the appointment is offered in error, and an important administrative meeting has to be cancelled to make room for the patient in the senior therapist's diary. In the room with the patient, the therapist starts the meeting: 'Thank you for coming in. I am very concerned to understand what has happened since we last met 3 days ago. We have 20 minutes to try ...'. The patient interrupts, in a state of high arousal: 'Twenty minutes, only 20 minutes! You expect to be able to offer meaningful support in 20 minutes. This is ridiculous and unethical. How can you expect me to even begin to tell you what happened in that short a time! This is cruel and mad! You are driving me crazy'. This was said with intense affect, and the therapist felt rage building in him. He said: 'I am afraid I cannot help you when you are shouting at me like this. I will leave now and come back when you calm down'. The therapist walks out. As soon as he is outside, he realizes that he has enacted something and, again following protocol, seeks immediate consultation from a colleague, to borrow a functioning frontal lobe, so to speak. But there is nobody about—everyone is in sessions or meetings. He goes to the day hospital. There is no one there either, as they are holding their reflective group. The only person available is the receptionist. So, the therapist goes to the receptionist and explains about the crisis, the phone call, the messed-up diary, the cancelled appointment, the 20 minutes, the shouting, him walking out, and so on. The receptionist looks up at him and says gently, nodding to the consulting room door: 'Doctor, perhaps you should go back in …'. The spare frontal lobe does not need decades of training to repair the rupture, just a little humanity and compassion.

3.7 AMBIT and non-mentalizing working contexts

How does AMBIT help to promote collaboration in helping systems? The AMBIT approach sets up systems that allow us to think together with other people and to take a broader perspective on our own thinking. We can question ourselves: is the focus of our joint intentionality such that it actually works in the best interest of our clients, or is it stymied by a distorting focus on internal network difficulties, anxieties, or politics? A network meeting—in which colleagues, helping professionals from more than one area, seek to discuss a particular client's situation and needs—is a clear example of a setting in which joint attention and the generation of the we-mode is called upon. The task for the workers, with their different perspectives—arising from both their personal understanding of the client and their different professional priorities and backgrounds—is to think together about the best interest of their client, who is, in this particular scenario, the object of the team's joint intention. These different perspectives and different areas of knowledge and understanding—whether they are those of a teacher, a social worker, a mental health nurse, a psychologist, or a housing officer—can be drawn together to create a valuable integration of the needs and demands of a complex social situation and the best strategies for responding to it. Joint intentionality allows the kind of complex social collaboration that Tomasello (2016) so accurately describes humans as being capable of. The network meeting should engage in cooperative or shared mentalizing processes, with the participants forming their impressions jointly with their colleagues. The convergence of mentalizing leads to more confidence when people take into account the (inferred) inner states of others, especially significant others. In a meeting like this, taking the perspective of others and adjusting the communication to a mutual understanding, or 'shared reality' (Echterhoff et al., 2009), can form and maintain social bonds within the group (Hardin & Higgins, 1996). To achieve a shared understanding with another, one has to 'tune' one's views towards the views of the other, clarifying their perspective through active listening, generating affiliative motivation towards the other, and enabling the opening of epistemic trust. The we-mode, if established in the network, is an experience that forms the basis of the epistemic trust necessary for cooperation and commitment to shared goals, and catalyses the development of joint action that is the ultimate goal of the meeting. The difficulty with the average network meeting, of course, is that while we do normally manage some form of joint attention and shared, we-mode cognition, most of the time—particularly in a large group—we are likely to do this in a suboptimal way. The experience of the we-mode is a mutual creation. It naturally comes and goes, it is lost in non-cooperative interactions, and we continually strive to restore it in the cultivation of epistemic trust. Often, this process is good enough, and although there are inevitably ruptures and misunderstandings that disrupt the we-mode, the process of group repair serves to generate epistemic trust. Perfect alignment may not only be unachievable but may also be undesirable from the point of view of establishing epistemic trust. It is likely that the rapid recognition and addressing (repair) of the misattunements and misunderstandings that inevitably arise does more to generate a common purpose, or we-ness, than perfect immediate attunement might have done. If agreement in the network meeting had been perfect to start with, it may have raised suspicions in many minds of 'groupthink' when the 'I-mode' never emerged, and therefore the 'we-mode' could not be felt as a genuine shared attainment. The we-mode must involve a recognition of the agency, separateness, and individuality of the other, and *voluntary* subsuming of the I-mode into a mode where the dominant goal is joint action and collaboration. The generation of an experience of feeling, thinking, and acting together thus entails an initial experience of having acted separately and where the 'I' sees itself as voluntarily transformed and the interpersonal landscape as becoming 'we-structured'.

Once trust is achieved in the group, there is a possibility that the different views of the participants, with their different professional backgrounds, can be listened to, and the potential is there for everyone in the network meeting to learn something about the client that they will feel is relevant to them, that they should remember, and that also provides information that they will individually be able to use in other contexts. It is through achieving the we-mode through mentalizing that they feel sufficient trust to modify their picture of the client and adopt a new understanding of the client's experience, perhaps even forgetting that it was not the view they had when the meeting was initiated. If all present at the meeting have similar experiences, then perhaps the meeting might have collectively created an image that is far richer and more complex than would be possible for one individual worker to have generated in isolation.

Difficulty arises when any form of joint attention and we-mode is unreachable. In such a scenario (and we have all been in meetings where this happens), various individuals may ostensibly be focusing and jointly attending to a shared issue, but there is no meaningful attempt to think together in an epistemically open way. We have described such a scenario previously, in clinical settings, as being one in which the client can hear but cannot listen, but it is also a common phenomenon among professionals.

As we have said throughout this chapter, epistemic trust is critical for a genuine change of view, based on someone else's perspective, to happen. To achieve epistemic trust, there must be a mutual understanding of perspectives, which can be broken down to a robust sense of self, presented sufficiently clearly to achieve social understanding. The social understanding, if perceived as sufficiently accurate by the other, will generate the match that creates the feeling of we-ness that catalyses the development of epistemic trust.

3.8 Implications

Establishing some degree of epistemic trust is a core objective for all aspects of the AMBIT approach. This is usually perceived as being related to the work that takes place between workers and clients, and is indicated when there is a greater sense of we-mode interactions in this area of work. But this chapter has also highlighted how we-mode thinking is also crucial in team and network relationships—and may be equally difficult to establish. Within a powerful service rhetoric of the value and desirability of inter-agency collaboration, it can be very difficult to even recognize the presence of epistemic mistrust in this crucial area of the work. In many of the subsequent chapters, there will be examples of the challenges that this presents and how different teams have developed their work across the networks in which they work. The theme is that there is no managerial formula for this, but a focus on relationship building between teams is how epistemic trust can begin to be fostered and strengthened.

References

Arnsten, A. F. T. (1998). The biology of being frazzled. *Science, 280*(5370), 1711–1712. https://doi.org/10.1126/science.280.5370.1711

Bateman, A., Campbell, C., Luyten, P., & Fonagy, P. (2018). A mentalization-based approach to common factors in the treatment of borderline personality disorder. *Current Opinion in Psychology, 21*, 44–49. https://doi.org/10.1016/j.copsyc.2017.09.005

Bateman, A., & Fonagy, P. (2016). *Mentalization-based treatment for personality disorders: A practical guide.* Oxford University Press.

Bevington, D., Fuggle, P., Cracknell, L., & Fonagy, P. (2017). *Adaptive mentalization-based integrative treatment: A guide for teams to develop systems of care.* Oxford University Press.

Campbell, C., Tanzer, M., Saunders, R., Booker, T., Allison, E., Li, E., O'Dowda, C., Luyten, P., & Fonagy, P. (2021). Development and validation of a self-report measure of epistemic trust. *PLoS One, 16*(4), e0250264. https://doi.org/10.1371/journal.pone.0250264

Csibra, G., & Gergely, G. (2006). Social learning and social cognition: The case for pedagogy. In M. H. Johnson & Y. Munakata (Eds.), *Processes of change in brain and cognitive development: Attention and performance XXI* (pp. 249–274). Oxford University Press.

Csibra, G., & Gergely, G. (2009). Natural pedagogy. *Trends in Cognitive Sciences, 13*(4), 148–153. https://doi.org/10.1016/j.tics.2009.01.005

Csibra, G., & Gergely, G. (2011). Natural pedagogy as evolutionary adaptation. *Philosophical Transactions of the Royal Society of London. Series B, Biological Sciences, 366*(1567), 1149–1157. https://doi.org/10.1098/rstb.2010.0319

Echterhoff, G., Higgins, E. T., & Levine, J. M. (2009). Shared reality: Experiencing commonality with others' inner states about the world. *Perspectives on Psychological Science, 4*(5), 496–521. https://doi.org/10.1111/j.1745-6924.2009.01161.x

Eisenberger, N. I. (2012). The pain of social disconnection: Examining the shared neural underpinnings of physical and social pain. *Nature Reviews Neuroscience, 13*(6), 421–434. https://doi.org/10.1038/nrn3231

Fonagy, P., Campbell, C., Constantinou, M., Higgitt, A., Allison, E., & Luyten, P. (2022). Culture and psychopathology: An attempt at reconsidering the role of social learning. *Development and Psychopathology, 34*(4), 1205–1220. https://doi.org/10.1017/S0954579421000092

Fonagy, P., Luyten, P., & Allison, E. (2015). Epistemic petrification and the restoration of epistemic trust: A new conceptualization of borderline personality disorder and its psychosocial treatment. *Journal of Personality Disorders, 29*(5), 575–609. https://doi.org/10.1521/pedi.2015.29.5.575

Fonagy, P., Luyten, P., Allison, E., & Campbell, C. (2017a). What we have changed our minds about: Part 1. Borderline personality disorder as a limitation of resilience. *Borderline Personality Disorder and Emotion Dysregulation, 4,* 11. https://doi.org/10.1186/s40479-017-0061-9

Fonagy, P., Luyten, P., Allison, E., & Campbell, C. (2017b). What we have changed our minds about: Part 2. Borderline personality disorder, epistemic trust and the developmental significance of social communication. *Borderline Personality Disorder and Emotion Dysregulation, 4,* 9. https://doi.org/10.1186/s40479-017-0062-8

Gallotti, M., & Frith, C. D. (2013). Social cognition in the we-mode. *Trends in Cognitive Sciences, 17*(4), 160–165. https://doi.org/10.1016/j.tics.2013.02.002

Gergely, G., & Jacob, P. (2012). Reasoning about instrumental and communicative agency in human infancy. In J. B. Benson, F. Xu, & T. Kushnir (Eds.), *Advances in child development and behavior, Vol. 43. Rational constructivism in cognitive development* (pp. 59–94). Academic Press/Elsevier. http://www.ncbi.nlm.nih.gov/pubmed/23205408

Hardin, C. D., & Higgins, E. T. (1996). Shared reality: How social verification makes the subjective objective. In R. M. Sorrentino & E. T. Higgins (Eds.), *Handbook of motivation and cognition, Vol. 3. The interpersonal context* (pp. 28–84). Guilford Press.

Kazdin, A. E. (2013). *Behavior modification in applied settings* (7th ed.). Waveland Press.

Luyten, P., Campbell, C., Allison, E., & Fonagy, P. (2020). The mentalizing approach to psychopathology: State of the art and future directions. *Annual Review of Clinical Psychology, 16,* 297–325. https://doi.org/10.1146/annurev-clinpsy-071919-015355

Luyten, P., & Fonagy, P. (2015). The neurobiology of mentalizing. *Personality Disorders: Theory, Research, and Treatment, 6*(4), 366–379. https://doi.org/10.1037/per0000117

Mascaro, O., & Sperber, D. (2009). The moral, epistemic, and mindreading components of children's vigilance towards deception. *Cognition, 112*(3), 367–380. https://doi.org/10.1016/j.cognition.2009.05.012

McAdams, D. P. (2008). Personal narratives and the life story. In O. John, R. W. Robbins, & L. A. Pervin (Eds.), *Handbook of personality: Theory and research* (3rd ed., pp. 242–261). Guilford Press.

McAdams, D. P., Anyidoho, N. A., Brown, C., Huang, Y. T., Kaplan, B., & Machado, M. A. (2004). Traits and stories: Links between dispositional and narrative features of personality. *Journal of Personality, 72*(4), 761–784. https://doi.org/10.1111/j.0022-3506.2004.00279.x

McLean, K. C., & Breen, A. V. (2009). Processes and content of narrative identity development in adolescence: Gender and well-being. *Developmental Psychology, 45*(3), 702–710. https://doi.org/10.1037/a0015207

Norcross, J. C., & Lambert, M. J. (2019). Evidence-based psychotherapy relationships: The Third Task Force. In J. C. Norcross & M. J. Lambert (Eds.), *Psychotherapy relationships that work. Volume 1: Evidence-based therapist contributions* (3rd ed., pp. 1–23). Oxford University Press.

O'Madagain, C., & Tomasello, M. (2019). Joint attention to mental content and the social origin of reasoning. *Synthese, 198*(5), 4057–4078. https://doi.org/10.1007/s11229-019-02327-1

Schaefer, J. D., Caspi, A., Belsky, D. W., Harrington, H., Houts, R., Horwood, L. J., Hussong, A., Ramrakha, S., Poulton, R., & Moffitt, T. E. (2017). Enduring mental health: Prevalence and prediction. *Journal of Abnormal Psychology, 126*(2), 212–224. https://doi.org/10.1037/abn0000232

Schulreich, S., Dandolo, L. C., & Schwabe, L. (2022). Sunk costs under stress: Acute stress reduces the impact of past expenses on risky decisions. *Psychoneuroendocrinology, 137*, 105632. https://doi.org/10.1016/j.psyneuen.2021.105632

Sperber, D., Clement, F., Heintz, C., Mascaro, O., Mercier, H., Origgi, G., & Wilson, D. (2010). Epistemic vigilance. *Mind and Language, 25*(4), 359–393. https://doi.org/10.1111/j.1468-0017.2010.01394.x

Sperber, D., & Wilson, D. (1995). *Relevance: Communication and cognition* (2nd ed.). Blackwell.

Tomasello, M. (2016). *A natural history of human morality.* Harvard University Press.

Vygotsky, L. S. (1978). *Mind in society: The development of higher psychological processes.* Harvard University Press.

Wilson, D., & Sperber, D. (2012). *Meaning and relevance.* Cambridge University Press.

4

Working out what is going on

Using the AIM cards with clients

Laura Talbot

4.1 Setting the scene

Supporting workers to create trusting relationships with clients who may struggle in their approach to help is a fundamental aspect of AMBIT. Once these relationships are established, it is important that they have the overall purpose of helping the client with their needs, even if these are not fully acknowledged or clearly understood in the early stages of the work. As we have discussed throughout this book, there are many understandable reasons why clients may not want help or see it as automatically trustworthy, and many challenges for workers in supporting a process of meaningful change in these contexts. Not least of these are the often very stark differences in perspective between the client, the worker, and others in the network about what help is wanted or needed.

This chapter will describe the *AMBIT Integrative Measure (AIM) cards*, a card-based activity designed to help a client and worker develop a relationship that is both trusting and purposeful. It will explain how the AIM cards help workers to develop an understanding with the client about how they see themselves and their circumstances, through a process that can support the development of epistemic trust and enable conversations about how purposeful activity might begin to take place. It will illustrate how the AIM cards can be used within a mentalizing stance and how the process fits with Active Planning, a concept that underpins the worker's stance in the client quadrant (as outlined in Chapter 2). The process will be described in depth because the work requires considerable care to avoid stimulating defensive reactions from client and worker alike. The chapter will finish by sharing some of the themes from a study that focused on understanding young people's experience of using the AIM cards.

4.2 Introduction

Establishing and maintaining purposefulness within a helping relationship is essential in promoting change. This process may be easier with clients who are actively seeking our help: usually, these are clients who may already have some trust in the helping process and who have been able to do some thinking about what they might want or need, perhaps on their own or with the support of trusted others. However, for many workers in AMBIT-influenced teams, the early stages in helping relationships with clients are characterized by high levels of mistrust and epistemic vigilance. Despite the worker knowing that they are approaching the client with good intentions, the client may feel equally certain that meeting with a worker is not going to be a good experience for a range of different reasons that may be more or less clear in their minds. These reasons may centre around being seen by the worker as the problem; being asked lots of questions about things they do not want to talk about; being told (sometimes in no uncertain terms) what they need to change and what the consequences will be if they do not do so; being asked to explain why they think, feel, or behave in certain ways, when they do not know this themselves; or generally feeling that they are being blamed, shamed, criticized, or not listened to. Sadly, not all of these fears will be products of the client's imagination, but most likely reflect experiences that they have had with others, including past or current helpers. As much as we may wish it to be otherwise, it is often these kinds of interactions that a client is exposed to when the systems around them become non-mentalizing. We must therefore remember that the stance and behaviour that we might see when we first meet a client may reflect the ways in which they have adapted in response to these experiences, in an attempt to keep themselves safe and minimize the possibility of further distress and harm.

Being faced with the prospect of trying to help a client who has become closed off to the possibility of help has an inevitable impact on how we feel and behave as workers. It can seem like an impossible task. Some workers tell us that they can easily feel very stuck with knowing how best to get started, particularly with clients who are expressing (perhaps very explicitly) that they do not want or need help. Other workers talk about feeling an overwhelming urge to rush in and do something, perhaps not always noticing that they have lost awareness of the difference between their own and the client's perspective about what is wanted or needed. During their first encounters with such clients, they might find themselves imposing their own ideas about what is needed, which often generates resistance or disengagement by the client. Alternatively, they may find themselves aligning too closely with the client's perspective when they say that 'everything is fine' or that 'nothing is going to change', as they do not know how to respond to these statements without risking upsetting the client or losing their engagement. In such situations, clients themselves may not see the point of meeting with the worker again, or a situation might emerge in which the worker and client continue to meet but without the meetings having a clear purpose.

It is not necessarily easier for workers to know how to help in contexts where clients have enough trust in the worker to be able to talk a little more freely about their difficulties, particularly when these difficulties are experienced as overwhelming or unmanageable due to their number, severity, or chronicity. At these times, there can be a sense for workers of being 'in the middle of the pond' with their client, immersed in the emotional intensity of the situation and unable to offer the kind of reflection or alternative perspective that might be possible when sitting on the bank of the pond. When there is this sense of the problems being 'lived' rather than 'named' by both client and worker, it is easy for responses to become reactive. This can create a pattern of 'fire-fighting' where the issues that fill the meetings between client and worker change from week to week and little real progress occurs.

As with many other aspects of AMBIT, our starting point in trying to address these various challenges is to recognize them as common and therefore to be anticipated, albeit to varying degrees for different clients. The task is to focus on supporting the worker with the challenges of attuning to the client sufficiently to help them feel understood, as well as nurturing the client's capacity for help-seeking in such a way that a relationship grounded in both epistemic trust and purposefulness emerges. The ideas in this chapter have been developed out of an experience of working with highly mistrustful and ambivalent clients, who often feel powerless and face outcomes that are undesirable to them. These clients include young people who are on the edge of care, custody, or an inpatient mental health admission, at risk of a breakdown in their foster care placement, facing permanent exclusion from mainstream education, or returning home following a period of secure or institutional care. These are young people who have had many failed experiences of help and very few reasons to trust. As you read this chapter, we ask you to imagine clients in these kinds of circumstances being guided through the process of developing a help-seeking relationship.

4.3 What are the AIM cards?

The AIM cards are a pack of 40 cards, approximately the size of a typical set of playing cards. Each card represents an area of a person's life and functioning. The AIM cards cover seven domain categories: daily life, socioeconomic factors, family relationships, social relationships, mental state, response to the situation, and a measure of complexity. In 2021, we added an additional domain, called 'Power and control', containing three items (experiences of discrimination, exploitation, and online life). Each card has a headline statement such as 'Getting angry' or 'Dealing with arguments in my family', followed by a short explanation of what this means. Each card also shows a scale from 0 to 4 (indicating *strength/not a problem* to *severe problem*) along the bottom so that, if desired, the client can rate each card.

The content of the AIM cards is taken from the AIM questionnaire (Fuggle et al., 2022). This questionnaire was an adaptation of the Hampstead Child Adaptation Measure (HCAM) developed by Peter Fonagy and Mary Target in their study of long-term outcomes of child psychotherapy at the Anna Freud Centre (Fonagy & Target, 1996). The original version of the questionnaire consisted of 40 items providing a holistic (or global) assessment of life and overall functioning. The AIM cards seek to convert the AIM questionnaire into a tool that allows young people to tell us which of the problems apply to them. At the time we developed the cards, we had no real conviction that they would be helpful, and it was something of a surprise when we discovered that the young people not only tolerated our explorations with them, but some actively liked it. We discovered that they could tell us the things that applied to them and, equally important, the things that did not. For some young clients it was a surprise to discover they did not have all the problems listed in the pack (e.g. 'Do some people really have hallucinations? That must be hard!').

The AIM cards can be used for a variety of purposes, including building a picture of a client's strengths and needs (i.e. as an assessment tool), building a shared understanding of how a client's difficulties have developed and connect with each other (i.e. as a formulation tool), supporting goal-setting, and as a way of measuring outcomes via the use of the rating scale. Teams are encouraged to make adaptations to the cards to fit their context, including creating versions using pictures (as has been done by a team working with adults with learning disabilities) or adding cards to cover additional areas. Teams that work with adults have found that the cards can be easily adapted from being a young person's tool by, for example, replacing terms such as 'school' to an adult equivalent such as 'work'.

4.3.1 A recap on mentalizing

An intention behind the AIM cards is that they should create an opportunity for the client to mentalize themselves and for the worker to mentalize the client. The conversations that happen when using the cards also help the client to accurately mentalize the worker's intentions in the prospective helping relationship. As we noted in the introduction, the initial stages of client work can present many challenges, which will inevitably impact both the client and the worker's emotional state and ability to sustain a mentalizing stance. For workers, the well-connected team (see Chapter 2) can help to provide the necessary support and containment to enable them to approach their client interactions within a mentalizing frame. It is through these experiences of being accurately mentalized that epistemic trust is triggered, signalling to the client that the worker is someone with whom it might be both safe and relevant to think, in order to learn more about themselves, others, and the world.

The next section will share some of the ways in which workers might use the AIM cards within a mentalizing stance and following an Active Planning process, to support the development of epistemic trust. Neither of these concepts (mentalizing stance and Active Planning) is designed to be used in a linear or procedural fashion; rather, different aspects of each may be more or less relevant to draw on depending on the context, purpose, and real-time dynamics of the interaction that is taking place. There is no strict protocol for how the AIM cards should be used; this should be adapted to each client and to the worker's style. We will take you step by step through a method of using the cards, in considerable detail, to illustrate the precarious nature of this process, where every step has the potential for the client to disengage.

4.4 Using the AIM cards with a client

4.4.1 Step 1: worker introduces the cards

As with any activity that we plan to undertake with a client, it is good practice to explain and check out with the client what we are proposing to do and why, so we will begin by thinking about how to introduce the AIM cards, with reference to Active Planning. The element 'Broadcasting intentions' in Active Planning refers to what we are doing when we share what is in our mind with someone else, for the purpose of trying to help them understand us. As workers, ensuring that we are accurately understood in terms of our purpose and intentions is key to developing and maintaining an effective helping relationship. We may do this naturally when we are mentalizing effectively—because we remember that people cannot read each other's minds—but when our emotional arousal is higher, our actions may not reflect this understanding. We might find ourselves doing things without sharing the thinking behind our actions, because we have forgotten that it is self-evident only to us or because we are not that clear ourselves about what is driving our behaviour in that moment.

Helping clients to understand our intentions assists us in establishing ourselves as trustworthy helpers. In the early stages, the need for the client and worker to be able to make accurate sense of each other is particularly acute but may also be challenging due to the emotional and relational context. The potential for misunderstanding is substantial. As workers, we can easily assume that clients will know the helpful intentions behind our actions and so fail to make these explicit. This kind of psychic equivalence (e.g. 'I think I am helpful and therefore I am'), combined with pressure to get into action, may lead us to skim over the process of sharing with each of our clients an explanation that helps them to make sense of who we are and why we are there. This gap in shared understanding may be filled by the client's expectations about what our intentions might be, which may lead us to be perceived as threatening, hostile, and, ultimately, untrustworthy.

Let us turn to thinking about the opportunity that using the AIM cards might give us to help these discussions get underway or to support those that have already begun. The aim here is for the client to be able to make sense of us and our ideas about trying out this activity with them and to reduce any potential for misunderstandings about it. To be able to broadcast our intentions, we first need to understand what those intentions are. This process is not something that should be taken for granted as happening automatically or intuitively for workers. Some of the introductory exercises in AMBIT training that involve broadcasting intentions have taken workers by surprise with regard to how much they have had to stop and think in order to be able to verbalize their intentions, whether in relation to trying to explain the purpose of their team or their specific role within it. These difficulties in self-mentalizing make sense to us given that the often fast-paced nature of the work can lead to many 'routine' tasks being carried out on autopilot, without much explicit attention being given to how they might be best contextualized for clients. To help kickstart the worker's mentalizing in relation to explaining the purpose of using the AIM cards with a client, some questions can be used to prompt reflection:

- Why do I want to use these cards?
- What are my ideas about why it could be helpful?
- How might using the cards link to who I am and what I am here for with this particular client?

We can also mentalize the client to help us work out how we might share our intentions in a way that connects with their specific circumstances:

- Do I know of any reasons that might make sense to my client as to why I might suggest that we look at these cards together? (Can I link it to something I already know they might be struggling with or want help with?)
- What might seem like an acceptable reason, from my client's perspective, to give these cards a try?
- What do I want my client to understand/not misunderstand about why I am using them?

These questions are intended to stimulate curiosity rather than to suggest that a worker must come prepared with an introduction to cover all of these questions. Below are some ideas of how these opening sentences might be worded in practice, with the expectation that they would be adapted according to the worker's style:

> I've brought some cards along that I use with lots of young people/families/parents when I'm trying to get to know them. These cards cover different areas of a person's life. Usually we look through the cards together and you help me understand how things are for you by sorting them into different piles. Would you be up for doing that sometime?
>
> I know things have been hard with your family/at school/you've been getting a lot of hassle from the police. These cards might help me understand a bit more about what's been going on for you.
>
> I've heard a lot from [family member/other professional] about what's been going on, but I don't feel as if people have heard that much from you, so I wanted to see if I could help put across how things are for you. I brought these cards with me today, as they might be able to help us with that.

4.4.2 Step 2: worker seeks agreement from client about using the cards

Having shared our ideas about why it might be helpful to use the cards, we next want to check out with the client what they think, to gauge how far our thinking about what might be helpful aligns with theirs. This connects to one of the balances we are trying to hold when working within a mentalizing stance, which is that between self and other. To do this, the Active Planning triangle (see Chapter 2) reminds us that broadcasting intentions (sharing our own thoughts) must be balanced with *sensitive attunement* (paying attention to the other person's state of mind) when trying to collaboratively develop and follow a plan. In any helping interaction, the aim is that both people's minds are acknowledged and understood. Where input is unequal, it can create a range of negative feelings and behavioural responses that undermine collaboration, such as one person actively disengaging from the interaction or more passively going along with what is being talked about, but without any genuine agreement. Many clients may feel unsure about whether it is safe enough to share what they really think and feel, particularly before trust is established in a helping relationship, even if this is not immediately evident to the worker from their behaviour. It is therefore critical that we consider how we might signal to a client that their perspective is actively welcomed and that our relationship can safely tolerate any differences in perspective that will inevitably arise between us.

In connecting this to the process of introducing the AIM cards, maintaining sensitive attunement is an important counterbalance to the efforts we have made to broadcast our intentions about why we are interested in using the AIM cards. Although checking out explicitly with the client whether they want to use the cards risks them saying no, this is preferable to them simply going through the motions of completing the activity without sharing anything meaningful about themselves (i.e. being in pretend mode):

> What do you think, is that something you'd be up for? If you're not sure, it doesn't have to be now—we could always come back to it another time or find another way of talking about what's going on for you.
>
> I don't know what you think about that as an idea. Does it seem like something that you'd want to try?
>
> If you're not sure, you can have a quick look at the cards now and then decide if you want me to bring them again another time—that's fine with me too.

4.4.3 Step 3: client decides how to look through the cards

If the client agrees to look through the cards, we can continue in the domain of sensitive attunement and ask them how they want to do this. Offering choice is important in order to support those clients who may struggle to read or understand some of the cards due to literacy or language needs (although, interestingly, this is not always as significant a barrier as workers imagine it might be). Depending on the client and stage of the helping relationship, the worker may phrase this in terms of knowing that some people prefer to look through the cards themselves, while others prefer the worker to read them out. It can be helpful *not* to explicitly link this choice to need or difficulty (e.g. not saying something like 'Some people prefer to have them read out as they find reading hard'), as requiring the client to acknowledge a need for help with the task upfront may trigger feelings of shame and vulnerability, which may feel too exposing and leave them not wanting to continue.

4.4.4 Step 4: client chooses labels for the piles of cards

The process of using the AIM cards involves the client sorting the cards into different piles, according to whether they feel the issues highlighted on each card are a strength or a need for them. Any cards that they deem not relevant to them can be discarded in a separate pile. Rather than assuming that everyone will be comfortable with the terms 'strengths' and 'needs', from the perspective of sensitive attunement, we might want to consider how best to describe these categories to each client, to increase the likelihood of them sorting the cards in a way that most accurately reflects their circumstances. Our choice of language and the extent to which it provides a good match with the client's current view of themselves is key, particularly for those clients who are the most ambivalent about seeking our help. While some clients may be able to proceed with the task no matter how it is described, for others it will be too emotionally dysregulating to undertake an activity that requires them to acknowledge (both to themselves and to another person) what their 'needs', 'problems', or 'difficulties' are. Instead, we might think about labels for the piles that are less explicitly deficit-focused, which tone down the significance of the problem (e.g. 'things that are not going so well', 'stuff that's not working right now'), or use a visual way to differentiate the piles (e.g. red/amber/green or emojis). All of these considerations may help to moderate the client's level of emotional arousal, helping to maintain their mentalizing and the connection between the client and worker. The language of 'strengths' might also be challenging for clients who do not readily see positives in themselves or their situation. Using more neutral terms for strengths, such as 'things that are going OK' or 'all right at the moment' might be less threatening. For some clients, additional piles might emerge as they begin to sort through the cards and come across cards that describe things they feel are only 'sometimes a problem' or 'a bit less of a problem' than some of the other cards they have chosen, in which case workers can help them add new labels accordingly.

Although these might seem like minor details, all of these considerations represent sensitive attunement in action. Using an inquisitive stance to find out what descriptions are most acceptable to the client may make the difference between them being able to engage in the task or not. Once agreed, the labels can be written on pieces of paper to make it easier to keep track of which pile is which during the card sorting that follows.

4.4.5 Step 5: client sorts the cards into piles

The idea is that the client takes the lead in sorting the cards and the worker takes a less active role during this part of the activity. The task of categorizing each card as a strength, need, or irrelevant (or whatever labels have been decided upon, as outlined in step 4) requires the client to be able to mentalize themselves—a process that may understandably need to be supported. There are several ways in which the AIM cards themselves and the worker's stance can facilitate the process of the client engaging in this reflective, sense-making process, which rests on them experiencing the process and the worker as non-threatening. Partly this occurs through the worker being aware of how such an activity might be emotionally dysregulating and taking steps to reduce the likelihood of this. We will now explore some of what this process might involve.

First, in sorting the cards into different piles, the client is invited to consider how things are for them across a range of different areas of life (e.g. family, education/work, mental health, friendships, risk behaviours). As we set out in Chapter 1, it is very common for clients who work with AMBIT teams to have multiple needs, which they often experience as inherently connected rather than as a series of separate issues. The experience of this is often overwhelming on both a cognitive and an affective level, which can make it difficult enough for the client to form a clear picture in their own mind of 'what the problem is', let alone to communicate it to someone else. Through the use of the AIM cards, this thinking process is supported by the client being invited to take up the position of being 'at the edge of the pond', to see themselves from the outside. This is helped by the fact that the AIM cards offer an external representation of a number of issues that might be forming part of the client's current difficulties; the client does not have to find the ideas and words themselves to begin to express how things are for them but can select what applies from the available options. While this process is not without its demands, clients often comment that it is easier to begin to work out what is going on for them using the AIM cards because the cards 'put the problems out there and not in my head'.

Second, the client can undertake the task of reflecting on themselves and their needs without this being tied up in a relational process. Such a process might ordinarily be experienced as aversive for many reasons, which may lead to fluctuations in the client's emotional state and lower their capacity for effective mentalizing. Furthermore, the breadth of topics covered by the cards means that the client is not restricted to being able to express their needs only in response to questions that are determined by the worker, who may have come with preconceived ideas about the client's problem or a service remit that does not allow them to consider the client's needs more broadly. The fact that the AIM cards reflect a range of areas increases the likelihood of the client having the experience of feeling mentalized rather than misunderstood in this initial process. There is less risk that they will feel that something very important to them is being missed, because *they* are in control of which cards they choose as relevant. Workers sometimes worry that clients will be overwhelmed by the number of cards in the pack, but this is not often borne out in clients' responses. Clients have commented positively on the number and variety of cards, for example, sharing that it felt good to be able to discard cards that were not relevant, as this indicated that they did not have 'all the problems you could ever have', or by being surprised about how the worker 'knew' which cards to include in the pack as there were so many that fitted for them.

Clients may still have dilemmas about whether they feel sufficiently trusting of the worker to reveal particular aspects of their difficulties even through the medium of the cards. However, the experience of seeing the range of issues on the cards can act as a signal to the client that these things might be something that the worker would be willing to hear about or help with at another time. This connects with other feedback from clients about using the cards: that it was easier to talk about something or bring it up having seen it on a card, because that gave them permission to do so or indicated that the issue must be one that other clients had experienced or got help with.

Third, another aspect of the process that may support the client to think about themselves reflectively is that they are being supported to consider their current circumstances from the perspective of both strengths and needs. This is an important example of *holding the balance*, one of the features of the worker's mentalizing stance (even though it is the cards rather than the worker facilitating this). Many clients with multiple needs have become accustomed to problem-saturated stories being constructed by others about their lives, meaning that only their problems are the focus of their discussions with others. Not only can this lead to clients feeling misunderstood and finding professional encounters aversive, this problem focus can also become self-fulfilling. Even though many helping approaches draw on strengths and exceptions as a process for creating change, it is understandable that these aspects of a client's life may receive relatively little attention when their multiple needs are exposing them to high levels of risk or harm. Despite wanting to promote a balanced approach with attention given to both strengths and needs, we must remember that talking about strengths may be a challenging prospect for a client for whom repeated negative relational and life experiences have undermined their capacity to acknowledge any positives in themselves or their circumstances. This issue highlights how holding the balance might intersect with sensitive attunement. As the client sorts the cards, we might begin to notice how manageable the task of acknowledging strengths feels to them, or how they respond when we show an interest in these. Simply holding the balance *equally* between problems and strengths may not be experienced as helpful, and we may need to bring strengths into focus in a more gradual way so as not to invalidate or dysregulate the client.

One final aspect of the process that may support mentalizing is that the client is afforded a space to think about how things are from *their* perspective, without this being clouded or invalidated by how things are viewed or understood by others. This experience offers an important counterbalance to the certainty that the client may have felt from others in their network about what the problem is and what needs to be done about it. All too often, the understandings that prevail within a network about what the problem is for the client have not been arrived at in dialogue with them, but this may be easy for a new worker to miss. There is then a risk that these understandings are imposed on the client without them being given an opportunity to arrive at and share their own ideas, undermining the development of a collaborative helping relationship. This highlights one of the most important balances to be held in client work: that of attending adequately to how things are for the client *from their point of view* before trying to introduce or elicit alternative perspectives.

We have understood from workers that this is not necessarily a stance that is easy to enact in practice, particularly when the worker may be anxious to get on with doing something to address the problems as they see them. For example, during AMBIT training, workers often express how difficult they find the parts of exercises where they are required 'only' to actively listen in response to someone else talking about a dilemma or challenge. Despite being very capable of actively listening, they report becoming strongly aware of—and sometimes unable to resist—the urge to problem-solve or seek to change the person's thinking in some way, even in the context of an exercise where affect (and the stakes) is relatively low.

This tension is often evident when workers are introduced to the AIM cards and hear that the client is given permission to sort them according to their perspective of the situation. Workers worry that clients will not give a 'true' picture or may 'deny' problems described by others, and sometimes ask whether they can remove any cards that they deem not relevant or 'correct' from how the client categorizes the cards. This highlights just how difficult it can be to hold a space for the client's perspective without it becoming overshadowed by our own ideas. While it is understandable that we want to reach a point of shared understanding so that we can move into much-needed action, this is not a process that can be rushed; it rests on the client having had their perspective validated and accurately understood by us, repeated experiences of which will increase the likelihood of epistemic trust being triggered, thus making the relationship feel like a safe space within which new or different perspectives and ideas can be introduced and explored.

4.4.6 Step 6: worker attunes to the client as they sort the cards

There are many ways in which the process of using the AIM cards can facilitate the development of epistemic trust, as it provides many opportunities for the worker to learn about different aspects of the client, which increases the likelihood that they can offer responses and reflections that the client will recognize themself within. This opportunity for learning is facilitated by letting the client take the lead in sorting the cards, which allows the worker to observe the process from the 'edge of the pond' rather than having to contribute to it more actively (as in a more traditional assessment process). From this more removed position, there are a number of things a worker can attend to, learn from, and be guided by in their attempts to offer attuned responses to the client.

For example, it can be interesting to notice how actively, or not, the client tries to engage the worker in the process of looking through the cards, as this may indicate their level of comfort with help-seeking in general and within this specific relationship. Some clients may involve the worker by asking questions, making comments, or explaining their choices aloud as they go, which gives the worker some natural opportunities to support, encourage, and facilitate the client's progress through the task. In contrast, others may seem to want to complete the task more independently, in which case the worker may feel that allowing silence and being as unobtrusive as possible is the most attuned response. For other clients, even if they are not initiating dialogue with the worker, completing the task without any active involvement from the worker may make them feel uneasy because they feel under scrutiny and unsure of what the worker is making of them. So, when faced with a client who is quiet, a worker may wish to offer some simple observations with the intention that they will affirm and validate the client's efforts (e.g. 'You thought a lot about that one'; 'Bit harder to know where to put that one?'; 'Hard work, this!'; 'You're getting through these quickly').

Whatever interjections the worker chooses to make, how the client responds to them will indicate whether more or less of the same will be experienced as helpful as the client continues through the task. Remaining humble and being willing to be corrected by the client is an important part of the worker's stance, as seeing the worker changing their mind will be affirming to the client of the worker's trustworthiness. All of these small but significant efforts to tune into the client can support the process of the client experiencing the worker as accurately understanding them, which will help with the process of establishing trust.

4.4.7 Step 7: worker and client explore how they have sorted the cards

The next part of the activity involves exploring each of the piles in turn to build a shared understanding about how the client has sorted the cards. Before embarking on this (i.e. continuing with *doing the plan* on the Active Planning triangle), the worker can show sensitive attunement to the client by asking how they have found the first part of the activity. The worker might have some of their own guesses, which they can check out. If it has taken the client some time to work through the cards, it may be helpful to let them know what the next steps are, to check out whether they want to come back to it another day. Establishing a shared understanding of how the client is feeling about the process can help the worker and client agree on how to approach the next phase, with the worker using this awareness to inform the stance they might take during the next section. For example, if the client has indicated that they found that some of the cards gave them a lot to think about, but they want to continue nonetheless, the worker can remind the client that they can stop at any time, and remain aware of any cues from the client that they may be experiencing the process as too emotionally arousing.

The client is asked to choose which pile to look through first, rather than the worker assuming whether the 'strengths' or 'needs' would feel better. It can be helpful to spread the cards from the chosen pile out on the table and move the other piles to one side. Let us imagine that the client has chosen to look through the problems first. Often, there are a number of cards in this pile, and the client may find it overwhelming to see them as individual issues and not in keeping with how they are experienced by the client, who may see them as very interlinked. To explore this, the worker can ask the client whether there are any links between the cards they have chosen and invite them to position them accordingly. The process of grouping the difficulties cards in this way usually reveals several smaller groups of cards. The worker can then ask questions to gain an understanding of why the client feels that certain cards go together and how the different piles of cards connect with each other.

When asked, clients usually have some reflections about what it is like to see their difficulties set out in this new arrangement. A common theme is that they had not really thought about how all the different problems fitted together before, but that it makes sense to see them like this. In terms of mentalizing, this part of the activity may be helping the client to begin to understand themselves better. What can emerge here is the start of a more coherent story about why things are the way they are, rather than the narrower and blaming narratives that have been frequently shared. The worker may wish to highlight these more mentalizing accounts arising from how the client has arranged the cards by reflecting them back:

> I can see you're trying to work out how all these things fit together; what happens that means that you break things sometimes? It's not just something that you do for no reason—it happens because you feel angry about the rules your mum has about when you can and can't go out, and this usually leads to a massive argument about some of the other things that don't make you feel good, and you just end up losing it?

The intention at this point is not for the worker to begin intervening, since a discussion about what the client might want the worker to help with has not yet taken place and there is a risk that the conversation could move too quickly to a point that the client does not feel comfortable with or is premature for this stage of the relationship. This may take a degree of discipline and restraint on the part of the worker, who may feel that all sorts of rich avenues for exploration are opening up before them. The worker does not need to do a 'full assessment' of what each of the chosen cards means to the client. Part of using the cards is about learning how able the client is to think about themselves and their situation, and how much they might be willing, able, and ready to accept some help with these matters. The client's need to feel comfortable and in control of the activity should be prioritized over the worker's wish or need to gather information and start intervening. These moments can always be returned to.

Whatever the client shares during this phase of the activity, the worker's emphasis should be on listening to understand rather than to solve. In reflecting back what the worker is learning about the client, any misunderstandings that arise are as valuable as those things they may get right. Even if the client does not indicate that we have misunderstood, it can be helpful to explicitly check out whether there is anything that has been missed out or that we have not quite got right. The more that the client has the experience that we are trying our best to understand them and experiences our attempts to understand as accurate, the more open they may feel to seeking or accepting our help as the relationship develops.

Looking through the 'strengths' pile can follow a similar approach. If the client has selected a number of cards, it might be affirming to ask the client what it is like to see so many cards laid out in front of them. If there are only a few cards, it might still feel supportive to explore this briefly, perhaps asking whether it felt harder to pick out strengths than difficulties. To normalize and validate this, the worker might share that other clients have also found this hard and that it is good that they could choose some cards despite this. The aim of exploring the strengths cards is to understand why these particular areas are going well for the client and to highlight what this might indicate about the skills, strengths, resources, and abilities that might exist within the client or their network. The worker should be mindful of tuning in to the degree to which they think the client can tolerate this level of exploration around a more positive focus, so that it is experienced as supportive, validating, and gently encouraging, rather than contrived or inauthentic. The worker may need to tread carefully with regard to not overstating the extent to which some of these aspects of the client's life are working well. Workers will no doubt have many ideas about how to do this, but some questions may include:

- Can you tell me a bit about why you picked this as something that's working OK at the moment?
- What is it about this card that's going well?
- How does this look when things are OK?
- How come you're able to do this?
- What helps this to go well for you?

Exploring the strengths pile, when managed with sensitive attunement, can also help with the trust-building process. The hope is that the client gets a sense that the worker is interested in them as someone with both strengths and difficulties, which may be particularly impactful if they are expecting a prospective helper to be interested only in their problems. Time spent focusing on strengths may also be a positive experience for the client in terms of the thoughts and feelings that it generates, helping them to feel comfortable in the relationship and potentially more open and able to move on to exploring more difficult aspects of their life.

Having an understanding of the client's strengths can be helpful in a number of ways to any work that may unfold, as the strengths can be drawn on to help with areas that the client is finding more difficult. For example, a worker might discover that the young person has an encyclopaedic knowledge of a football team, which provides a useful example of their capacity to learn that may be in contrast to how they are getting on with learning at school. This could be usefully explored and built upon if school difficulties are chosen as a focus for the work.

In concluding this part of the activity, it can be helpful to check with the client whether there is anything important that has been missed. Not all of life's problems are captured by the cards, and perhaps there was a topic that they were hoping to see on a card that has not come up. Including some blank cards where any additional topics can be jotted down can be helpful.

4.4.8 Step 8: exploring whether there is anything the client might want to be different

Not making any assumptions about help-seeking is an important part of the worker's initial stance when using the AIM cards, even though to do so may cause the worker some anxiety, as they are likely to perceive a number of issues the client would benefit from receiving help with. Given that many clients of AMBIT-influenced teams have not directly sought help, there is a need to balance validating their state of mind around this with also looking for opportunities to influence it, given the level of need and risk that is often present in their circumstances. In such contexts of client ambivalence, help-seeking is a process that we need to nurture, not something that we just wait for in the hope that it spontaneously occurs. How this works is exemplified in approaches such as motivational interviewing (e.g. Miller & Rollnick, 2012), which offers a way to supportively guide clients through a process of change by actively working with their ambivalence. In our experience, following the step-by-step process of using the AIM cards set out here fits with the intention to nurture help-seeking. So far, the worker has been primarily focused on attuning to the client's state of mind, offering support and validation, and aiming to give the client an experience of feeling understood, all in the pursuit of the gradual development of trust. This relational context can form a good foundation for progressing to the next, perhaps more challenging, step of exploring the client's ideas about help.

The worker can begin by commenting on and summarizing how much they have learned about the client from using the cards so far and expressing their appreciation that the client has been able to share things with them, to the extent that this feels contingent and appropriate. The next step is to consider whether the client might wish to see a difference in any of the areas that have come up when sorting the cards. This is deliberately distinct from asking the client whether they want help with anything or suggesting that the worker may have a role in this at this point. The worker can refer back to the groupings of 'difficulties' cards and share that having heard how things are for the client, they are interested to know:

- Are there any of these areas that you would want to be different?
- Is there anything here that you would want to change if you could?
- Is there something here that, if it was going better, would make your life a bit easier?
- Is there stuff here that you would want to be feeling is a bit better than it is now?

Another way of approaching this is to ask the client whether there are any cards in the difficulties pile that they would have wanted to be able to put in the strengths pile. It may feel relevant to acknowledge that thinking about things being different may not be easy if the problems have been around for a long time. This is just about understanding whether the client would want things to be different, rather than for them to get bogged down in thinking about how or whether this could actually happen. Here, there are further opportunities for the worker to validate and express understanding around any cards that the client chooses ('Yes, I can see how getting more sleep would make things a lot easier right now'; 'Having fewer arguments would give you a bit of a break', etc.).

In this part of the activity, the cards that the client chooses may not align with things that the worker (or others in the network) thinks are important to address, which may understandably raise concern and anxiety in the worker. Unfortunately, challenging the client's choices directly (as the worker may feel an urge to) is unlikely to be productive before the client's trust has been gained. We do, however, recognize that it is important that the worker feels equipped with a plan for how they might be able to begin to influence this in the future, and this is covered later in this chapter. In the moment, an alternative response could be for the worker to take an inquisitive stance and show curiosity about the difficulty cards that have *not* been chosen by the client as things they would want to see a difference in, to understand the client's choices better ('There are some cards here that describe things that are hard for you at the moment, but you've not picked them as ones you'd want to be different—I was wondering a bit about why that might be?').

If the client does not pick *anything* that they would like to see working differently at the moment, this clearly presents a dilemma for the worker. While being in this position may feel worrying and frustrating for the worker, they should take seriously this important feedback about the client's current state of mind around help-seeking. We can make sense of the worker's options for managing this with reference to the Active Planning triangle. If the client *had* been able to name some areas they would like to see a difference in, the worker could have straightforwardly progressed to step 9 described below (i.e. exploring whether the client might want help from the worker with any of these cards), which itself naturally leads the client and worker into the territory of '*setting/doing the plan*'. However, without the client naming anything that they wish to be different, there is not such an obvious route for getting into planned action. In terms of the triangle, this leaves the worker with the choice of whether to proceed by taking up a position of *sensitive attunement* to further understand the client's state of mind or first sharing something about their own state of mind by *broadcasting their intentions*.

In terms of *sensitive attunement*, the worker could tentatively explore more about the client's reasons for not choosing any cards highlighting issues they would want to be different at the moment. Approaching this in a spirit of genuine curiosity, in order to be able to make sense of this with the client, is the primary aim here; the client should feel mentalized by the worker's efforts and *not* that they are being interrogated, criticized, or persuaded to take a different view. If this process is not managed well, the client could easily feel that the worker has been disingenuous in their attempts so far to understand them ('You were just pretending to care; you're just trying to tell me what to do like everyone else') if the worker cannot also take on board and respond sensitively to the client's feelings about help, which are of course likely to be highly interconnected with the other needs that they have shared.

Having validated the client's state of mind, the worker could *broadcast* some of their own state of mind, being cautious as to what the relationship can safely tolerate at this point. They might restate how helpful it has been to learn about how life is for the client, but that they understand that the client is not necessarily feeling ready to think about things being different at the moment. Again, the client could very easily feel that there is an undercurrent to this—that the worker is angry or disappointed in them for this being the case—so it may be important for the worker to let the client know that they can see why they feel this way. It can be helpful for the worker to share that there is something else they would like the client to know—that other young people/parents/families do sometimes ask for their help to make changes with some of the problems on the cards, and that if the client felt as if they might want to do this in the future, the worker would be happy to help. The idea is not to add any extra stress or pressure to the client's life, which again may need to be explicitly stated.

The worker may be wondering how to bring the meeting to a useful close at this point, without having established a clear reason to carry on meeting the client. It might be that a discussion takes place about what another meeting could look like—with the worker holding in mind that the priority here will be to continue to develop the client's trust through focusing more on low-threat engagement activities (e.g. getting something to eat or drink; thinking of something concrete and useful they could offer to do for the client; doing something together around one of their interests). If the client agrees, this can become the '*plan*' for now and the worker can look for future opportunities to revisit a more explicit conversation about what the client might want their help with as the relationship develops. They might also pay attention to whether the client begins to seek their help implicitly through talking more about particular issues the more they get to know each other (e.g. sharing more about how things are with their family; talking about problems at school). Sometimes this feels like a more manageable and less shameful route into help-seeking than for the client to say 'I want your help with this, can you help me?', which in their mind may risk the possibility of the worker saying no. In these circumstances, particularly given that the worker will have repeatedly broadcast their intention to want to help through the process of using the AIM cards, the worker can perhaps assume a little more about what the client may be intending in repeatedly talking about particular issues when meeting with them, and experiment with beginning to offer some help with some of what is brought. They can take their cue from how the client responds to this, rather than trying to broker the client's explicit agreement to offer help before doing so, which may lead the client to back off again. This is the fragility of the helping process and, for some clients, it being named as such is something that can happen only retrospectively, once some more trust has been built through the client seeing that the worker has been able to be helpful.

4.4.9 Step 9: exploring who can help with the chosen cards

Let us return to imagining a scenario where the client has been able to pick some cards that they would like to see being different in the future. The next step is to explore whether the client might want any help with the issues described on these specific cards, and from whom. The worker can make explicit that they would be willing to help out with any of the chosen cards:

> I know we don't know each other very well, but I'd really like to make things a bit easier for you if I can. So if there were any cards here that you wanted help with, I'd be happy to give that a bit of a go with you? Just in case it's helpful to know, some of the things here are things that I've helped other (young) people with before. Is there anything here that you'd be up for talking about a bit more together?

Having managed to participate in the process this far, more often than not, the client is able to identify some cards at this point, even if only a small number. The worker may wish to double check whether or not there is anyone already helping with any of the chosen issues, or someone who the client already knows who they would prefer to get help from:

> I'm definitely happy to help out with these if I can—but also I don't want to assume you want help from me with this stuff! Sometimes people have already got loads of workers trying to do things with them. Is there anyone already helping with any of the cards you've picked? Or anyone that you would prefer to help instead of me? I'm happy to let them know if that would be useful.

Sometimes at this point, the client may share that they do have other workers, some of whom may not already be known to the worker. An option here is to use the Pro-Gram (introduced in Chapter 2) to map out the client's view of the professional network they already have, checking for the client's understanding of *who is helping with what*, which can vary considerably and may contrast with what the worker has understood from any communication they have already had with the client's network. This may present a useful opportunity for promoting integration with the network, which could take many forms, including the worker:

- Offering to clarify any helping roles that are unclear to the client (e.g. 'Why does that mental health worker keep sending me appointments?')
- Offering to share the map of who is helping with what with others in the network, so that everyone understands
- Offering to let people in the network know what the client has chosen from the AIM cards, so that other people do not try to keep talking with them about these things too.

The goal of this part of the process is to agree a provisional plan with the client for who is going to help with what. The client and worker can discuss how they are going to work together from this point and which of the chosen issues the client might like to have help with first.

4.4.10 Other ways of using the cards when there is more significant ambivalence about help-seeking

At several points during the above description of the process, we referred to the fact that sometimes clients are not able to move through the activity in such a way that results in them selecting cards that they wish to get help with. This is to be anticipated sometimes and a sure sign of the need to continue to build trust with the client. In motivational terms, the client may be in a state of precontemplation or contemplation (Prochaska & DiClemente, 1984) with regard to seeking help, and it may be within the worker's role and skillset to take a role in trying to address the client's ambivalence in the hope that this moves them closer to seeking help. This is skilful work that takes time and is not without risk. The worker must hold the balance between continuing to build and sustain a relationship with the client and making progress towards developing a purposeful focus on some of the risk or safety issues that need attention. So, how might this look?

One option is for the worker to acknowledge the client's expressed wish for nothing to change at the moment and share that this leaves them with a dilemma because they are worried about the client. They can use the AIM cards to help the client to mentalize them or others in the network with regard to what they might see as the problem. The client could be asked to sort the cards into piles as if they were a particular worker or a member of their family who was being asked to say what they thought the difficulties/strengths were for the client. This may help to draw out the contrast in perspectives between the client and others, which can then be explored. Useful questions might include:

- What would these people pick as problems for you? What would they say are your strengths?
- How come people have different ideas about this?

- Which cards do you most agree with from the ones [family member/other worker] might choose, even if it's only a very small amount?
- If you had to compromise, would there be one card from the other person's choices you would be willing to talk about?
- Would there be one card here that would get other people off your back for a bit if you picked it?
- What would the advantages/disadvantages be of trying out getting help with a card that someone else has chosen?

These questions may create conversational openings that help move the dialogue forward. Again, this is careful work that should not be experienced by the client as pushy. It will be successful only if the worker manages to balance this exploration with maintaining sensitive attunement.

Another option arises when a worker is faced with a situation where discussion of a particular aspect of the client's difficulties is non-negotiable, often due to risk and/or their professional responsibilities. Many workers will be accustomed to such situations arising with clients and may have existing ways of approaching this. In mentalizing terms, all that we might add to this is an acknowledgement of the difference that exists between the perspective of the worker and that of the client. It can be helpful for the client to see that the worker recognizes that this is an issue that they do not currently want to get help with or focus on, and that the worker's push for this is coming from their own professional role and responsibilities. Given this, the worker might ask how best they can make a conversation feel manageable for the client in these circumstances and do their best to offer a clear and predictable way in which such issues will be explored in the sessions. The worker can do their best to proceed with sensitive attunement around as many aspects of the process as possible.

4.4.11 Summary

This description of the sequence of interactions that may arise from using the AIM cards may inadvertently convey that it always happens in a straightforward way. Of course, even with this carefully considered process, there are ways in which it might veer off course. The skill is to go as slowly as possible so as not to stimulate the sense of threat that such an activity may evoke in the client. In some ways, the problem with the AIM cards is that they can sometimes potentially be *too* effective in opening up dialogue. A positive session may be followed by a series of missed appointments if this is not recognized by the worker sufficiently for them to help the client to regulate their emotions through the process. Close connection with team members is essential for the worker to avoid the feeling that they have come to have a unique understanding of their client that no one else has previously managed. This is why AMBIT cannot be done by individual workers alone, as none of us is free from the attraction of feeling extremely helpful to our clients.

4.5 What do clients say about using AIM cards?

In 2016, Jo Carlile completed a doctoral study that included detailed interviews with eight young people and ten workers about the use of the AIM cards (Carlile, 2016). The service contexts from which the sample was drawn included a youth offending team, an intensive outreach service in children's social care, and a youth mental health outreach service. The qualitative analysis of these interviews generated three main themes with additional subthemes, some of which are summarized here. It is very interesting to see the degree to which young people's experiences of using the cards overlap with some of the intended benefits as we see them.

The first theme described the cards as *a useful tool for young people to work out what is going on for them*, helping them to break down their issues and explain what difficulties look like from the outside. Young people reported that it helped thinking and reflection: 'It helped me realize what is actually going on in my life and what is relevant'; 'You can really think about how badly it is affecting you'. This process of reflection was related to both behaviour, 'I don't really think before crimes and it made me think sometimes before I do things', and identity, 'It actually helps you understand who you actually are'. Within this theme were also reports of how these difficulties 'wouldn't even enter my head' without the cards, 'because I never really thought about it but when I saw it there, I had to think about it'. They also reported that it was 'much easier than heavy-going thinking' as the cards are 'not confusing for the user, it's just one simple question and you can just put them into categories'.

This positive feedback was balanced with some comments about what was not helpful. Some young people commented, 'For the little things it's useful but for the bigger things it's not that useful', and 'The thing is, the stuff on the cards I probably would have told him, so it might not have made a difference'. There was also a comment about the negative emotional impact that using the cards might have ('They might make someone upset').

A second main theme in Carlile's study was that the young people reported that using the cards *helped to give them more control over their life*. One client described that it was like 'playing a game of goals' where the young person chooses ('cause it ain't my YOT [youth offending team] worker assuming what is best for me, it's me choosing what is best for me'). For others, it helped to clarify their motivation, with one young person reporting, 'It was helpful for me to see what … what I actually care about in my life and what my motives and goals are'. Four young people referred to the helpfulness of the ratings, for example, 'It's like all the numbers are an easy way for you to put where you are on the scale, easier to set yourself goals'.

It also helped them to solve their own problems. One young person said, 'Before I had the cards and the mentor, I would go around doing bad stuff, now I have other ways to deal with it', and then explained, 'I understood that breaking things is not the way to release my anger, like breaking things or hurting others, so I would just talk to my mentor at school, so I found ways to calm myself'. There was a sense from young people that the cards influenced their ability to solve their problems and make changes: 'The cards say that is why I got angry and then you try and resolve around it'; 'I have made a few changes in my life because of the cards, you know'.

The third theme was that *playing with the cards was easier than just talking*. This theme is more focused on the cards as being helpful in fostering communication between the young person and the worker. Young people said it was helpful to see things and 'having them all out in front of you'. They described the cards as better than having a worker telling or asking them something. There was also the benefit of reading through the cards on their own, with one person commenting, 'It's better reading them 'cause then you can picture them in your head', and another explaining, 'You are going to read it from your point of view, how you understand it'.

Participants also described the cards as being helpful for young people to communicate to their worker what was on their mind without having to speak: 'I think it's useful if I had got a problem and I don't want to talk about or say anything about it … can you just bring the cards again and we can do that'. One young person said, 'They have personal questions, but they are easier to talk about on the cards than just saying it through your voice', and another said, 'Maybe I would tell him eventually, but the cards made me tell him quicker'.

The young people also described that the cards helped the worker understand them, with one young person commenting, 'She would know what to talk to me about, and then she can help me and advise me … because of the cards, if she hadn't, she would have made assumptions'. Another described that 'The worker could understand what I was saying and the emotions that I feel'. These conversations were also linked to supporting help-seeking, with one young person reflecting that 'We talked about why I chose these cards and then it's also a way to, like, get you going on to a conversation and advice to be given to see what you need to work on'.

The detailed feedback from Carlile's study appears to be broadly consistent with a number of the ideas set out in this chapter, in that the young people's experiences of using the AIM cards with a worker helped them to understand themselves better and supported their help-seeking. We would welcome further studies or evaluation to help us understand these issues further.

4.6 Implications

All interventions addressing health and social needs require a degree of engagement between those providing the services and the clients. Such engagement can involve being warm, friendly, compassionate, and efficient. For some projects working with young people there can be the assumption that engaging young people in positive activities alone will lead to real engagement in addressing their life problems. What we have learned in AMBIT, however, is that real engagement requires an effort to communicate about difficult matters and to really enquire about what is happening for a client. Our experience is that young people do not in general shy away from this, despite our predictions that they probably would. We have discovered that the complicated verbal language of mental health is hard for young people to connect with. We need to provide much more scaffolding to enable young people to make sense of what we are trying to do. One element of this is to use more concrete, visual, and easy forms of exchange to build a shared understanding of what the young person is experiencing. This is not a matter of abandoning evidence-based methods for creative methods, but of using creative methods to access well-tested ways of understanding and helping clients with mental health needs. It is the concepts of mental health that are 'hard to reach', and the benefits we have found from using a simple method such as playing cards are an indication of how much we need to move away from our heavy dependence on the intricate language of mental health. In the following chapters, we will begin to learn about how AMBIT has been applied to a series of teams in different countries around Europe. The first of these, Chapter 5, will describe how AMBIT-trained teams were established in Barcelona and will share the profound challenges of introducing AMBIT to a complex helping system.

References

Carlile, J. (2016). *Exploring engagement and the usefulness of the AIM Cards with 'hard to reach' adolescents; hearing views and experiences from young people and clinicians* [DClinPsy Thesis, University College London]. https://discovery.ucl.ac.uk/id/eprint/1516119

Fonagy, P., & Target, M. (1996). Predictors of outcome in child psychoanalysis: A retrospective study of 763 cases at the Anna Freud Centre. *Journal of the American Psychoanalytic Association, 44*(1), 27–77. https://doi.org/10.1177/000306519604400104

Fuggle, P., Bevington, D., Fairbairn, J., Talbot, L., Cracknell, L., & Smith, R. (2022). *A practitioner guide to the AMBIT Integrative Measure (AIM)*. Anna Freud National Centre for Children and Families.

Miller, W. R., & Rollnick, S. (2012). *Motivational interviewing: Helping people change* (3rd ed.). Guilford Press.

Prochaska, J. O., & DiClemente, C. C. (1984). *The transtheoretical approach: Crossing traditional boundaries of therapy*. Krieger.

5

Getting started with AMBIT

The ECID project in Barcelona

Mark Dangerfield

5.1 Setting the scene

In this chapter, we will learn about the setting up of an AMBIT service that began in September 2017. The service was radically different from the clinic- or hospital-based psychiatric services already available to young people in the region and it was led by Mark Dangerfield, a clinical psychologist based in Barcelona. We first met Mark when he came to London to attend the first international AMBIT training that was organized in 2014. It was an inspiring week for us as we worked with a group of psychiatrists, psychologists, nurses, and managers from as far afield as Perth (Australia), New Orleans (USA), Barcelona (Spain), and Amsterdam (the Netherlands). Although their service contexts were very different, the problems of the young people they worked with, and the way services struggled to work together to address their needs, were strikingly similar. At the end of the week's training, the participants went back to their respective services enthusiastic but daunted as to how they were going to implement what we had discussed and explored together for five very intensive days.

This chapter tells the story of how Mark went about creating a team based on AMBIT principles and practice in Barcelona. The chapter is structured so that each of the four parts of the AMBIT approach described in Chapter 2 is considered in turn, but it also describes how the approach built on existing expertise, resulting in local adaptations crucial to the local context. In particular, Mark draws on his clinical background to develop an understanding about the nature of the young people's difficulties, which he calls adverse relational experiences (AREs), and shows how these are embedded in family and parental dynamics. He describes his early contacts with one young person and how having this understanding of the young person's needs helped him to see the young person's behaviour as making sense rather than just as oppositional to others. The chapter goes on to describe how the first team was set up and how they established relationships with other teams working with young people with similar needs. The chapter includes some of the key outcomes of their work, and these impressive results have resulted in wider interest in health services in this region.

5.2 Introduction

'But Mark, are you really a psychologist?' I smiled and felt hopeful when John asked me this interesting question after a few weeks of visiting him in his room, where he had been since retreating from the world almost a year before. It made me think that the door to epistemic trust (Fonagy & Allison, 2014) between us had cracked open; he was starting to show curiosity towards me, as if communicating: 'I am interested in you because you have consistently shown interest in me'. 'Yes, I am a psychologist', I replied. He then paused the video game we were playing together, looked at me and said in a funny way, 'Well, you're a pretty weird psychologist, man!'

John had been referred to the day hospital for adolescents where I worked before starting the AMBIT-influenced ECID project. He had dropped out from school and from life, spending all day at home playing video games in his room. He presented a clinical picture compatible with an at-risk mental state, characterized by a highly persecutory experience of relationships outside his home, especially with his peers, and with significant difficulties in the modulation of his emotional life that led him to experience moments in which he was overwhelmed by intense anxiety. This state of mind increased his need to retreat into his room, dissociating himself from the outside world through very long video-gaming sessions. Prior to the day hospital he had been referred to the local child and adolescent mental health service (CAMHS) but had attended only once and refused to return. The day hospital did not make much difference; it must have been the same thing in his mind, I thought: 'Just grown-ups trying to fix me ...' So, he refused to go there as well.

A mental health day hospital for adolescents is an intensive outpatient centre that works with adolescents with severe mental health problems, such as psychotic states, suicide attempts, at-risk mental states, severe depressive disorders, or severe behavioural disorders. Young people referred to the day hospital must be willing to accept their need for help and go to the centre to follow the treatment plan that has been designed for them. But what happens to the group of young people who do not want to go to a mental health service? This group of young people, who are often referred to as non-help-seeking, were our main concern at the day hospital for adolescents, and the reason why we looked to AMBIT.

After attending a conference at which Dickon Bevington introduced AMBIT to the Barcelona mental health community for the first time, I thought that what he described made so much sense, and seemed to so appropriately address the difficulties we encountered in our daily work with non-help-seeking adolescents, that I felt the need to learn more about what this group of professionals were doing at the Anna Freud Centre in London and, hopefully, get some training in AMBIT.

In retrospect, I felt quite accurately mentalized by Dickon as he told us about the challenges one must face when working with adolescents who present complex problems and do not seem very interested in the help offered by mainstream services. I identified with the difficulties and challenges he described and was struck by what was apparently a simple but effective way of applying mentalizing principles, theory, and technique to our work with this group of young people. A concept I found extremely valuable was that of applying these principles not only with our clients, but also with our team, the wider network, and the process of learning at work: the four quadrants of the AMBIT wheel (described in detail in Chapter 2).

The AMBIT and mentalization-based treatment (MBT) training sessions had a big impact on me, as they challenged my ways of organizing care around these adolescents. It triggered my own questioning of some of the principles that supported my practice: the work setting, the way of being with the young person, some of the ways we organized and approached our team and the wider network, and so on. But it made so much sense and, as I said, it made me feel that it so helpfully addressed the issues I had to face in my daily work, that I dedicated my efforts to organizing a project based on these ideas and this new way of thinking about care in the mental health field. Six years later, together with the Fundació Vidal i Barraquer and the support of the Fundació Nous Cims in Barcelona, we have started three AMBIT-influenced teams: the ECID project, which is named for the acronym for 'Home Intervention Clinical Team' in Spanish (*Equipo Clínico de Intervención a Domicilio*).

We currently have two ECID teams at the Fundació Vidal i Barraquer, and a third team has been set up with another institution in Barcelona, the Hospital Clinic. We have the support of the Catalan public healthcare system and various private foundations that have contributed to commissioning the project, as well as the interest generated among the network and other professionals in Spain. I think that all these developments that have taken place in such a short period of time are clear evidence of how much sense AMBIT makes, and how appropriately it proposes new ways of organizing our systems of care, especially for the high-risk group of young people.

In this chapter I will go around the AMBIT wheel to describe the process of how our practice changed with the implementation of AMBIT. This implementation process and the changes we made were based on long years of experience of different professionals working in mental health services in the Catalan public healthcare system. We used AMBIT as the building blocks with which to scaffold the project, following careful observation and assessment of both the limitations we encountered within mainstream services and the therapeutic factors that AMBIT helped us to identify and develop as core aspects of our work.

We know that AMBIT is not a therapy in the usual sense. However, our experience and outcomes confirm that AMBIT contributes greatly to facilitating a therapeutic relationship, allowing the organization of a system of care that implies a reconsideration of what can really be helpful for the young people and families with whom we work. This process started with a shift in our intentions: instead of having in mind the idea of how to facilitate change in the young person's mind in order to improve their life, AMBIT invited us to consider what we should change in our own minds as professionals and what we would have to change in our teams, institutions, and healthcare network to facilitate the establishment of a relationship with this group of young people, who do not expect anything good to come from a relationship with another human being and, understandably, much less from a relationship with a mental health professional.

5.3 Working with your Client

John presented high psychopathological risk and was at high risk of social exclusion, as well as having a very poor prognosis considering his reluctance to accept the different therapeutic proposals that had been offered from mainstream care services. The conditions in which he lived, withdrawn from the world in his room, implied a risk of worsening and chronicity of his mental and physical state due to his severe isolation, as well as the dysfunctional relational dynamics in which his family had been trapped for many years.

John's mother described him as a smart and happy child, although he had significantly changed in the past couple of years. She said they were very concerned because when he started secondary school (which happens at the age of 12 in Spain) he had gradually begun to lose interest in his schoolwork and behavioural problems began to surface, especially at home. They did not understand why John had changed so much, and why he was not reacting to their firm disciplinary measures, consisting of cutting back his privileges. Disagreements between John's parents had also started to emerge, and conflicts and tensions at home were a daily problem. The family felt trapped in a relational dynamic that seemed only to reinforce their despair and lack of understanding of each other's perspectives and feelings. They all felt very alone and misunderstood by one another, situations that led to mutual accusations, certainties about others, and more frequent conflicts.

Both parents had personal stories marked by AREs (Dangerfield, 2020) in their childhood—stories of suffering and neglect that had marked their lives and conditioned the way they had to organize psychically to be able to survive in a relational world lived with high levels of distrust and hypervigilance. This relational pattern marked the family dynamics, which obviously had an important impact on John's psychological development.

Mainstream services such as primary mental health services and day hospitals usually require some preconditions for treatment to be initiated: the young person must accept their admission to the facilities and, thus, have a minimal sense of needing help. Throughout many years of our work in different mental health services, the group of professionals who started the ECID project had witnessed how valuable these clinical settings can be for a considerable group of children, adolescents, and their families, but also how they fail to offer the help required for a specific but numerous group of adolescents: those for whom it is highly adaptive to keep away from the helping relationships we offer.

When encountering young people presenting difficulties like John's, the inpatient unit for adolescents was the only option we would have to start offering some help, although we also knew that it was not the best way to try to engage a highly distrustful adolescent in a therapeutic relationship. This is especially true as it would most likely imply getting him to the inpatient unit in an ambulance, after dragging him out of his room and medicating him: this does not seem like the best way to establish epistemic trust.

I would argue that inpatient units for adolescents are necessary and helpful only in certain specific situations: after a suicide attempt; when there is severe self-harming behaviour; in an acute psychotic breakdown that overwhelms the containing capacities of the closest relational environment; and in life-threatening cases of anorexia nervosa. In many other situations in which a young person presents high psychopathological risk and risk of social exclusion, as well as a lack of interest in seeing a mental health professional, an AMBIT-based outreach approach that takes the therapeutic perspective to the young person and family's daily lives is much more convenient. This was the starting point of the ECID project.

From our perspective, we consider the problem of this group of non-help-seeking young people not as a specific difficulty of adolescents who reject help, but as a problem derived from the fact that helping systems are not always designed or organized to facilitate young people's engagement with the treatments they offer. We could even say that mainstream mental health services are systems that seem designed to exclude this group of young people (Beale, 2022).

Following AMBIT principles, one of the main ideas we had in mind when designing the ECID project was that instead of continuing to ask young people to adapt to the treatment proposals made by the different mental health services, we should be the ones who tried to adapt to their limited and damaged attachment capacities, that is, we should take our therapeutic stance wherever they can feel safe accepting our presence. To achieve this, we started going to their homes to initiate therapeutic processes, with an emphasis on the relationship already established between the young person and the professional who assumes the role of the keyworker.

Our main goal in the ECID teams is to facilitate a relational experience that allows the development of epistemic trust (see Chapter 3) that can, hopefully, be generalized to the wider relational and social network around the young person. We aim to offer a relationship in which the young person can revisit the psychological developmental process that leads to a sense of agency and trust, which in turn facilitates mentalizing (Malberg, 2013, 2019). We try to provide a different relationship model for both the young person and the systems that surround them, to facilitate a generalization of this different emotional experience to the young person's relational environment (family, friends, school, etc.). This generalization is the final objective of our intervention, since our experience shows that it is this condition that determines the therapeutic effect of our team's intervention.

The ECID is a pioneer mental health project, since it is the first project that was accepted as part of the Catalan public healthcare system, in July 2017, to work with young people who present with significant difficulties in attending mainstream mental health services.

5.3.1 Understanding adverse relational experiences as an impediment to relationships

We know that human development is driven by genes but sculpted by experiences, especially those that happen during the sensitive and critical first few years of life (Teicher et al., 2016). There is strong evidence showing the consequences of attachment styles with parental figures in the developmental process (Fearon et al., 2010; Grossmann et al., 2005; Slade, 2014; Steele et al., 1996), as well as extensive evidence (Artigue & Tizón, 2014; Bendall et al., 2008; Dangerfield, 2012, 2020; Kessler et al., 2010; Merrick et al., 2019; Shevlin et al., 2008; Sørensen et al., 2010; van der Kolk, 2015; Varese et al., 2012) on the psychopathological consequences of adverse childhood experiences, or AREs as I prefer to call them, and the transmission of transgenerational trauma (Dangerfield, 2020), as John's case clearly exemplified.

According to Teicher et al. (2016), adverse experiences in childhood related to relational trauma appear to be the leading preventable risk factor for mental disorders and substance abuse. Emerging evidence suggests that maltreatment alters trajectories of brain development 'to affect sensory systems, network architecture and circuits involved in threat detection, emotional regulation and reward anticipation' (Teicher et al., 2016, p. 652). These brain alterations, Teicher and colleagues argue, should be regarded as adaptations:

> Specifically, we propose that childhood abuse alters the development of particular brain regions, in an experience-dependent plastic manner, to facilitate survival and reproduction in what seems, so far, to be a threatening and malevolent world. From this perspective, what we construe as psychopathology reflects evolutionarily selected alterations in cognition, affect and behaviour that in the past have facilitated reproductive success in certain environments.
>
> The diathesis–stress [the damage caused to the developing brain by toxic stress] and plastic-adaptation hypotheses are not mutually exclusive. Some experiences might be so severe as to damage the brain. However, virtually all of the reported biological and behavioural alterations can be construed as adaptations. (Teicher et al., 2016, p. 653)

We could argue that the position of retreat from the world adopted by some of the young people we work with can be understood as a survival mechanism or adaptive response to dysfunctional attachment relationships that constitute an early experience of a neglectful, threatening, and confusing relational environment.

Regarding terminology, I consider it more pertinent to use the concept of AREs (Dangerfield, 2020) instead of the usual concept of adverse childhood experiences. I believe that using the term 'relational' makes it more explicit and emphasizes the importance of the level at which these adverse experiences occur in childhood— that is, the relationship. Furthermore, if we think about what makes it difficult for these young people to access therapeutic interventions, we see that it also has to do with their difficulties in being able to feel trust in relationships with healthcare professionals. For these reasons, making the relational dimension more explicit in the helping process is one of the fundamental goals of the ECID project. This is manifested at different levels:

- Understanding the difficulties and strengths of young people and their families from a relational perspective.
- Understanding the relationship between the young people, families, and professionals involved. This includes understanding the impact on the professionals and the different teams of our clients' relational and emotional difficulties.
- Understanding the young person's current clinical picture from a developmental perspective, including an adequate assessment of the AREs throughout the developmental process.
- Assessment of the presence of AREs in the parents' developmental process, as well as the transgenerational transmission of relational trauma and its relationship with the young person's current clinical picture.
- Understanding the relational difficulties between different services in the healthcare network, which frequently come about when we are all trying to help young people and high-risk families.

Our experience shows that this group of young people cannot trust that relationships with others will be benevolent because they have not had enough good experiences to allow them to expect that good things will come from others. Being able to trust that their emotional needs will be met in a human relationship is not part of their life experience. Tolerating dependence and the need for affection is something that is often experienced as catastrophic, due to their lack of trust in a sufficiently available and reliable relationship. With these young people, it is frequently observed that being in contact with another human being is something that evokes fear of a traumatic repetition of the experience of emotional neglect in relationships, or of experiences of abuse. An experience of not existing for others or a deep distrust in human relationships has accompanied them almost always and this, in turn, makes them feel a great anger towards the world, something that, understandably, also terrifies them.

For a young person like John who has not known any other option in his life, the world is unreliable and has become an inhospitable place in which he survives by building a sort of cocoon where he hides and feels safe, but which also hides his enormous emotional and relational fragility and shortcomings. For young people who have suffered severe AREs, their emotional experiences have not been recognized and contained, but rather have been neglected or even despised, so their adaptive response is to remain in a position of epistemic mistrust or hypervigilance, maintaining a safe distance that protects them from another round of AREs that they expect to have in new relationships. These AREs have damaged the organization and development of their thought processes, their ability to modulate emotions, and their capacity to mentalize.

All of this has an anti-integrative function in their mind, something we know to be a high-risk factor for serious mental disorders (Quijada et al., 2010). In very general terms, and independently from the manifestations at the clinical-phenomenological level, AREs during childhood can be considered relational traumatic experiences that have caused significant damage in the organization of the emotional sphere, affecting the ability to modulate emotions and to make sense of one's own emotional experience, and the capacity to mentalize (Dangerfield, 2016, 2017, 2021).

We have met many young people like John, who have experienced intense suffering and severe emotional isolation, which has configured an internal world full of pain without words. This has important implications at the healthcare level, since this group of young people often does not ask for help; it is very difficult to connect with one's own emotional needs if one has not had a minimal experience of a 'good-enough' available relationship. Such young people tend to feel deeply distrustful and hopeless when faced with what human relationships can offer, and we think it is essential for helping services to take this into account when organizing mental healthcare. In John's case, our initial approach was to respect his need to not be forced to leave his room and go to a mental health centre, validate the potentially intrusive nature of our presence in his home, and be explicitly curious about his interests and his life at home. This facilitated a containing experience that helped to diminish his persecutory anxieties and let him start feeling some curiosity towards me. We know that the experience of feeling seen and understood, especially about one's painful emotions, is one of the stepping stones to a trustful relationship.

Despite the wide range of disorders that are compatible with the broad spectrum of clinical presentations that this group of young people present, when observed through a developmental lens we see that practically all of them have suffered AREs in their childhood (Dangerfield, 2020)—something that is very frequent in adolescents with mental health disorders, as shown by the extensive empirical evidence described above. Adolescents who have grown up in relational environments where AREs have continuously and severely prevailed are dominated by intense non-mentalized anxieties and by the predominance of emotional voids in their psychic lives; a very intense suffering without words predominates in their internal world. They desperately need help but it is common to see that contact with their emotional needs is very threatening, as it destabilizes their fragile survival system.

Throughout their years of practice in mainstream services of the Catalan public healthcare system, the various members of the ECID team have gathered extensive clinical evidence of the difficulties of engaging with this group of young people who accumulate AREs. We found that there was a need to change the way we approached these young people, and AMBIT seemed to offer resources that would lead us to finding better ways to do so. We were also aware of the alarming evidence that these adverse events in childhood are insufficiently assessed by mental health professionals. This can interfere with the possibility of establishing a relationship with truly therapeutic effects, since young people with a history of these experiences who are assessed on only a symptomatic level will not feel adequately understood and their real needs are unlikely to be properly addressed. This situation can lead to a high risk of making things worse, especially if an accurate assessment of AREs in both the young person and their parents is absent from the therapeutic plan. We know, for example, that stories of abuse are often overlooked (Cavanagh et al., 2004; Read et al., 2018) or unassessed (Dangerfield, 2020).

Based on our experiences of working with high-risk adolescents and the evidence on the impact of AREs, we describe our work at the ECID project as a mental health approach based on a deep understanding of family dynamics and family history, with an explicit need to participate in the daily life of the family to get a first-hand experience of what it means to live in that home. We are convinced that this level of understanding is impossible to achieve in outpatient or partial hospitalization services, where there are understandable limits to what can be assessed, as well as difficulties in actually seeing the young person because of their reluctance to come to the service. Van der Kolk (2015) describes how research has consistently shown that child maltreatment disrupts brain systems dedicated to assessing risk and safety, resulting in lasting difficulties regulating biological homeostasis and emotional responses to it throughout life. The author comments that despite the numerous studies and the solid evidence collected over the past 30 years that show its devastating effects on mental and physical health, the role of trauma, referring more specifically to relational trauma, continues to be of little account in both our diagnostic classifications and our therapeutic programmes.

Clinical experience and research (Dangerfield, 2020) show that parents of these young people have also suffered AREs in their own childhoods, which has an impact on the organization of their emotional and relational life as well as their capacity for mentalizing. Parents' poor mentalizing capacity inhibits their ability to provide an experience of mutuality and reflective curiosity about the inner experience of their children's relationships. Furthermore, parents' inability to regulate their own affective states creates an unpredictable and inconsistent relational environment for their children to grow up in. The transgenerational transmission of relational trauma is evident and facilitated in this context. Fraiberg et al. (1975) understood that the problem for these parents was the presence of what the traumatic relational experience had left in them: the so-called ghosts in the nursery. Fonagy et al. (1991) later demonstrated that mothers' ability to mentalize their own early attachment experiences predicted infant attachment security more than 16 months later. Following this evidence, they proposed that mentalizing plays an important role in the transgenerational transmission of attachment, proposing an intergenerational pattern in which mentalizing, and the ability of parents to imagine what their baby's behaviour is communicating about what they feel, need, and want, underlies sensitive responses and promotes attachment security (Fonagy & Target, 1997).

Parental mentalizing promotes secure attachment. In turn, the development of better mentalizing capacities occurs in the context of a secure attachment relationship, when babies discover their minds through a relationship with someone who treats them as someone with a mind. Reflective functioning is seen as an underlying sensitive response, helping mothers to mentally put themselves in the baby's shoes and imagine the baby's experience (Fonagy & Target, 1997). Following this idea, there is evidence that the reflective functioning of parents regarding their own attachment relationships, both past and present, underlies sensitivity in the interaction with their own children; furthermore, higher reflective functioning is associated with fewer negative behaviours (Ensink et al., 2016; Slade et al., 2005; Suchman et al., 2010). Ensink et al. (2014) found that the relational difficulties in women who had suffered AREs in their own childhood have more to do with an absence of mentalizing specifically in relation to trauma than an absence of mentalizing in general. They reported that that women with a history of childhood abuse and neglect did not show a generic lack of reflectiveness (mentalizing) but rather showed difficulty considering traumatic experiences in mental-state terms (i.e. *trauma-related* mentalizing).

Ensink et al. (2016) also describe how better awareness helps mothers detect their own negative, intrusive, aggressive, and withdrawn responses that undermine the development of attachment security and organization in their babies. These authors state that mothers with a greater capacity for reflective function can be better at filtering their own affects of aggression, anxiety, and fear, protecting their babies from negative behaviours, because they are more aware of their own mental states and how their affect and behaviour might be experienced by others, including their babies. Mentalizing also involves an implicit understanding that affects become less intense over time and can be changed through thinking and viewing situations differently, and this can help mothers with greater reflective functioning to tolerate difficult feelings. There is empirical evidence of the multigenerational transmission of trauma and psychopathology, identifying connections between parents' own childhood experiences and the relational and caring styles they display, which, in turn, affect the wellbeing of their children (Lyons-Ruth & Jacobvitz, 2016).

5.3.2 Implications of adverse relational experiences in our work: what AMBIT offers with our clients

After realizing that John was not going to come to see us at the day hospital, my colleague and I started visiting his home on a weekly basis. To facilitate the establishment of a relationship with our young clients and their families, AMBIT helped us to take a very active role that, among other things, implied that we would be the ones going to see them where they were, to initiate a therapeutic process with a specific focus on the supporting the relationship established between each young person and their keyworker. This shift in our work setting implied putting ourselves in a more vulnerable position. We would be faced with higher levels of anxiety, which had to be acknowledged and supported by the other team members.

We started organizing what would become the building blocks of the ECID project: an intensive outreach mental healthcare team for young people presenting severe mental health problems and not attending mainstream services, and their families.

When working with young people, we consider it indispensable to also work with the parents. In the case of John, one of my colleagues took charge of working with his parents while I worked with John.

As mentioned before, our goal is to facilitate a relational experience focused on the development of epistemic trust and, more specifically, to offer a relationship in which the young person can experience a sense of agency over their own life and of trust that, in turn, facilitates mentalizing (Malberg, 2013, 2019). The process always begins with a phase of assessment and formulation of the case. Unlike the usual mental health interventions, this phase can be prolonged over time, going well beyond the initial three or four assessment visits. This is because there is no demand for help from the young person, so we dedicate as many visits as necessary to achieve the establishment of a minimal relationship of trust. Obviously, these visits also provide a lot of information, especially when they are carried out at home, which is always a very good way to get an idea of aspects of family life and the relational dynamics that are often invisible when working at an outpatient service or a hospital.

Working with parents is a central aspect of the ECID teams' work. Following Malberg (2015), when working with parents, our main goal is to help them develop a mentalizing stance—that is, one that is characterized by perspective-taking, curiosity, and learning from each other. To facilitate this, we must first try to find a way to be available enough and explicit in our understanding of the challenges they are facing as parents. It is essential to thoroughly assess their personal histories as well as potential psychopathology. We need to develop an understanding of how their own relational histories and AREs have determined their relational patterns and capacities to deal with their own and their child's emotional life. By doing so, we will be able to offer an experience in which they can feel mentalized by us, particularly in relation to the difficulties and suffering arising from the complex problems that their child presents.

We know that epistemic trust is a fundamental concept to understand therapeutic work (Fonagy & Allison, 2014). In our therapeutic work with parents, epistemic trust is stimulated by the parents' understanding that the therapist has connected with them in a manner marked by authenticity and empathy. This empathic connection, arising from the parents' experience of having been adequately mentalized, is what allows them to feel that they can trust what the therapist will offer in terms of knowledge. It will allow the parent to learn about themselves and the way they relate to their child through the mind of someone they trust. This is what organizes our work with parents as an ECID team. First, we must empathize with and validate the parents' feelings of despair. By doing so, we can facilitate the development of epistemic trust with the therapist, modelling a way of being with the other that facilitates a reparative approach to the damaged or conflictual relationship they may have with their adolescent child. From a mentalizing-informed framework, the therapist's main goal is to help parents generalize this different way of being with the other towards their children.

As Bateman and Fonagy (2004, 2016) describe, non-mentalizing cannot be addressed with mentalizing. We must first try to help modulate the levels of emotional arousal, to try to facilitate the recovery of the capacity to mentalize, and this is what we must keep in mind when working with parents: our goal is to *help them understand the value of this way of being with the other in a relationship by offering them a relationship in which they feel mentalized.* In the ECID team we understand that we cannot do this in a rational or intellectual way; instead, we must offer an emotional experience where parents can feel the transforming value of being adequately understood, which can facilitate perspective-taking and learning from each other in a way that improves their mentalizing capacities and will invite them to take a more genuine interest in what lies behind their child's behaviour, which in turn will better serve their child's social and emotional needs and improve their relationship. The therapist's capacity to mentalize the parents seeks to facilitate this new attitude in the parents, characterized by higher levels of flexibility, curiosity, and genuine openness towards their child.

A helpful reminder which AMBIT embodies is the importance of being explicitly humble when approaching the young person, which means organizing the professional's stance towards the young person and the family away from the position of the 'expert'. We have learned that it would be somewhat contraindicated to adopt a position in which the professional *knows* too much about what may be happening to the young person. A neutral or distant position is also contraindicated, since it will only confirm the young person's persecutory experience of relationships with the professional. For a young person who has suffered a predominance of AREs in childhood, it is not safe to approach the mind of another person, as they have never had a predictable and consistent experience of attachment. Therefore, we must adopt a stance that takes this into account and focuses on the young person's psychic developmental process.

As mental health professionals, we understood that we should take a position in which we made our own need for help explicit towards the young person and the family. Because of the young person's difficulty in tolerating their own need, we think that the professional must be responsible for assuming it and making it their own. The professional will make explicit their own need for help to be able to understand the young person's situation: how they live, how they feel, what they think, what they do, the music they listen to, what video games they play, what it is like to live in their family, and so on.

As we look through these lenses, the professional's attitude offers a model that makes implicit thought processes explicit. In particular, we model an awareness that we are not perfect, that we are aware that there are limits to our knowledge and are confident enough to acknowledge it: 'I'm curious because I know I don't know'. We also offer a model of interest in our own and others' mental states, reflecting on how we might feel or what we think about a certain situation and wondering aloud how the other person might feel and think, checking with the young person to see if what we are wondering makes sense to them or not.

I want to stress the importance of the first contact with the young person and how decisive it is for the rest of the process. The active role of the professional implies meeting the young person wherever they are; that is, in a place where they feel safe. This facilitates the relationship, but it also makes for a considerable impact, especially in the initial meeting. Therefore, we try to focus on making the young person feel seen and understood by us from the very beginning. We must validate the young person's initial rejection or distrust, especially if we show up in their home without them having made any request for help or agreeing to our visit. Often this means several weeks of home visits in which our sole purpose will be to validate the young person's discomfort as it is triggered by our presence. In such a scenario, our goal is for them to feel adequately recognized by us in what they are feeling and in what we are contributing to provoking in them. It is through this process that we seek to facilitate the establishment of a certain relationship of trust; the purpose is to generate an experience in which the young person can feel understood through us explicitly showing our curiosity about their life, as well as the limits of our own knowledge that justify this explicit need for their help to understand.

5.3.3 ECID goes live

We will now return to the case of John. On our first visit to John's home, we were struck by his fragile, emaciated physical appearance. We were also struck by the vulnerability and suffering he conveyed, albeit non-verbally, at first. He seemed quite surprised by our arrival. Even so, he did not utter a single word, or come out of his bedroom. John remained there, playing a war-themed video game. A colleague from the ECID had come with me on this first visit to this household, a clean, well-kept flat in a working-class neighbourhood. John's mother welcomed us. She expressed her appreciation for our visit to them in their home, and immediately began to share her desperation about John's situation. Her mood was depressive. She said she was exhausted and that she had been struggling for years to offer her son a better life than she had. It was exasperating for her to find that John did not even want to leave the flat.

John presented a high risk of psychopathology and social exclusion. Furthermore, his prognosis was poor, considering his reluctance to accept any of the numerous therapeutic options that the mental health services had offered him. His living conditions, withdrawn from the world in his bedroom, implied a high risk of his physical and mental condition worsening and becoming chronic.

ECID protocol establishes that two professionals always go on initial home visits. One professional usually remains as the professional of reference for the family, and the other as the keyworker for the young person. Both professionals are almost always present at family visits, too, as these visits are more demanding, and it is easier for one of the professionals to remain in an observer role throughout the entire interaction and come to the rescue in those inevitable moments when the other professional loses their mentalizing capacity.

After our preliminary conversation with John's mother, she took us to his bedroom. John was sitting in front of his PC, in a room lit only by the glow of the screen. The only window had the blinds pulled all the way down. We were surprised to see that his room did not look like an adolescent's bedroom. Rather, it appeared as if frozen in time several years ago in the course of John's childhood. The PC occupied a prominent place, as did a comfortable-looking 'gamer's chair' where John sat, continuing to play his war-themed video game. His answers to his mother's remarks and introductions came in monosyllables and grunts.

I introduced myself and asked John if it was all right for me to come into his bedroom. He said yes, without ever stopping his game, although his tone and non-verbal language seemed to suggest the opposite: a certain unease caused by my presence, and what I imagined to be an understandable mistrust. I told him that I did not know how he felt at that moment, but I guessed that me coming to his home, and now being in his room, was a little surprising. Perhaps it was making him feel uncomfortable or somewhat upset. I wondered out loud if what I was saying made any sense to him. He said that it did, and that he did not like psychologists. I apologized. I said that I was sorry if I was making him upset, and that it was not the intention of my visit. I said I had come wanting to get to know him and find out how he spent his time. I told him that I would like to ask him about this; that he could help me get to know him a little better, and that I would like him to get to know me. Then we would see if it was possible to come up with a work plan together. I said I was sorry to be causing him discomfort, and that I understood if he wanted me to leave. John said I could stay, but that he would keep on playing his video game. I thanked him and asked about the game he was playing.

In the same way that at the ECID we adapt to the external working circumstances, going wherever the young people and their families are, we must also adapt to the level of relationship they can tolerate with us. Here, the act of attaching more importance to the process than to the content of the patient's discourse, as proposed by MBT, proves its worth. Considering that our goal is to establish epistemic trust, we must focus on the process and attempt to promote an experience in which the adolescent feels recognized, especially in their suffering. We must also acknowledge how our presence may only contribute to increasing their unpleasant emotional states, as a way of validating the impact that our intrusion into their homes may produce.

Rather than trying to get them to adapt to our model, our interest is in being able to accompany the young person as they develop their mentalizing capacity. Therefore, we adapt to focus our attention on the areas where the adolescent feels most secure. In John's case, this meant keeping our shared attention on the virtual world of his video game. We know that we cannot approach non-mentalizing with direct attempts to mentalize 'at them', as this only contributes to greater anxiety and dysregulation of the young person. Stimulating mentalizing in areas where it is more tolerable facilitates the experience of shared attention, in which the professional and young person meet each other to start observing, identifying, modulating, and expressing the shared emotional experience in the here and now—even if it means being in the virtual world of the video game for several weeks, as occurred in the case of John.

The ECID professional will make the effort to try to maintain a mentalizing stance at all times, with the intention of modelling a new way of approaching emotional and relational life, although it is done within the limited focus that the young person can tolerate. This is what happened in John's case. The virtual scenario of the video game, and the quantity and intensity of powerful relational moments that arose in it, were used by me to gradually convey to John what was going on for me in that moment, what I felt and thought about the experience I was living during these video-game sessions, in addition to asking about what John was feeling and thinking as he played the game.

The professional thus approaches areas of the young person's life with a mentalizing stance, but at a level of intensity that can be tolerated. This approach implies explicit curiosity, something like an invitation for the young person to flexibly move through the various poles of the dimensions described by Lieberman (2007): mentalizing of self versus other, mentalizing in relation to internal versus external characteristics, and cognitive versus affective mentalizing.

The professional seeks to stimulate effective mentalizing, always seeking to keep a balance across these dimensions and inviting the young person to apply them in an appropriate way depending on the context. In the case of John, this meant everything that happened, and happened to us, while we shared the video game. The work is done by focusing shared attention on mental states, using plain language, a humble attitude, and explicit curiosity based on recognizing the fact that we need the young person to help us understand them, while we professionals assume this necessity, which is quite unbearable for them to acknowledge.

The goal of this position is to work towards better management of emotions—to what Jurist (2005, 2008, 2018) defines as *mentalized affectivity*, a process that seeks to improve the capacity to identify, modulate, and express emotional states. The process involves being able to accompany patients in progressively tolerating contact with painful emotions, for as long as it is possible and appropriate. Jurist (2018) under-scores that this process enables us to observe and reflect on emotions without feeling driven to act on them. Mentalized affectivity helps us understand that mentalizing is not exclusively cognitive and implies an acceptance of how emotions can be confusing and hard to identify.

With John, our initial focus of attention was the video game we were sharing. As could have been expected, my video-gaming skills turned out to be quite limited, and for that reason, my character in the game was unable to survive in the complex virtual world with enemies around every corner. My character was regularly killed within seconds of beginning play. My gaming incompetence exasperated John. I took it with a bit of self-deprecating humour, and often used these opportunities to seek his help so I could learn to manage better and defend myself from all the imminent dangers.

On one visit, John surprised me by launching the game in a mode in which there were no enemies. He told me he had chosen a much easier 'training mode', to teach me how to move around the virtual world of the game. I thought that this might also be understood as a piece of valuable communication of his own needs. Perhaps he was informing me of his need to feel that we could have some time together, in which we could move around a safe environment, before having to deal with more complex and threatening realities of the outside world, as well as his own fears of facing them.

Obviously, I said nothing to John about these hypotheses, because inviting him to mentalize about the experience I was imagining would have been premature at that point. Such a movement would have meant spurring him into contact with an intolerable external reality and his own emotional needs that had to be addressed in order to face it. At that time, this would have probably triggered an inhibition of his mentalizing capacity. In addition, at that time John was showing a highly satisfactory capacity to mentalize me, as shown in his decision to adapt the demands of the game to my limitations, with the aim of helping me extend my character's life expectancy in the world of the game. I thanked him for his help, telling him I felt very well understood by him, which was helpful to me. I told him that his ability to understand my fear and difficulty in the video game had made me feel more secure and confident in my potential to learn how to handle myself in the virtual world.

At that stage of the therapeutic process, it was I who had to assume the more vulnerable and fragile position. At the ECID, we see this as a key aspect of the process with this group of young people, who have understandable difficulties accepting being positioned as the one who needs help. The ECID professional takes this position from the very beginning. By doing so, we model a new way of approaching our own mental states, capacities, and limitations. We also model the importance and value of the need for help, which facilitates possibilities for managing one's emotional and relational life.

Despite the absence of enemies in the mode of play John had chosen, due to my utter lack of skills in the virtual world, my character continued to die frequently. John was surprised, and actually dismayed, by my clumsiness and deficiencies in video gaming. He was, however, patient enough to help me improve a bit, and my character managed to stay alive for a few minutes. I attempted to make very specific remarks regarding my fear and confusion, which were all too real in certain stages of the game. I also spoke to him of my need for him to help me learn to survive and carry on when I faced challenging circumstances. At that same time, I concentrated on mentalizing this moment of our relationship, making continued, specific references of recognition and appreciation of his ability to effectively mentalize me, and of the value this had in the process.

This was a valuable part of the initial sessions in John's home for a number of reasons that characterize the work of the ECID: the professional is willing to meet the young person wherever they feel safe; the professional holds explicit curiosity about whatever interests the young person; the professional initially takes the more vulnerable role and specifically states their need for the young person to help them understand the young person's world; and, most importantly, the professional can feel comfortable in the not-knowing stance and acknowledge this need for help, with explicit humbleness that moves them away from the 'expert' position.

At the ECID, professionals model this new or different way of being in relationships, towards others and intrapsychically. We believe it is difficult to carry out this phase of the therapeutic process in hospital or outpatient environments. This is because such facilities initially place the young person in the position of 'patient' and the professional in that of 'expert'. This is an unequal relationship, worsened at some centres by the use of white coats and desks, which are, incomprehensibly, still in use at some CAMHS centres.

In John's case, being placed in the position of a patient needing help had contributed to the failure of previous treatments. They failed because this meant asking him to tolerate facing his difficulties without this preliminary phase of modelling, and prematurely asking him to accept the role of the one needing help. Furthermore, at the ECID we also believe that our position of directing the therapeutic outlook and work towards the daily lives of the young people and their families can contribute to reducing the stigma of seeking and receiving help in ordinary mental health services.

After a few weeks of my visiting him in his room, John asked me the question I quoted in the introduction: 'But Mark, are you really a psychologist?' 'Yes, I am a psychologist,' I replied. He then paused the video game we were playing together, looked at me and said in a funny way, 'Well, you're a pretty weird psychologist, man!' I then wondered aloud what his idea of a psychologist was. He said that I did not talk like a psychologist, because I had never made him talk about his problems, nor had I ever focused on the need for him to go back to school and resume his education. He added that whenever he had been seen by other psychologists, all of them had wanted to talk about these difficulties, something he could not stand.

The therapeutic process with John continued developing until we could begin to widen the focus of our shared attention, leaving the virtual world and approaching his internal world and external reality, as well as the significant difficulties that John had in those areas. A process began in which we were eventually able to change the focus, begin to address his own difficulties, and face life and the external world. We worked together to be able to leave his bedroom and return to life outside the home. John tolerated this exchange of roles, with him being the one who could acknowledge and accept his need for help in facing life, and me taking the place of the person who facilitated that process for him, just as he had very effectively done for me in his virtual world.

We have met many young people like John, who have lived in a very emotionally isolated manner, in situations of intense suffering, which configures an inner world rife with speechless pain. Our initial focus with John respected his need to not be forced out of his room to be taken to a mental health facility. It was also very important to acknowledge and validate the impact that my presence in the household had on him, as well as being explicitly curious about his interests and life at home. This process facilitated an experience of containment that helped to reduce his persecutory anxiety and enabled him to begin expressing some curiosity about me as a professional. We know that the experience of feeling seen and understood, especially in relation to one's painful emotions, is key to establishing a relationship of epistemic trust.

We like to describe our work at the ECID project as a mental health focus based on a deep understanding of the family dynamic and history, which leads us to participate in the family's daily life and gain first-hand knowledge of what it means to live in their household. We are convinced that this level of understanding is impossible to reach in outpatient and hospital settings, where there are understandable limitations to what can be valued and understood in each case, as well as also understandable limits to professionals' fields of intervention.

5.3.4 Professional's stance

What we learned from the AMBIT model was much more than a set of techniques. Above all, it was a different way of being with the young person. In this sense, the role of the professional is not so much about having the ability to always read the young person's emotional states accurately, but rather a way of approaching relationships that reflects the expectation that thoughts and feelings will be enlightened, enriched, and modified by learning about the mental states of the self and others (Bateman & Fonagy, 2019). At the same time, we made our curiosity explicit, and maintained our awareness of the impact of emotion and that the young person's mind is opaque, while modelling an ability to take different perspectives on the same reality. More than anything else, our intention was to promote an atmosphere of epistemic trust that restores the young person's capacity for agency and hope.

Our main task is to try to offer a relationship in which young people can have the experience of someone who is genuinely interested in them, who has their mind in mind and makes them feel that they matter as human beings, while showing how professionals try to respond contingently in a wide range of different situations. We must also bear in mind that for many of these young people, getting closer to thinking about certain aspects of their past and present is quite unbearable. John told me that he didn't like talking about his life, which I respected, as it only triggered intense anxieties that would interfere in my goal of facilitating the development of his mentalizing capacities. I understood that it was important to give John time to try to develop mentalizing in an area where it was more tolerable and safer: the video game. We also found that this could be more easily achieved if we approached mentalizing from the most primitive level of the different sensory experiences found in this virtual world that we were both sharing, as well as the emotional experience shared during the game.

What we also found essential was the idea of scaffolding existing relationships: the process of identifying, valuing, and supporting the help that the young person may receive beyond what we can offer. The work of scaffolding involves being curious about and respectful of what others can offer, and being humble about the fact that we are joining a system of help that may already exist around the young person, but that the young person may not be prepared to trust. Instead of seeing the solution to the young person's situation as coming only from us, we must acknowledge and help to identify the value of relationships with other people in their relational and professional environment. There may be people who, from the young person's perspective, are more accessible to them and can play a decisive role in the therapeutic process—people with whom they already have a previous relationship or who they may already trust, albeit in a limited way—although we need to keep in mind the need to manage the risk that could be associated with these relationships.

In John's case, both of his parents were very clearly the most valuable relationships that we needed to scaffold, and this would be indispensable in the process of re-engaging John with life and with a life project. This also implied risks, because of the dysfunctional family dynamics that were very explicit and that we witnessed very often during the home visits. Despite their good intentions and what we understood was an honest concern about John's situation, his parents very frequently struggled to see beyond John's retreat into his room and his video games, to consider the intense anxieties and painful feelings underlying them. This predominant relational pattern led to very frequent situations in which they were not able to see John's suffering, fear, intense feelings of threat, and despair, and they usually reacted to John's behaviour in ways that further dysregulated him rather than helping him to feel understood and, thus, supported and contained. This is what, from a mentalizing perspective, is described as non-mentalizing vicious cycles, in which John and his parents functioned most of the time. The very powerful and unpleasant emotions experienced by each family member reduced their capacity to mentalize, which in turn made it harder for all of them to understand each other's behaviours or intentions, and increased their feelings of despair, rage, sadness, and isolation. This situation also implied an increased psychopathological risk because of the intense levels of suffering in all of them, lived in sheer isolation.

As I have briefly described above, when working with John's parents our goal was to offer a relational experience where they could feel seen, understood, and validated in relation to the difficulties they faced, which they experienced as overwhelming. Our intention was to develop epistemic trust with them, to model a different way of being in a relationship that facilitated a reparative approach to the highly damaged and conflictual relationship they had with John. Our goal was to help the parents generalize this different way of being in their relationship with John, in order to facilitate a different experience in family interactions characterized by higher degrees of curiosity towards each other's underlying emotional states, with the idea of strengthening their relationship and increasing the possibility of John feeling greater support from them, to help him face the challenges of life outside his home.

As the situation improved and John felt confident enough to start considering the possibility of going back to school, we supported him to reconnect with the school by asking John to help us identify the teacher who he could remember as being more helpful and understanding towards him. To our surprise, he said that the maths teacher was the only person he liked there, because she had approached the moment when he started dropping out from school in a way that felt different from the others, in that it seemed that she really did care rather than being demanding and judgemental about the obligations John was failing to meet. He said that the maths teacher was the only person who really understood him. This was a very helpful communication, as we then contacted her and organized initial meetings at the school, at which John and I spent some time with her planning John's gradual return to school. At the same time, John also reconnected with some old classmates, whom he had begun to meet when leaving school, as well as resuming playing video games together with them, instead of doing so in the isolation of his room.

5.4 Working with your Team

AMBIT had a powerful impact on the group of professionals who made up the first ECID team: Anna Oriol, Jordi Artigue, Marta Montaner, Valentina Bruno, and me. I was very lucky to be able to engage such an experienced and well-trained team of mental health professionals in the project. This was a group of people with the emotional and relational resources that I think are essential for this kind of approach: humility and curiosity, both towards others and themselves, and also towards finding new ways of working. They also have the capacity and courage to challenge what supports their professional identity, to change their way of working, to tolerate the anxieties implicit in the not-knowing stance, and to move away from a hierarchical organization, which has not always been easy. But above all, it was a group of people with whom we were comfortable enough to start sharing our fears, anxieties, and hopes in relation to the new professional challenge we were embarking on.

When we started working together, our main goal was to become a well-connected team—something that is easier said than done. We believed that this could be achieved by feeling confident enough to be honest about our fears, anxieties, and other unpleasant emotions related to our work and, at times, our lives. It took a while, but I think they would all agree that we have proved capable of doing this. It is worth remembering the initial idea that we often return to, and which helped us throughout: we should worry when we do *not* feel anxious in our work. This was also possible when the second team joined us: David López, Elsa Coll, Laia Ferrer, Lina Gutiérrez, and Oriol Canalias.

We consider epistemic trust to be the key organizing concept in ECID's work, as it is with the client and network quadrants of the AMBIT wheel. As we know, it is facilitated by the experience of being adequately understood by the other. This is what we have always tried to achieve in our team: to help our co-workers feel seen and understood by others, as a way of supporting them in their work. It also offers the team a way to model what we know our clients, and the professionals working in the various teams of the wider network, need. However, no matter how much training and experience one may have, a salient difficulty for those working in the mental health field is the capacity to be truly available to the young people and families with whom we work. This availability has to do with our emotional capacities to tolerate this position, as well as our capacity to stand the intense suffering that is conveyed to us by the people we try to help. This is particularly difficult when we are working with young people who do not really want to work with us, no matter how much we know that this sometimes active rejection of our presence in their homes—with the young person shut in their bedroom when the professional arrives, or showing an active reluctance to talk to or even look at the professional—may be a highly adaptive response.

Therefore, in our experience, the technique of 'Thinking Together' (described in Chapter 2) became one of the AMBIT model's key contributions to our work. By Thinking Together, we can work to regain our capacity to mentalize, which is inevitably overwhelmed by the intensity of the emotions we experience in our daily work.

5.4.1 Design of the ECID team

We decided we needed to start a team that would be clearly different from the existing mainstream services. This is why we thought it was essential to be seen from the outset as a new service that would be part of the local mental health network. We did not want to be a programme of an already existing service, like CAMHS or the day hospital, as we thought that this would mean eventually being taken over by their dynamics, which would not allow us to develop based on a new way of organizing care. Following AMBIT, we decided that the best way to start the ECID project was by working with young people and their families at home, in the streets, or wherever they felt safe. This shift implied that the professional assumed a more vulnerable position by leaving the containment offered by the office and the institution. Adopting this model required a significant shift in our way of organizing our work as a team, and it resulted in the professionals who started doing the outreach work encountering higher levels of anxiety. However, we still thought that, in principle, we would have better internal resources than the young people we work with to deal with these new and challenging relational situations, so it made sense to take this more active role in trying to engage with them in a therapeutic relationship, and not continually ask them to take the active role of coming to find us.

Traditionally, the young people we work with were labelled as 'hard to reach' because they did not come to our services. AMBIT helped us to realize that it was actually *us* who were hard to reach, and that our lack of flexibility was the reason why this particular group of clients showed little engagement in the therapeutic process. Consequently, we realized that it was our responsibility to change in order to make mental healthcare truly accessible for all young people who need help, and not only for those who can tolerate needing it and are capable and patient enough to find their way to the services. In addition, we had learned that asking young people who are at high risk and who have fragile resources when it comes to managing their emotional and relational life to meet a mental health professional (an unknown adult) in a mental health centre or hospital often represented an impossible demand that made our interventions fail.

Despite our team's enthusiasm and commitment to this new way of organizing help, during the initial process of implementing the approach we found that no matter how well equipped our mental health professionals may be, with ample training, personal therapy, and extensive clinical experience, because of the levels of anxiety inevitably triggered by the outreach work it was essential to organize support and containment for the team on a regular basis. As a team, our goal was to try to minimize the impact on us of all the new situations we encountered in this totally new work setting.

Leaving mental health centres, hospitals, or institutions was a stimulating but challenging experience that put us face to face with the difficult and demanding task of working with a complex group of young people and families in sometimes frightening or threatening environments. Another chief concern was the risk of professional isolation. We had decided that the initial visits to homes would always be done by two professionals, but we could not hope to maintain this set-up throughout the whole therapeutic process. Therefore, our concern was the risk of professional isolation, which we all knew was a common aspect of our past experiences in mainstream mental health services. Overall, the group felt concerned about the higher chances of feeling isolated due to outreach work, and we all agreed that AMBIT could offer an extremely helpful and valuable tool to counter this: Thinking Together. We agreed that the main goal of our work as a team should be to offer support and containment in relation to the inevitable anxieties experienced by each one of us on a daily basis if we were really available to the young people and families we work with, and to try to organize this team containment in a structured or even protocolized way. We all had extensive experience of clinical supervision, clinical sessions, or team meetings in which we could share our work with other team members, but we had also all had experiences where this kind of teamwork had not really addressed our anxieties or difficulties.

We started by assessing how we felt after a team meeting, with the goal of determining whether our level of anxiety or discomfort when leaving the meeting was lower than before it began. We thought that this was a good way of assessing whether we were truly addressing the core aspect of what we had been taught as the main function of the Team around the Worker or a well-connected team: offering support and containment to the worker in relation to the emotional impact of the work, which can interfere with their capacity to mentalize and, consequently, their capacity to provide appropriate help to the young person through adequate mentalizing of the young person's situation.

In the ECID team's first year of working, the technique of Thinking Together became well embedded in our practice. We worked together to develop our new project and implement what AMBIT was offering. The team was quite adept at acknowledging anxieties and the need for help and working together to not feel ashamed about expressing anxiety, fear, or confusion relating to this new way of working. We also thought that our difficulties in being sufficiently available to receive and modulate the anxieties and pain of the young people were often related to the isolation in which professionals work day to day, despite working in teams, and we were aware that the intense suffering of young people is not communicated to us only with words. On home visits, we are impacted by other sensory pathways—what we see, hear, smell, and feel—all of which increase the difficulties we encounter when trying to make sense of the whole home-visiting experience and adequately mentalize the young person and the family's situation.

Identifying non-mentalizing modes proved productive in situations of higher emotional impact. These higher levels of emotional arousal clearly interfere with our ability to mentalize, moving us to function in different inappropriate ways to try to regain control of the situation. We begin to have certainties about the young people and their families (psychic equivalence), we tend to simplify explanations of what is happening by using diagnostic labels that reassure us because they give us a false sense of control over the situation. Feeling in possession of a truth, we make theoretical reflections on what we suppose we are understanding (pretend mode), and we tend to carry out concrete actions as if they were a quick solution to a much more complex and multidimensional problem (teleological mode). For these reasons, the team needed to develop an approach to teamwork that provided the support and containment that enabled the recovery of mentalizing capacity for the team members.

Mentalizing is a relational capacity: it is gestated and develops in the context of the attachment relationships with our primary caregivers (Allen, 2013; Allen et al., 2008; Fonagy, 2004; Fonagy et al., 2002; Sharp & Rossouw, 2019). We also know that it is fragile, and that we all lose our capacity to mentalize in situations of emotional arousal. After an encounter that has overwhelmed us, we all need a relationship that can help us modulate our emotional experience and recover an adequate capacity to mentalize the experience. When establishing the ECID project, we took this basic theoretical concept as a core organizing principle. It even influenced the choice of our team's headquarters: we did not choose an ordinary facility that might remind us of a mainstream mental health service, with different offices for each professional. Instead, we settled on what would be a collaborative workplace, with a large main room and only two separate offices, with the idea that the space would limit professional isolation, foster collaboration, promote learning together as a team, and nurture a strong team culture. However, we soon found that we needed to find a way to balance our main goal of being a well-connected team with moments of private time, even if it still meant sitting in the large main room. We found ways of marking off these moments of private time, and made sure that when Thinking Together we would all close our laptops and silence our phones.

Following the AMBIT model, any professional from the ECID team can be the keyworker for a young person. This was a very important shift in the way mental health services are organized in Barcelona and the rest of Spain, as there is still a predominant hierarchy in the services—only psychologists or psychiatrists can be considered keyworkers, and the other professionals will intervene in the case as needed. This classical organization divides professionals into clinical and non-clinical teams. We believe that this organization does not contribute to a well-connected team. The ECID project was committed to a different team dynamic, with a horizontal team in which any of us—psychologists, psychiatrists, social workers, or nurses—could be the keyworker of any case. The rest of the workers are organized as a team around the keyworker with two main functions: to provide containment for the emotional impact experienced by the keyworker in their daily work, and to offer support to the keyworker from each of our specific professions or specialities.

The keyworker was able to convey to the young person the various contributions of the co-workers, based on the specific changing needs of the case. Thus, the young person will be assisted by a multidisciplinary team, but through their unique relationship with their keyworker. Obviously, this involves modelling a humble stance, relinquishing the position of omniscient professional, and explicitly admitting to our need for help from other members of the team. On occasion, this help can be requested in front of the young person; this also models the value of being able to tolerate our need for help, which is essential for these young people who live predominantly in epistemic mistrust. As professionals, we model a position that involves feeling safe uncertainty or tolerating a not-knowing stance. The capacity to tolerate this professional stance has to do with how much we feel supported and how much we trust our co-workers.

5.5 Working with your Network

To illustrate our experience in the network quadrant of the AMBIT wheel, I will use another clinical vignette from the day hospital, before we started the ECID project. Laura was a 16-year-old young woman who presented with serious long-standing conduct disorder and chronic truancy, spending most of her time on the streets. She often ran away from home and got involved in high-risk situations. She self-harmed frequently and used different kinds of drugs and alcohol to manage her despair and intense anxiety. She lived with her mother and a younger sister, and for some time they had received interventions from social services, the child protection service, both CAMHS and adult mental health services, the police, and a long list of different professionals and services within the care and justice network.

Laura had been referred to the day hospital for adolescents by the local CAMHS team after having been admitted to the adolescent inpatient unit several times because of the high risk she presented and the fact that they could not offer any treatment at the CAMHS due to her irregular attendance. Not surprisingly, her attendance at the day hospital was also very irregular. She would occasionally show up and spend a few hours with us, but there was no way to get her to join any regular therapeutic process.

She came in one morning and told me that the day before she had been at another centre talking to a professional, although she was confused and could not tell whether they were a social worker from the child protection service or from social services. She told me that she saw so many professionals that she got muddled up, having to remember so many people. I said that I thought she was right, that I imagined that it was very confusing for her to have to see so many different professionals, and that I had the feeling that we were not helping her this way, and asked what she thought about this. She told me that the woman she had seen the previous day was nice and that the people here, at the day hospital, we were also nice people, but no matter how often she came here or occasionally went to see other professionals, we were not helping her and things were getting very bad for her. I told her that I was sorry that this was the case and asked her to help me understand what she thought we could do to try to help her. She said, 'Do you really want to help me?' I said that I would like to try, but that I needed her to help me understand how to do it in a way that would work for her. She then said, 'If you really want to help me, you have to come to my house and find out what it is like to live there'.

Laura's statement made sense and connected fully with what I thought AMBIT was trying to convey. Our experience with high-risk young people has taught us that one of the most common problems we encounter is that the more serious the case, the more services intervene, all of them with the best intentions, but in a very disintegrated way. The young person is asked to see different professionals from different services, who work with different objectives, using different treatment models or interventions that focus on different aspects of the young person's life, using different theoretical models to understand and name the young person's situation. In spite of the best intentions of all the professionals involved, we very often witnessed situations in which the experience of the young person in this unconnected system of help is similar to a repetition of the neglectful experience lived out in their family environment. Moreover, if we consider the difficulties that this group of young people present in their mentalizing capacities, as well as their disorganized lives (on both external and internal levels), we could probably mentalize their experience with our network as: 'Do I, a fragmented and disorganized young person, with a disorganized life and disorganized family, have to integrate everything that you professionals haven't been able to integrate and organize in so many years?' Seen this way, it is easy to understand that our way of offering and trying to convey help is almost guaranteed to fail.

For an adolescent with significant attachment difficulties and who is dominated by epistemic mistrust, sustaining just one intense relationship with a single professional is difficult enough. However, these young people are still asked to engage with multiple professionals from numerous services, and to integrate and make good use of the various inputs received from so many different sources. Our proposal for the network in which we worked was to adopt a model whereby one keyworker acted as the single professional responsible for each case and was also responsible for the integration of what the different services could offer. This proposal was readily accepted by the network. The keyworker role could be taken by any member of the ECID team; in Barcelona, a mental health nurse or a social worker could now be the leading professional in a young person's therapeutic process, a different approach to that used elsewhere in Spain. This was quite an achievement!

Following the principle that guided us throughout the implementation process, our goal was the establishment of trusting relationships among professionals in the wider network. To achieve this, we initiated a programme for getting to know each other before working together on a complicated case. We held 'house-warming' meetings, in which we would invite teams to our facilities and also visit them in theirs, with the intention of offering them the experience of being understood by us in relation to the particular difficulties they had to face in their daily work. We also tried to restructure our expectations about networking, anticipating the differences, misunderstandings, and inevitable conflicts with other services that might come up whenever our mentalizing goes offline.

In the end, we did this in a more or less professional way, as we managed to design a service that offered support to teams working with high-risk young people and were able to secure some funding for it. This facilitated our rapid integration into the network, as we were actually sharing our experiences of thinking together and mentalizing as ways of managing our own difficulties within our team. The humbleness and acknowledgement of our own mentalizing difficulties that we strive to demonstrate when working with our clients was equally valuable in establishing good-enough relationships with the wider network. This may sound simple, but the tricky part has proven to be acknowledging and accepting the moments when we are taken over by non-mentalizing modes as individuals, as teams, and in our work with the wider network.

5.6 Learning at Work

As the ECID project began as a pilot project in the Catalan public healthcare system, we knew from the very beginning that outcome measures would be an essential part of our work. Our institution was already using routine outcome measures, so it was simple to implement outcomes monitoring in our work. However, we thought that these measures did not assess what we considered to be the main indicator of successful work: the re-engagement of the young person with their school.

All the young people we work with at ECID have dropped out of school and are not attending the mental health centre to which they had been referred. For these reasons, we thought that two very important measures that would show the effectiveness of our work would be (a) the number of young people who we managed to engage in a therapeutic process with an ECID professional and (b) the number of young people who returned to school during the process of our intervention.

These are the Badalona ECID team's results for these two measurements during 2019:

- Ninety-five per cent of all the young people we worked with during 2019 engaged in the therapeutic process. This is an important measurement, as all the young people we work with present serious mental health issues and were previously referred to mainstream mental health services, although they did not attend these services. We think that this clearly shows how our new way of organizing care, based on AMBIT, effectively conveys help to those young people who had been labelled as 'non-help-seeking'. This confirms our idea that the problem is probably not so much in this group of young people, but in the way mainstream services insist on asking them to adapt to what the services can, or want to, offer.

- Sixty-two per cent of the young people went back to school during their work with their ECID keyworker. This is another important parameter because of what it implies about the important shift in the young person's attitude towards life and their future. It is a clear improvement that shows a recovered interest in life and their future.

The purpose of this chapter is not to give a detailed account of our outcome measures, so we will not burden the reader with further data. However, this process of making our implicit work processes more explicit is an essential part of what we have learned in the implementation process of this AMBIT-influenced team. Due to our clinical background and roles, the idea of investing time in research and outcome measures was not a part of the work that excited us. We acknowledge this, share the impact it has on us with our co-workers, and keep on doing it as we know it is essential for the future of the ECID project. We recognize that the only way to consolidate this AMBIT-influenced way of organizing care is by supporting our impressions and our clients' experience with objective data. Our commissioners will listen to us and support the development of our project and future plans of opening new teams throughout Spain as long as we can clearly demonstrate the real impact that our team is contributing to.

In addition to the importance of this part of our learning-at-work process for the future of our project, other aspects of the Learning at Work quadrant have become valuable for our team. As a team, we have found that manualizing contributes to generating a greater sense of cohesion. Thinking together about what we do and the difficulties we encounter in our work encourages mentalizing. Bringing together different perspectives, different minds, and different experiences in a safe environment enriches our creativity as a team and strengthens the sense of a well-connected team. It has also allowed us to develop an ongoing 'team culture' whose collective memory and experiences can be drawn on when we encounter difficulties. It also allows us to share our knowledge and experience with other colleagues or teams. However, manualizing is still sometimes difficult, as we tend to be quite demanding of ourselves when faced with the task of writing—this keeps on happening no matter how much we have reminded each other that we are not writing a scientific paper. The act of asking ourselves how we do things, why we do them the way we do, and the impact of this way of working on the young people with whom we work is very helpful to prevent us from going into defensive ways of organizing help. Our capacity to mentalize depends precisely on the possibility of keeping our curiosity active in order to continue learning from our experiences and developing better ways of dealing with the various situations that we face on a daily basis. To that end, we continually maintain this explicit assessment of our experiences, reaching consensus about what can lead to a genuine improvement of the well-connected team's work.

5.7　Implications

This chapter has described how, since 2017, AMBIT has become established in Barcelona in the work of the ECID project and the promising results it has produced. For us, it is an inspiring account of how the process of change needed to take place at many levels at once—for individual therapists who started doing things they had not previously done, for teams to function in new ways, and for the relationships that the new team established with other teams to be properly recognized and attended to. It offers a rich description of how we might go about holding a mentalizing stance across *all* aspects of the work. The stance of being curious, of acting with humility, of being willing to express the need for help, and of being open to being helped by others is as evident in ECID's approach to forming relationships within their own team and with professionals across the network as it is with their clients. It also runs through the team's approach to learning, which is one of an ever-evolving understanding of what it might take to do the work in the most helpful way, with the acknowledgement of this being a continual process of discovery that is enriched by the multiple perspectives of those in the team, as well as holding value in the perspective that routine outcome monitoring can offer.

Throughout this chapter, the focus has been on putting relationships first. The emphasis on relationships was applied from the very first stages of setting up the project. But the ECID team has also done something more, in that the focus on relationships has linked the AMBIT approach to understanding the nature of the young people's difficulties with insight into the family relationships in which such difficulties arise. Metaphorically, they have connected the AMBIT wheel to their own engine; this 'engine' is the enormous depth of psychotherapeutic knowledge and experience, drawn from psychoanalysis and attachment theory, about the needs of young people who are the target of the AMBIT approach. This brings a rich and heartfelt theoretical understanding of the minds of young people and provides the fuel to drive the AMBIT approach to produce new forms of help for the young people ECID serves. All of this knowledge was in place long before AMBIT came along, and AMBIT does not seek to replace it; rather, the chapter gives an eloquent account of the AMBIT principles and tools that the team felt would usefully enrich their existing approach and how they began to embed them in their practice.

But this is not the only engine that can be connected to the AMBIT wheel. Some readers may be thinking of different groups of clients, such as those involved in violence and gangs, those who have a chronic illness, or those with learning difficulties. As we mentioned in Chapter 1, we have discovered, to our surprise, that when teams working with many different areas of need hear about AMBIT, they can see how it applies to them. This is very welcome. But, as Mark has shown in this chapter, it is vital that each team can connect their own engine to the AMBIT wheel, and that their existing knowledge and experience is validated and not replaced. For example, teams working with adults with learning difficulties will have a rich understanding of the nature of learning difficulties, and the specific systemic factors of discrimination, powerlessness, stigma, and social disadvantage that these clients face, which need to be fully expressed within the AMBIT framework. However pragmatic the AMBIT approach may appear to be, it grows out of the existing bed of professional expertise balanced with humility and respect for the knowledge of clients about their own lives. For the development of AMBIT, we were fortunate indeed to link up with such a creative and inspiring team of professionals who did just that.

References

Allen, J. G. (2013). *Restoring mentalizing in attachment relationships: Treating trauma with plain old therapy*. American Psychiatric Publishing.
Allen, J. G., Fonagy, P., & Bateman, A. W. (2008). *Mentalizing in clinical practice*. American Psychiatric Publishing.
Artigue, J., & Tizón, J. L. (2014). Una revisión sobre los factores de riesgo en la infancia para la esquizofrenia y los trastornos mentales graves del adulto [Review of risks factors in childhood for schizophrenia and severe mental disorders in adulthood]. *Atención Primaria, 46*(7), 336–356. https://doi.org/10.1016/j.aprim.2013.11.002
Bateman, A., & Fonagy, P. (2004). *Psychotherapy for borderline personality disorder: Mentalization-based treatment*. Oxford University Press.
Bateman, A., & Fonagy, P. (2016). *Mentalization-based treatment for personality disorders: A practical guide*. Oxford University Press.
Bateman, A., & Fonagy, P. (Eds.). (2019). *Handbook of mentalizing in mental health practice* (2nd ed.). American Psychiatric Publishing.
Beale, C. (2022). Magical thinking and moral injury: Exclusion culture in psychiatry. *BJPsych Bulletin, 46*(1), 16–19. https://doi.org/10.1192/bjb.2021.86
Bendall, S., Jackson, H. J., Hulbert, C. A., & McGorry, P. D. (2008). Childhood trauma and psychotic disorders: A systematic, critical review of the evidence. *Schizophrenia Bulletin, 34*(3), 568–579. https://doi.org/10.1093/schbul/sbm121
Cavanagh, M.-R., Read, J., & New, B. (2004). Sexual abuse inquiry and response: A New Zealand training programme. *New Zealand Journal of Psychology, 33*(3), 137–144.
Dangerfield, M. (2012). Negligencia y violencia sobre el adolescente: abordaje desde un Hospital de Día. *Temas de Psicoanálisis, 4*, 1–29. https://www.temasdepsicoanalisis.org/2012/06/19/negligencia-y-violenciasobre-el-adolescenteabordaje-desde-un-hospital-de-dia/
Dangerfield, M. (2016). 'Sense un lloc a la teva ment, sense un lloc al món.' Aspectes tècnics del treball amb adolescents desatesos ['Without a place in your mind, without a place in the world.' Technical aspects of working with neglected adolescents]. *Revista Catalana de Psicoanàlisi, 33*(2), 99–239. https://raco.cat/index.php/RCP/article/view/326316/416855
Dangerfield, M. (2017). Aportaciones del tratamiento basado en la mentalización (MBT-A) para adolescentes que han sufrido adversidades en la infancia [Mentalization-based treatment (MBT-A) contributions for adolescents who have suffered adversity in childhood]. *Cuadernos de Psiquiatría y Psicoterapia del Niño y del Adolescente, 63*, 29–47. https://www.sepypna.com/documentos/articulos/psiquiatria-63/03-dangerfield.pdf
Dangerfield, M. (2020). *Estudio de las consecuencias psicopatológicas de las adversidades relacionales en la infancia y de la transmisión del trauma transgeneracional* [Study of the psychopathological consequences of relational adversities in childhood and the transmission of transgenerational trauma] [PhD Thesis, Universidad Ramón Llull, Barcelona].
Dangerfield, M. (2021). Working with at-risk mental states in adolescence. In T. Rossouw, M. Wiwe, & I. Vrouva (Eds.), *Mentalization-based treatment for adolescents: A practical treatment guide* (pp. 151–165). Routledge.

Ensink, K., Berthelot, N., Bernazzani, O., Normandin, L., & Fonagy, P. (2014). Another step closer to measuring the ghosts in the nursery: Preliminary validation of the Trauma Reflective Functioning Scale. *Frontiers in Psychology*, 5, 1471. https://doi.org/10.3389/fpsyg.2014.01471

Ensink, K., Normandin, L., Plamondon, A., Berthelot, N., & Fonagy, P. (2016). Intergenerational pathways from reflective functioning to infant attachment through parenting. *Canadian Journal of Behavioural Science*, 48(1), 9–18. https://doi.org/10.1037/cbs0000030

Fearon, R. P., Bakermans-Kranenburg, M. J., van Ijzendoorn, M. H., Lapsley, A. M., & Roisman, G. I. (2010). The significance of insecure attachment and disorganization in the development of children's externalizing behavior: A meta-analytic study. *Child Development*, 81(2), 435–456. https://doi.org/10.1111/j.1467-8624.2009.01405.x

Fonagy, P. (2004). Psychotherapy meets neuroscience: A more focused future for psychotherapy research. *Psychiatric Bulletin*, 28, 357–359. https://doi.org/10.1192/pb.28.10.357

Fonagy, P., & Allison, E. (2014). The role of mentalizing and epistemic trust in the therapeutic relationship. *Psychotherapy*, 51(3), 372–380. https://doi.org/10.1037/a0036505

Fonagy, P., Gergely, G., Jurist, E., & Target, M. (2002). *Affect regulation, mentalization, and the development of the self*. Other Press.

Fonagy, P., Steele, M., Steele, H., Moran, G. S., & Higgitt, A. C. (1991). The capacity for understanding mental states: The reflective self in parent and child and its significance for security of attachment. *Infant Mental Health Journal*, 12(3), 201–218. https://doi.org/10.1002/1097-0355(199123)12:3<201::AID-IMHJ2280120307>3.0.CO;2-7

Fonagy, P., & Target, M. (1997). Attachment and reflective function: Their role in self-organization. *Development and Psychopathology*, 9(4), 679–700. https://doi.org/10.1017/S0954579497001399

Fraiberg, S., Adelson, E., & Shapiro, V. (1975). Ghosts in the nursery. A psychoanalytic approach to the problems of impaired infant-mother relationships. *Journal of the American Academy of Child Psychiatry*, 14(3), 387–421. http://www.ncbi.nlm.nih.gov/pubmed/1141566

Grossmann, K. E., Grossmann, K., & Waters, E. (2005). *Attachment from infancy to adulthood: The major longitudinal studies*. Guilford Press.

Jurist, E. L. (2005). Mentalized affectivity. *Psychoanalytic Psychology*, 22(3), 426–444. https://doi.org/10.1037/0736-9735.22.3.426

Jurist, E. L. (2008). Minds and yours: New directions for mentalization theory. In E. L. Jurist, A. Slade, & S. Bergner (Eds.), *Mind to mind: Infant research, neuroscience and psychoanalysis* (pp. 88–114). Other Press.

Jurist, E. L. (2018). *Minding emotions: Cultivating mentalization in psychotherapy*. Guilford Press.

Kessler, R. C., McLaughlin, K. A., Green, J. G., Gruber, M. J., Sampson, N. A., Zaslavsky, A. M., Aguilar-Gaxiola, S., Alhamzawi, A. O., Alonso, J., Angermeyer, M., Benjet, C., Bromet, E., Chatterji, S., de Girolamo, G., Demyttenaere, K., Fayyad, J., Florescu, S., Gal, G., Gureje, O., . . . Williams, D. R. (2010). Childhood adversities and adult psychopathology in the WHO World Mental Health Surveys. *British Journal of Psychiatry*, 197(5), 378–385. https://doi.org/10.1192/bjp.bp.110.080499

Lieberman, M. D. (2007). Social cognitive neuroscience: A review of core processes. *Annual Review of Psychology*, 58, 259–289. https://doi.org/10.1146/annurev.psych.58.110405.085654

Lyons-Ruth, K., & Jacobvitz, D. (2016). Attachment disorganization from infancy to adulthood: Neurobiological correlates, parenting contexts, and pathways to disorder. In J. Cassidy & P. R. Shaver (Eds.), *Handbook of attachment: Theory, research, and clinical applications* (3rd ed., pp. 667–695). Guilford Press.

Malberg, N. T. (2013). A caged life: A girl's discovery of freedom through the co-creation of her life's narrative. *Journal of Infant, Child, and Adolescent Psychotherapy*, 12(2), 59–71. https://doi.org/10.1080/15289168.2013.791132

Malberg, N. T. (2015). Activating mentalization in parents: An integrative framework. *Journal of Infant, Child, and Adolescent Psychotherapy*, *14*(3), 232–245. https://doi.org/10.1080/15289168.2015.1068002

Malberg, N. T. (2019). Psychodynamic psychotherapy and emotion. In L. S. Greenberg, N. T. Malberg, & M. A. Tompkins (Eds.), *Working with emotion in psychodynamic, cognitive behavior, and emotion-focused psychotherapy* (pp. 13–52). American Psychological Association.

Merrick, M. T., Ford, D. C., Ports, K. A., Guinn, A. S., Chen, J., Klevens, J., Metzler, M., Jones, C. M., Simon, T. R., Daniel, V. M., Ottley, P., & Mercy, J. A. (2019). Vital signs: Estimated proportion of adult health problems attributable to adverse childhood experiences and implications for prevention—25 states, 2015–2017. *Morbidity and Mortality Weekly Report*, *68*(44), 999–1005. https://doi.org/10.15585/mmwr.mm6844e1

Quijada, Y., Tizón, J. L., Artigue, J., & Parra, B. (2010). At-risk mental state (ARMS) detection in a community service center for early attention to psychosis in Barcelona. *Early Intervention in Psychiatry*, *4*(3), 257–262. https://doi.org/10.1111/j.1751-7893.2010.00192.x

Read, J., Harper, D., Tucker, I., & Kennedy, A. (2018). Do adult mental health services identify child abuse and neglect? A systematic review. *International Journal of Mental Health Nursing*, *27*(1), 7–19. https://doi.org/10.1111/inm.12369

Sharp, C., & Rossouw, T. (2019). Borderline personality pathology in adolescence. In A. Bateman & P. Fonagy (Eds.), *Handbook of mentalizing in mental health practice* (2nd ed., pp. 281–300). American Psychiatric Publishing.

Shevlin, M., Houston, J. E., Dorahy, M. J., & Adamson, G. (2008). Cumulative traumas and psychosis: An analysis of the National Comorbidity Survey and the British Psychiatric Morbidity Survey. *Schizophrenia Bulletin*, *34*(1), 193–199. https://doi.org/10.1093/schbul/sbm069

Slade, A. (2014). Imagining fear: Attachment, threat, and psychic experience. *Psychoanalytic Dialogues*, *24*(3), 253–266. https://doi.org/10.1080/10481885.2014.911608

Slade, A., Grienenberger, J., Bernbach, E., Levy, D., & Locker, A. (2005). Maternal reflective functioning, attachment, and the transmission gap: A preliminary study. *Attachment and Human Development*, *7*(3), 283–298. https://doi.org/10.1080/14616730500245880

Sørensen, H. J., Mortensen, E. L., Schiffman, J., Reinisch, J. M., Maeda, J., & Mednick, S. A. (2010). Early developmental milestones and risk of schizophrenia: A 45-year follow-up of the Copenhagen Perinatal Cohort. *Schizophrenia Research*, *118*(1–3), 41–47. https://doi.org/10.1016/j.schres.2010.01.029

Steele, H., Steele, M., & Fonagy, P. (1996). Associations among attachment classifications of mothers, fathers and their infants. *Child Development*, *67*(2), 541–555. https://doi.org/10.1111/j.1467-8624.1996.tb01750.x

Suchman, N. E., DeCoste, C., Leigh, D., & Borelli, J. (2010). Reflective functioning in mothers with drug use disorders: Implications for dyadic interactions with infants and toddlers. *Attachment and Human Development*, *12*(6), 567–585. https://doi.org/10.1080/14616734.2010.501988

Teicher, M. H., Samson, J. A., Anderson, C. M., & Ohashi, K. (2016). The effects of childhood maltreatment on brain structure, function and connectivity. *Nature Reviews Neuroscience*, *17*(10), 652–666. https://doi.org/10.1038/nrn.2016.111

van der Kolk, B. (2015). *The body keeps the score: Brain, mind, and body in the healing of trauma*. Penguin Books.

Varese, F., Smeets, F., Drukker, M., Lieverse, R., Lataster, T., Viechtbauer, W., Read, J., van Os, J., & Bentall, R. P. (2012). Childhood adversities increase the risk of psychosis: A meta-analysis of patient-control, prospective- and cross-sectional cohort studies. *Schizophrenia Bulletin*, *38*(4), 661–671. https://doi.org/10.1093/schbul/sbs050

6

Connecting psychotherapy to the streets

The Malmö approach

Ernst Dahlquist

6.1 Setting the scene

This chapter will describe the way that a team in Malmö, Sweden, adapted the AMBIT approach to their own local context and specific aims. As the author emphasizes in this chapter, the team's introduction to AMBIT did not replace what they were already doing but built on their work of many years. AMBIT merely helped them along a journey they were already on. This journey is extremely impressive, and in this chapter they will share with you their highly creative and deeply thoughtful approach to enabling young people who would never consider having psychotherapy as a way of addressing their needs to enter into conversations where this type of help becomes accessible to them. They have created an integrated model combining intensive outreach work and psychotherapy. The approach is highly relational in that it places at its heart the need to create trusting relationships that are supported by psychotherapeutic expertise. Although the focus here is on psychotherapy, the ideas could also be applicable to other forms of help. The key is that an existing relationship of trust was used to support a young person to engage in another helping relationship. This required both workers to adapt how they might usually practise to work jointly to support the young person so that the young person could receive the benefits of both of the helping approaches.

6.2 The team today

The C & E Mind team is an outpatient team that has worked with young people since 2010. The target group is children and young people with severe psychosocial problems that society has had difficulty reaching through previous interventions by child and adolescent psychiatry, social services, and schools. We receive referrals from social services, and we provide a combination of concrete support in everyday life and psychotherapy in various forms. We work with the young person individually as well as with their family and the professional network. Since 2016, we have started to apply aspects of the AMBIT model to our work. The team consists of two psychotherapists (one of whom is a psychologist and the other a social worker), three youth treatment workers, and a social worker who works as a parent support worker. We also provide psychotherapy and supervision within the framework of these activities.

The business is private and is owned by two of the team members, one of whom is a psychotherapist/social worker (ED) and the other a social worker/youth treatment worker (CB). Our treatment model is based on 8 hours per week per client, which also includes time spent on things that are not direct client work. We adapt, in consultation with the referring social worker, the model to the individual client's needs, which means that sometimes there are more and sometimes fewer hours per week. Each youth treatment worker is responsible for an average of four clients, and each client is also linked to a psychotherapist. Our treatment processes are relatively long, usually 1–2 years but sometimes even longer. In some cases, we do not manage to establish contact and then they naturally become much shorter. The fact that we are a private business makes us sensitive to the attitudes of social services towards us. Having a good reputation is important, and we are also sensitive to political or ideological fluctuations both nationally and regionally. We have premises that we rent centrally in Malmö, which contain consultation rooms, offices, and a large coffee room where we also have our treatment conferences every week. The youth treatment workers and the parent supporter spend much of their time out in the community, meeting clients, participating in meetings with families, schools, social workers, and so on. The psychotherapists also provide regular psychotherapy with private clients and supervise different staff groups in the treating professions.

6.3 How it started

In 2009, I (ED) worked at the Child and Adolescent Psychiatry (*Barn- och Ungdomspsykiatri*; BUP) service in Ystad, Sweden, in a team with a strong family therapy focus, whereas my own psychotherapeutic education was psychodynamic. Before joining BUP, I had worked for 6 years in adult psychiatry and received supervision from a psychoanalyst. At this time, there were a lot of conflicts in the psychiatric field regarding method and theoretical orientation, and I was seeking to integrate different perspectives into my work with families, children, and young people. I had also developed an interest in mentalizing theory and attachment theory, as these perspectives seemed to me to be helpful in integrating, and adding something completely new to, the prevailing theoretical scene. At the same time, CB was working in a residential institution for boys with major behavioural problems. She had previously worked at another institution for girls. Her therapeutic knowledge consisted of courses in functional family therapy.

In the institution where CB worked, there was a 16-year-old young person for whom CB was the contact person. He had a diagnosis of attention deficit hyperactivity disorder (ADHD) and serious problems with crime, hypomania, dissociation, aggression, and self-harm. The institution referred the young person to BUP for treatment. In addition to medication for ADHD, he was also referred for psychotherapy. The psychiatric team assessed the young person and concluded that psychotherapy was not appropriate for him, partly because of the degree of his difficulties and partly because the young person was not at all interested in it. So, for these reasons the referral was rejected. However, the department stood its ground, saying that it was unreasonable for a psychiatric childcare team to be completely dismissive of treatment other than medication of a young person with such serious problems. This led us to rethink. Their arguments were reasonable, but at the same time we were not sure how we could be helpful.

We decided to meet with the team at the institution to talk about it. This meeting clearly revealed that the young person was indeed not in the least interested in psychotherapy, but also that he had built up a trust in CB, who was his contact person, and that she was eager that he should receive psychological help. She was also confident that she could persuade the young person to come to the psychiatric clinic if anyone there was prepared to meet with him. We then decided that CB would bring him and that they together would meet with me (ED).

At BUP, we had already developed a method for having tripartite conversations. For example, it could be a psychotherapist who invited a doctor to a session. The doctor interviewed the therapist in the presence of the patient, and then proceeded to examine what the patient thought about what the therapist said. The aim was sometimes purely therapeutic, but the conversation could also, at the same time, constitute a medical assessment. Another variant was that a therapist met with a young person, for example, three times, and then, together with another therapist, met the young person and their parents. At this meeting, the second therapist interviewed the first therapist about how they had understood the young person and then discussed what the young person and the parents thought about what was said. Inspiration for this type of conversation came from various systemic therapists, of whom Tom Andersen (1991) and Jim Wilson (1998) were perhaps the most influential. Wilson had for some time served as supervisor for the team at BUP.

Since I was interested in mentalizing and attachment theory, it seemed suitable to me to apply such a perspective to this type of dialogue. I felt that it was the missing piece of the puzzle to clarify the aim of working in this way. I read books on mentalizing theory (Bateman & Fonagy, 2019; Fonagy et al., 2002) and started using the concepts of *psychic equivalence*, *pretend mode*, and *teleological thinking* to understand and progress my psychotherapeutic thinking. Mentalizing became both the goal and the means of psychotherapy, and I was now able to apply my new knowledge to the tripartite discussions we had within BUP and let them complement and deepen my previous understanding from the psychodynamic and systemic theoretical perspectives.

In systemic family therapy, it is assumed that emotional ties exist between the family members and that the therapist's contribution will be to create new understanding among the members with the help of questions. One could also say that the therapist helps members to get in touch with and express feelings and thoughts in a way that increases mutual understanding and security. In other words, efforts are made to increase mentalizing between the family members. In psychodynamic psychotherapy, interest is focused on the relationship between patient and therapist. The psychodynamic perspective is not uniform but consists of a collection of theories and practices with some common denominators. One such common denominator is the interest in the relationship between patient and therapist. A classic way to use the relationship is that the therapist tries to pay attention to when the patient attributes to the therapist characteristics, thoughts, or feelings that originate in the patient's internal unconscious or conscious expectations, rather than in reality (transference). These mostly negative expectations of others can usually be linked to the difficulties that have brought the patient to treatment, because they also arise in the patient's relationships outside the consulting room, and they often originate in relational experiences with important others during childhood. The therapist tries to make the patient aware of this by simply reflecting on what the therapist understands, through interpretations or other interventions. In this way, the therapist challenges the patient's beliefs and at the same time gives the patient a new experience of a relationship that can contrast with their previous experiences. An important part of psychodynamic psychotherapy is thus to allow the development of a strong emotional bond between patient and therapist, and that the patient working in this relationship gets the opportunity of experiencing something new, challenging the internal destructive patterns of relationships emanating from their earlier life. Expressed from a mentalizing theory perspective, one could say that the patient, within the framework of a secure relationship, becomes mentalized by the therapist and at the same time develops their own capacity to mentalize. In research, the term 'corrective emotional experience' is used to describe this process and it is considered to be one of the common factors involved in psychotherapy. I will come back to this concept later on in this chapter.

The thoughts that I had in preparation for the meetings with CB and the young person were that the main therapeutic attachment was between them, and would continue to be so. From a family therapeutic perspective, one could say that I regarded the young person and CB as a system. CB had been of real help to the young person, helped him practically, helped solve conflicts, and did fun things with him. They had thus built up a trusting relationship. My job would be to make room for and support CB's mentalizing of the young person and the relationship between them, as well as the young person's mentalizing of CB, himself, and others, to the extent that this would be possible. Theoretically, these ideas were thus influenced by systemic thinking, mentalizing and attachment theory, and psychodynamic theory, as described above.

6.4 The first meeting

I (ED) began by confirming to the young person that I knew he did not want to come for therapy, but that I was glad that he had agreed to come with CB after all. I also said he did not have to say anything in the conversation, but if he wanted to, it would be very welcome. In addition, I explained the background of our meeting, that is, that many around him, including CB, thought he needed psychotherapy. The young person answered in a few words and gave a rather dismissive impression, but still accepted being there. I then asked CB what made her want to come with the young person to meet me.

CB told me that she had been a contact person for the young person for about a year. She felt that the young person often put himself in difficult situations and that afterwards he could feel really bad. She also told me that he had grown up in difficult circumstances (including being a street child and in orphanages in a poor country) and that she believed he had experienced many traumas. The young person was adopted by a Swedish single woman and came to Sweden at the age of 7. CB thought that many of the young person's problems were related to the abandonment he had experienced as a child. I asked CB what she thought was the biggest problem right now. CB then told me that the young person, when together with the others at the institution, could be aggressive and sometimes very angry and lose control of his anger. This led to incidents that made the young person become self-destructive and hurt himself. CB also told me that she was anxious and concerned about how the young person felt and what would happen to him.

At this point, I turned to the young person and asked if he wanted to say anything about what CB had said. He had been watching CB the whole time during the conversation. He said he was surprised that CB had so many thoughts about him. That was something he had not understood at all, and he agreed that he often messed up when he was angry and lost control. However, he did not think it had anything to do with his childhood. He felt that there were others at the institution that behaved badly and that was the reason he often was angry. CB confirmed this, saying that there were others there who could be provocative and that they knew it was easy to make the young person angry. I also confirmed this to the young person and said that I could understand that he was angry.

CB described an occasion when the young person and some of the other youngsters sat and watched TV and a discussion had started. CB told me that early on she realized that this might become difficult, and she had noticed that the young person started to lose control. The discussion led to a major brawl in which the young person, who was the one acting most violently, was blamed and punished for what happened. That same night, the young person cut himself on his leg with a razor blade. I asked CB what she thought was happening inside the young person after the incident. CB told me she thought he felt ashamed. She also thought that the person with whom the young person had been fighting was one that he really wanted to make friends with, and that this might also have had something to do with the cutting. I turned to the young person and asked him what he thought about it, and he said he didn't think the cutting had anything to do with what happened. It was just something he did, and he didn't want to talk about it. I confirmed to him that if he didn't want to talk about it, we would respect that, but I also said that I could understand how CB was thinking and that she was concerned. Then I said that at least it seemed that they both thought it was a problem that he sometimes could not control his anger and I wondered if we could try to talk about how he and CB together could help with this. This conversation resulted in an agreement that CB would give the young person a sign with her hand when she noticed that he was about to lose control. The idea was that he would thus be mirrored and hopefully also be able to take control of his emotion. The two would also try to notice the types of situations in which the young person became angry, so that we, in our meetings, could increase our understanding of what had happened.

CB and I continued to meet with the young person every 2 weeks for about 6 months, and he became more and more comfortable in these three-way conversations. His ability to control his anger increased, his self-destructive behaviour decreased, and his trust in the staff at the institution grew. We believed that the young person gained a new relationship experience with CB—that is, with someone who mentalized him and helped him put his feelings and needs into words. This in turn helped him feel confident and developed his own mentalizing skills. The meetings offered a space for reflection for both CB and the young person.

6.5 How our thinking developed

Based on the above experience, CB and I began to contemplate developing a method for working with young people, combining and integrating social work and psychotherapy. The target group would be young people not reached by the usual psychiatric or existing psychosocial treatments. Working at BUP, we often received referrals from social services regarding young people who lived in chaotic social conditions. We rarely managed to establish any fruitful contact with them. In some cases, we tried to reach them through family therapy, but often the parents were also difficult to reach, and our effort came to nothing. At the same time, their needs were enormous. Besides, there were often conflicts within the professional network around these young people.

Our thoughts developed into a model in which a social worker would work intensively to create a therapeutic attachment relationship with the client. This relationship would in itself have a therapeutic value, while at the same time aiming for external objectives such as improved physical health, school attendance, and/or meaningful leisure activities. We believed that the external objectives should be formulated together with social services and the client, based on an assessment of risks and protective factors. We thought that the type of tripartite conversation focusing on mentalizing described above would be included in this overall approach. The purpose of these tripartite meetings would be therapy for the client, but they would also be of help for the youth treatment worker. Through the tripartite meetings, the youth treatment worker would be securely anchored with the therapist, and, together with the therapist, would be able to share their thoughts and feelings, and thus avoid ending up in—or get help to get out of—the 'pond' (see Chapter 2). At the time, we were not familiar with AMBIT and did not use the 'pond' metaphor, but we were well aware of the high risk for the youth treatment worker to lose perspective and 'drown' in the case. The terms we used then, and to some extent still do, were all anchored in psychodynamic theory—parallel processes, splitting, countertransference, and primitive defences—and they provide a rich theoretical basis for this familiar experience.

6.6 The beginning

Based on the thoughts discussed above, CB and I started a company and applied for permission from the Swedish National Board of Health and Welfare to provide psychosocial treatment to cases referred to us by social services. We got the necessary permit and then created a website that we hoped would reach the social services that we thought we could work with. This is how we explained how we worked:

Our treatment model combines concrete psychosocial support and psychotherapeutic interventions. The method is primarily based on mentalizing, but also has its base in attachment theory and knowledge about health-promoting factors for children and adolescents. Mentalizing is a term that describes the ability to understand and reflect on how one's own and others' internal mental states interact with behaviours. This ability normally develops in interaction with attachment figures. Many psychosocial difficulties can be understood from a perspective of mentalizing and a lack of the ability to do this. During the treatment, our aim is to increase the child's or young person's mentalizing skills, which makes up an important part of creating a better everyday life and living for the youngster. The Anna Freud Centre in London has developed evidence-based methods of psychotherapy and psychosocial work based on mentalizing. The model we have developed is as follows.

The youth treatment worker works supportively and intensively with the young person. The youth treatment worker meets the young person frequently and regularly in the home and local environment, and works according to the young person's needs and the objectives of the assignments. Risk and protection factors are an important component that provides direction in this work, while the therapeutic goal is to create a safe and supporting relationship. These two objectives are equally important and interact with each other. Together with the youth treatment worker, the young person also meets one of our psychotherapists in what we call reflective talks. In these talks we focus mainly on three areas:

- The concrete objectives set for the young person.
- The alliance and the relationship between the young person and the team.
- The young person's and our own understanding of the inner emotional state of the young person's sense of self and understanding of others, how these lead to certain behaviours, and what this means for the young person. Through our three-way method of talking, the young person is also mirrored by the youth treatment worker and given the opportunity to listen to how the youth treatment worker perceives them in the above-mentioned regard.

We know from experience that a trusting relationship with the young person is a prerequisite for being able to help them both emotionally and in achieving sustainable development. The relationship between the young person and the youth treatment worker thus forms the basis for both the therapeutic and the structuring and supportive work.

When we started our business, we went to London and took a 2-day course in mentalization-based family therapy at the Anna Freud Centre. Now we were prepared and longed to test out our thoughts in practice. We had a clear idea of how we wanted to work, a theoretical foundation, and long experience. I had worked in different social work and therapeutic settings for almost 20 years and CB had worked with young people in an institution for 10 years. The only problem was that no one knew we existed, so we needed to make social services aware of us and somehow make them understand and believe in our method. We invited ourselves to several different social service departments to tell them about us and what we wanted to do. This was not easy, and sometimes we were met with scepticism and suspicion. Eventually, however, social workers started to contact us and make referrals to us.

6.7 Our first clients

One of our first clients was Anna. She was 16 years old and lived with her mother in one of Malmö's suburbs. Anna and her mother had a highly emotional (conflictual?) relationship that sometimes also turned violent. At school there were problems that involved Anna becoming aggressive and difficult. She was in her final year of school, and it was doubtful whether she would be able to get a graduation certificate. CB was with her as a support in school during some lessons and also spent time with her outside school, when they both went to the cinema, had their nails done, went for coffee, and so on. At the same time, CB, Anna, and I met every week for reflective sessions. Even in these sessions, Anna could lose her temper, and on one occasion she rushed out of the room and slammed the door. The relationship between Anna and her mother became at times untenable and, during certain periods, Anna was temporarily placed in foster care while we continued our work. CB and I also had meetings with Anna and her mother together, with a focus on their relationship. These meetings fell into an unconstructive pattern. The mother wanted to convince us how badly Anna behaved and was at times disparaging about her, which in turn made Anna angry. What happened at home was thus repeated with us, but now both parties tried to get us on their side. However, we felt that Anna now had a secure therapeutic attachment to CB. She sent CB text messages when she was upset about something and was then supported by CB in dealing with the situation. She never failed to attend planned appointments and she was happy when they did things together. She even began to speak the same dialect as CB.

We understood that Anna's mother felt that we did not really understand her and that she probably also felt criticized by us. She wasn't completely wrong. Even though we tried to hide it, we felt annoyed at her when she spoke disparagingly about Anna. At the same time, we thought that it was of course painful for her that Anna was able to relate to CB. We thought about how we could help the mother and came to the conclusion that it would be good if someone could meet the mother and take an interest in just her, in the same way as we were interested in Anna—someone she could feel mentalized by—and then we could meet them together, when both Anna and her mother had someone with them who they felt understood them.

CB had worked a few years earlier with E, a woman who worked in a business supervising foster homes. She knew that E wanted a new work challenge, and she also knew that E very much shared our thoughts about treatment. As a result, we hired her as a parent supporter. E began to meet Anna's mother in her home and, using a mentalization-based approach, focused on offering a supportive stance towards the mother's life experience. The mother was burdened with poor finances and mental and physical health problems. She felt helped by the support provided by E, although she was initially suspicious. We had decided that E should *not* try to educate the mother about how she should be as a parent but should primarily take an interest in the mother's own narrative. Of course, the relationship with Anna also became part of what they talked about. At the same time, E was able to help the mother to trust CB's efforts and good intentions. Relatively quickly, without even having time to have joint conversations, the relationship between Anna and her mother improved. A year later, when we finished our work, the two travelled together on a long journey and Anna was completing her high school studies.

From this experience we formulated the following: if we want someone to be able to mentalize someone else, that person first needs to feel mentalized themselves, have a sense of feeling understood, a sense of really being listened to by someone who is genuinely interested in them. It also became clear to us how important it was to strengthen the relationships that already existed and that would continue to exist when we were no longer there. Anna acquired a form of therapeutic attachment to CB in which she felt mentalized. At the same time, the mother gained the same in her relationship with E. When both had had this experience, it was easier for them to meet. That is how we understood the improvement that took place in their relationship.

6.8 We become a team

After our first completed treatment, we started to receive more requests from social services and decided to hire additional youth treatment workers and one more psychotherapist. We have now become a team of seven people. What CB and I strive for and constantly try to maintain is that we and the team should be the employees' 'safe base'. Working as a youth treatment worker is at times very stressful, lonely, and tough.

You get rejected by clients, embroiled in affective conflicts, criticized, and questioned. Through all this, you need to continue to try to keep a cool head and avoid losing your own mentalizing stance. This requires that you are securely connected to your own team (i.e. part of a well-connected team) and that there is a space for care and mentalizing for the youth treatment worker. There also needs to be a clear acceptance of 'failures', as these are an inevitable part of the work with our target group.

Neither CB nor I are authoritarian in nature, and we neither want to nor can exercise that kind of leadership. We think that if we can create a workplace with a culture that is mentalizing and based on trust, then this will bring about a positive parallel process—our employees will feel safe and respected, which in turn will have positive consequences for the work they do. Sometimes CB and I get into role conflicts when, on the one hand, we are colleagues with our employees and work together with clients, and on the other hand, we are employers and managers. The same applies to the employees.

6.9 AMBIT

I can't really remember exactly when we first became aware that AMBIT was developed at the Anna Freud Centre, but I think one of the employees first read something about it. Anyway, we found an article on AMBIT (Bevington et al., 2013). When we read it, we felt that it was a way of working that would suit us. CB and I explored the possibility of going to the Anna Freud Centre to learn more about AMBIT. We thought that it might give us the opportunity to develop what we did so that we had a clearer structure, and at the same time draw upon the experience and knowledge of others who worked and developed mentalization-based treatment with clients who are 'difficult to reach'. In 2016 we completed the 'AMBIT Train the Trainer' course at the Anna Freud Centre. We have since integrated large parts of AMBIT into our working method—a process that is still in progress and in which we have had ongoing supervision from the team in London.

One of the more comprehensive changes we have made since we began integrating AMBIT into our work is illustrated by the AMBIT wheel. Seeing the whole complexity of working with our clients, with mentalizing at its core, helped us realize the importance of working in the different domains in a more pronounced way. Our previous work was more client centred, so to consider the other parts of the wheel as equally important was an eye-opener for us. I would say that this has made us much more systemic in our way of working than before. On a more concrete level, we have started to use several of the methods and approaches contained in the basic AMBIT manual (I will come back to this later in this account). A further change is that we have begun to formulate our own way of working more clearly, both generally and in relation to specific problems, and we have started to formulate our methods on the internet-based wiki manual ('Learning at Work') (see Chapter 2). For example, we have manualized a way of working with deep conflicts between family members, based on the experiences we had with Anna and her mother, as described above. In this way, our implicit working methods become clearer to us, explicitly formulated, and something that we continue to use.

6.9.1 Theoretical aspects

The method that we had already developed was not in any way contrary to AMBIT, because mentalizing was from the beginning a fundamental part of our way of working. Even the integrative approach to theory and practice was part of what we already applied. One method that we are not so familiar with is cognitive behavioural therapy. We believe that there is a lot for us to learn there and perhaps one of us will deepen our knowledge in this therapy, just as we are open to other methods and theories that do not conflict with a mentalizing approach. Something that we really appreciate in AMBIT is the view of the team and its work as a process of continuous development. AMBIT also has a built-in and formalized way to take advantage of the team's creativity and experience through the interactive manual. The participation and responsibility that this entails for team members, we believe, promotes genuineness in meeting our clients, colleagues, and networks. This is in contrast to more strictly manualized methods, which can leave practitioners feeling as if they are part of an already finished and rigid production apparatus. In this way, I think that AMBIT is structured in a way that gives room for the mentalizing of both the team as a whole and the team members, which leads to a sense of meaningfulness that in turn benefits the clients.

6.9.2 Working with your Client

In the previous sections I have described our process and development since we started our business. I hope this has given the reader an understanding of how we think and work. For this chapter we have been asked to write in particular about the 'Working with your Client' quadrant of the AMBIT wheel. For us, the content of all four quadrants of the AMBIT wheel has changed our way of working since we started integrating AMBIT into our work. However, we have also benefited greatly in our work with clients from the approaches described in the first AMBIT book (Bevington et al., 2017) and in the AMBIT wiki manual (https://manuals.annafreud.org/ambit).

When it comes to 'Working with your Team', which is intimately associated with 'Working with your Client', we derive great benefit from 'Thinking Together'. When we first started applying this method, we made it explicit and also trained with role-playing. After a while, however, the steps in Thinking Together became so integral to the way we helped each other that we began to perform them more implicitly. We no longer marked that 'now we are going to Think Together', but still followed the steps in the model. Lately, we have again started to use the method more explicitly, partly because we noticed that we were starting to lose the steps, but also because we gained new employees who were not familiar with the model.

The dis-integration grid belongs to the quadrant of the AMBIT wheel that deals with 'Working with your Network', but in our experience, it also helps the youth treatment worker to get a clear picture of the context they are in with the client. This in turn facilitates understanding of what efforts may be needed to achieve the formulated goals. We have now decided that as a rule we will use the dis-integration grid at our own treatment conference 1 month into the treatment.

As I have described already, our way of working is based both on concrete help to create salutogenic environments for the young person (functioning schooling, living, leisure, etc.) and on therapeutic work with the aim of promoting the mentalizing of the young person and their network. In AMBIT terms, we are seeking to 'work in multiple domains' by offering help in a number of different areas of the young person's life. Common to all these efforts is that the youth treatment worker, with the help of the team, strives to maintain, or perhaps rather to constantly re-establish, a mentalizing approach. In this, both Thinking Together and the 'pond' metaphor are very helpful. We see the youth treatment worker's commitment as the most important helping factor, and we want to avoid demands for some kind of perfectionism in 'having a mentalizing attitude'. On the contrary, we expect that this is not possible because of how immersed the youth treatment worker becomes in their relationship with the client (i.e. when they are forming a strong keyworker relationship with the young person). There must therefore be continuous work in which the youth treatment worker is given space for their feelings and thoughts by maintaining links to a well-connected team. Working with your Team is therefore intimately associated with Working with your Client in our work. The three youth treatment workers and the parent supporter have daily contact with each other; this may be about discussing something that has come to mind or some difficulty they have found themselves in, but it can also relate to more acute dilemmas. We strive to maintain a team culture in which the workers feel that they can always contact each other.

In the following sections I will give some descriptions of tasks that we think are important in the work of Working with your Client. The text is structured so that the task is described and linked to theory/thoughts and sometimes case histories. Several of the tasks overlap, and the division is therefore to some extent constructed.

6.9.2.1 Create contact: establishing epistemic trust

Our target group are young people who are difficult for society's usual care institutions to reach. This means that the most difficult task is simply to connect with the young person. Generally speaking, we usually say that we need to meet the client where they are, both in concrete and in emotional terms. Their epistemic trust is often low and we need to show in different ways that we want to be of real help. In the beginning, we often need to want this more than the client. Many clients initially find it difficult to think of the relationship itself as something helpful and often associate us with social services, which they often have negative experiences of. Many have also grown up with insecurity in their early years, which means that they have insecure attachment patterns and associated difficulties in receiving help. It can therefore be a major challenge for the youth treatment worker to try to reach out with good intentions and for these intentions to be accurately understood by the client. As is shown in the example below, this may require persistence on the part of the youth treatment worker.

We think that strong external and/or internal insecurity often leads to teleological functioning, that is, the client sees no point in a helping relationship per se but cares only about the concrete consequences of it. For example, this could be expressed as: 'What good is it for me to come and talk to you?' In fact, it may also be that the way in which the young person lives requires action before therapy. We therefore have a conscious idea that those who are most difficult to reach may sometimes need to be met at a teleological level. At the same time, such a response becomes alliance-building.

Example
We get a referral for a 16-year-old girl, Wilma. She lives with her mother, but the relationship between them is chaotic and the mother has some problems with alcohol abuse. Wilma is rarely at home but is usually with her boyfriend and his family. The youth treatment worker tries to meet Wilma at the mother's house, but either she is not there or there is such a big fight between Wilma and her mother that it is impossible for the youth treatment worker to make contact with her. Instead, Wilma is clearly dismissive of her. A short time after we get involved, Wilma becomes pregnant. The following text conversation between Jessica, our youth treatment worker, and Wilma results in the first reasonably trusting contact.

JESSICA: Hi Wilma,
   My name is Jessica. I just met your mother. Too bad you weren't home. Because I'd love to see you. Mom has misunderstood because I don't work at soc [social services]. I work with young people and help them when they have problems. I don't decide anything. It's soc that decides things. I'm for you and I listen to whatever you want. I'd love to meet you (your boyfriend can come along if you want). I can buy you a cup of coffee. Food. Would that be OK? Take care of yourself. Jessica
WILMA: I don't want to see anyone. and I've already said that. Goodbye
JESSICA: I know your situation. That you don't want to stay at home and that you are pregnant. I have met other girls in your situation. It is absolutely you who are in charge of your body. I also know that soc won't leave you alone. If we meet, I can help you get soc to listen to you. Otherwise, there is a risk that they place you somewhere. We can just meet so you can see who I am. If you want someone you know to come with you, it's OK. Think about it, I'm here. You can text at any time if you have any questions.

WILMA: I've talked to social services once and said I don't want to see anyone. Now they say otherwise man. Why should I see you? I don't need help from anyone. I can't talk to anyone about my situation. Leave me alone and don't tell me that kind of stuff, that you're going to put me somewhere, because you're making me worse with your talk.

JESSICA: We're not going to place you! We're not soc. Maybe we can help you so that you don't get placed. I'm sorry if I annoyed you. Just want to see you. We don't even have to talk. We can go and do nails together if you would like.

WILMA: Yes, OK we can meet and talk a bit. I like doing my nails, so it sounds good to me. We can meet on Wednesday if it's possible.

JESSICA: I can do Wednesday at 2 pm so then we can make an appointment. So much fun!

Wilma meets Jessica a few times, but after several months she is still dismissive. She does not want to participate in reflective sessions. At one time when Wilma experiences complications with the pregnancy and acute pains, she calls Jessica, who accompanies her to the hospital and stays with her there for several hours. When the baby is born, Wilma is placed in an assessment unit that assesses her parenting skills and when she, her boyfriend, and the baby are to be discharged from there, she wants to have contact with Jessica. The small family has greater needs than Jessica can meet, but in collaboration with the social worker, the contact starts again, now with the intention that Jessica will motivate Wilma and her boyfriend to receive more intensive and comprehensive support from social services. Eventually, Jessica succeeds in motivating Wilma to receive such expanded support.

6.9.2.2 Care planning and linking to the network

Although our first concern is the young person, in another way our client is always social services. In Sweden, there is a system for outpatient care within, or on behalf of, social services. The assessment is carried out by the social secretary. In Sweden, a social secretary is like a social work case manager and is responsible for a child or young person making progress and achieving results in line with their care plan. This plan contains the overall objectives that need to be addressed. It can sometimes be the social services' own outpatient care, family home care, or something similar, that carries out the work, but it can also be other private healthcare providers—the category to which we belong. If we are contacted, we usually meet the social secretary together with the young person and possibly the parent(s). If the young person and the parent(s) want to have contact with us, we will initiate a contact. Often, depending on the problem, the introduction may look completely different, for example, as described above in the description of Wilma's case. We might then get an assignment that in the beginning is just about making contact.

Regardless of how the contact starts, within a month we have to formulate an implementation plan. In the implementation plan, we formulate our plan for *how* we will meet the goals of the care plan. As far as possible, we make the implementation plan together with the client and, where appropriate, with the family. After that, we have regular follow-up meetings with social services and the client/family. These follow-up meetings become a form of evaluation in each case. Often the implementation plan needs to change as new circumstances arise, in a way that is consistent with 'Active Planning' (see Chapter 2), so that plans are checked to see if they are sufficiently attuned to the current context and adapted accordingly. We often feel that we need to go back to the implementation plan to keep the direction and not lose ourselves in everything that can happen in the lives of our clients and their network.

This requires us to pay attention to one of the key aspects of the mentalizing stance, namely 'holding the balance'. Our approach involves recognizing the importance of providing both concrete support and thinking support (i.e. the reflective conversation sessions) alongside each other rather than in sequence (i.e. deal with social care needs first and then come for therapy). Second, we balance attention to what the client sees as important with what others see as important, as there are commonly different views about what needs to change, and basing the plan solely on the client's views may continue to expose them to risk. However, these things cannot be rushed. Third, we try to balance being helpful with promoting agency in the client, which ultimately will lead to more sustainable change.

6.9.2.3 Concrete targeted support

Providing concrete support in everyday life is a big part of the youth treatment worker's work. This part of the work is to a large extent about '*doing*'. The direction and objective of this work is formulated in external objectives for the young person such as 'attending school', 'creating meaningful leisure time', or 'not disappearing from home for several days'. Examples of such efforts can be to help the client to get a customized course of study or to agree with the client to pick them up and drive them to school. It can also be about being helpful in contact with other healthcare bodies or authorities, but also in more everyday activities such as helping to furnish a room or doing homework. Further examples are to help the client to get involved with a leisure activity by seeking information and helping them to get started. Sometimes, for example, the support might be that you go to the gym and work out with the client, which can both be a help in daring to do something new and at the same time give an experience of doing something together. In providing concrete support, we think it is important to be sensitive to the client's own perspective. For example, the young person may feel that the demands to attend school are coming strongly from the network and also from the youth treatment worker. Not infrequently, this objective is also included in the care plan from social services. There is then a risk that the youth treatment worker will start pushing the client in a certain direction in a teleological (quick-fix) kind of way, which can have destructive consequences for the alliance. At the same time, the young person may need to be challenged. Therefore, the balance between tuning in to the client and challenging them is very much present both in the structured conversation situations and in daily contact. The youth treatment worker's anchoring in the team is an important part of maintaining this balance.

Similarly, we try to maintain a balance between, on the one hand, being helpful when needed, and, on the other hand, encouraging the client's own abilities. An important therapeutic endeavour is to help the client feel agency in their own life, so that the client gets a realistic sense of how they can achieve things through their own actions. It is important not to curb this development by providing more support than is necessary. There may also be others in the client's network who can be helpful, and in these cases we strive to support these pre-existing relationships, which, unlike us, will remain in the client's life.

6.9.2.4 Emotional support

The emotional support is, of course, deeply entwined in the concrete support. On a theoretical level, however, one could contrast the two by defining emotional support more as 'being' and relating as opposed to the 'doing' of concrete support. Much of what is included under this heading also applies to the approach we seek to use in our reflective sessions, and these can also be regarded as an essential part of the emotional support. Emotional support can have several different meanings. It can be about reflecting and mentalizing feelings that the client has difficulty formulating, and it can take place virtually anywhere—in the car, by text message, or in a waiting room. Not infrequently, such conversations take place between the youth treatment worker and the client in the car on the way from one of the reflective sessions where a psychotherapist has also been involved. An important aspect is that emotional support is also about challenging, and thus supporting, the constructive side of the client. At other times, it may be about helping the client to deal with strong affect in a highly aroused situation. Sometimes such situations can be difficult for the youth treatment worker, for example, when the client or other family members may want to draw the worker into taking a stand in conflicts. The fact that this type of support often takes place by phone or sometimes even by text message does not make it easier.

6.9.2.5 Coexistence

By coexistence, we mean the aspect of the youth treatment worker's relationship with the client that is not linked to any external, concrete goal, but only has to do with being together. This gives the experience of 'being with' someone in the intersubjective sense. Stern (2004) describes intersubjectivity as a separate motivational system that is similar to, but not the same as, the attachment system. For example, a drive or a walk can be a situation where the client is given the opportunity to be together with the youth treatment worker and gain the experience of the mutual attunement that such a moment can entail. At the same time, this type of intersubjective experience is something that permeates the entire relationship, even when doing activities or solving problems.

Example 1

We meet Anna 6 years after the end of our work with her. One of the things she re-members with pleasure is one day when she and the youth treatment worker got up early, drove 100 km to a ski slope, and skied all day. She talks about how she enjoyed the drive in the car as much as the skiing.

Example 2

Niklas has grown up with a mother who constantly controlled him. The mother herself has some kind of psychiatric problem and has difficulty mentalizing around Niklas. In his process of seeking more freedom during his teenage years, the situation becomes untenable, with very violent quarrels between them. Niklas has also on several occasions run away and stayed away from home for several days. We get connected with Niklas but the situation does not improve, and he is placed by social services in an on-call accommodation. Our efforts continue, and the youth treatment worker picks up Niklas on some mornings and takes him to school. During a reflective conversation session, the youth treatment worker says she has been thinking about something. She tells us that she and Niklas do not talk at all in the car when she drives him to school. She thinks that it has become a kind of tacit agreement that feels quite OK for her, and she thinks Niklas thinks the same. Her feeling is that Niklas doesn't want to talk in the mornings and that he knows that the youth treatment worker knows this and therefore is silent. She wonders what Niklas thinks about it. He nods in agreement and says that he is unable to answer questions in the morning and that he understands that the youth treatment worker understands this. This quiet, implicit attunement from both parties became explicit in the conversation, but we think that the experience as such has value in itself and contrasts with Niklas's past experiences of socializing, which were characterized more by control than by attunement.

In a wider perspective, we think that these intersubjective experiences help the client to be able to be in other relationships as well. This type of relating is, and usually remains, implicit, but it is still something that we deliberately try to create space for and that we value.

6.9.2.6 Reflective conversations

The young people we work with have often grown up in precarious environments and have insecure attachment styles. Our youth treatment workers' overall goal is to create a supporting relationship with the young person, which can be thought of as a thera-peutic attachment relationship. In the 1940s, Alexander and French (1946) wrote a book on psychoanalytic psychotherapy in which they formulated the term 'corrective emotional experience'. This term has since come to be used to describe one of the most important factors for successful psychotherapy, a so-called common factor that in some psychotherapy research has been shown to have greater significance for the outcome than the method of therapy used (Luborsky et al., 2002). A corrective emotional experience is about the patient having a new emotional and relational experience in relation to the therapist that changes the patient's inner and relational life. This is of great importance because many people with mental illness have both unrealistically negative expectations of other people and a negative self-image.

The theory of mentalizing offers a perspective on how this manifests itself in practice and, together with attachment theory, it makes it possible to understand how such negative images of oneself and others can develop in precarious attachment relationships. Through insecurity in attachment, lack of marked congruent mirroring, and possible trauma, unmanageable emotions arise and the development of a cohesive self-image is disrupted (Fonagy et al., 2002).

In working with the young person, the youth treatment worker strives to build a secure therapeutic attachment, within which the young person can have some new emotional experiences that make a difference. In ordinary psychodynamic psychotherapy, the frames and therapeutic 'abstinence' are important ingredients—this means, for example, that psychotherapy takes place in the therapy room and that the therapist does not act to help the patient outside of this setting. The young people who we meet would probably find it difficult to work with this type of psychotherapy. Often, they lack the ability to forge an emotional bond with a psychotherapist who they meet for 45 minutes once a week, and if clients come to these sessions after all, it can be difficult for them to meaningfully connect what happens in the therapy room with what is going on in their life outside.

As described above, we always begin our treatment efforts with the youth treatment worker trying to create trust in the client. When the youth treatment worker feels that the relationship with the client is 'holding', we begin the reflective conversations. This means that the *client, together with the youth treatment worker*, begins to see one of the psychotherapists every week or every 2 weeks. Sometimes the reflective conversations can start right from the start, but on many occasions the youth treatment worker first needs time to create security in the relationship with the client. Many of the clients function on a teleological level and they therefore need to feel helped in a very concrete way in order to build trust in the youth treatment worker.

The reflective conversations may differ depending on the client's age, problems, current situation, and personality. We constantly strive to apply a mentalization-based approach as described in this book. Sometimes we find it difficult to find ways to make meaningful conversations, but we always try to think creatively and to adapt the conversation situation so that we can get there. For example, if the young person does not want to talk, the therapist and the youth treatment worker talk to each other, and the young person is allowed to listen. I don't think it has ever happened that the young person hasn't started to get involved during such conversations.

In the conversations, our goal is to create mentalization-based stories about things that happen in the client's life, by investigating what the client is involved with, who is involved, and how feelings and thoughts are related to behaviour. These may include relationships with family members and friends, or between the youth treatment worker and the client. We focus primarily on the client's current situation and daily life, but it happens that the conversations also process trauma or other painful experiences that the young person has had. Sometimes our clients find it difficult to talk and reflect on themselves and others, simply because they are too young, in terms of their actual age, developmentally, or because of trauma. For these young clients, their capacity to mentalize is still forming, and for the young person it can be either as painful or frightening to talk about difficult things as experiencing them (psychic equivalence), or there is an absolute difference between what is being talked about and reality (pretend mode). Then we use creativity and play (which one can see as an area between these two extremes) as a way in which we, together with the young person, can approach their inner world. In such therapeutic work we use images, drawings, retelling of films or TV series, and so on. Sometimes the youth treatment worker and the young person see a film together and we talk about it. Gently, we can then try to connect the playful or fictional to the young person's reality.

Some of the benefits that we see with this type of conversation, compared with individual psychotherapy, are:

- *Security*: the young person has the youth treatment worker with them, with whom they feel safe in the conversation situation
- *Integration*: the youth treatment worker is helpful in taking aspects of the young person's life into therapy, and taking things we work with in therapy into the young person's life
- *Deepening*: the conversations are often perceived to lead to a deepening of the relationship between the youth treatment worker and the young person
- *Mentalizing*: with three participants present, it is easier to make it clear to the young person that you can perceive things differently
- *Help for the youth treatment worker*: the youth treatment worker gets close to the client in daily work, and in doing so runs the risk of losing perspective and getting caught up in countertransferences or 'falling into the pond'. The third person, that is, the therapist, can help the youth treatment worker to get out of or avoid such situations
- *Epistemic trust*: the youth treatment worker shows, through their own trust in the therapist, that one can receive help.

Although we see many advantages of this type of trialogue, we can also see some problems that we have to deal with. Some of our clients have not managed to make these conversations meaningful at all, and with them we have decided to meet very occasionally and then mainly as a sort of follow-up meeting to help the youth treatment worker feel less alone. Yet, we still think that these meetings have served as a learning model in receiving help, and as a way to increase epistemic trust. In some cases, the clients come to the conversations on their own and the youth treatment worker is there only occasionally.

Another problem with these trialogues has to do with ourselves. It can sometimes be difficult for the youth treatment worker to 'switch' from being on the move and arranging things to being more reflective in the conversations and taking an interest in taking different perspectives on what is happening. This is especially true when it comes to young people who are living a destructive life or in periods when there is a lot of conflict in the network. Other challenges or problems may include:

- *Insecurity*: our most common impression is that our clients feel safe when the youth treatment worker is involved, but we have also experienced the opposite. Some clients seem to experience a loss of control and become afraid in the situation. They may feel it is 'two against one'
- *The collaboration between therapist and youth treatment worker* is important, and it takes time to establish and find forms for the common pursuit of a mentalizing attitude.

In our quest to maintain a mentalizing approach in the conversations and to take a curious, not-knowing stance, there are two clear trenches that we try to avoid: 'mind-reading' and 'psychobabble' (Bevington et al., 2017). 'Mind-reading' is a form of psychic equivalence that the youth treatment worker or therapist can, for various reasons, get into, in which one is too sure of what is going on within the client. This may be perceived by the client as invading, but it can also be a more or less deliberate attempt to 'save' a client who has difficulty mentalizing. However, such a 'rescue' does not always promote the client's own ability to mentalize. Some clients have such great difficulty in mentalizing that they may need to be assisted with their own hypotheses in order to take a mentalization-based perspective. One must then constantly pay attention to the slightest signs that the client shows of self-mentalizing and try to catch it and encourage further development. Whether the client's understanding of the situation that is being mentalized seems likely or not is less important. 'Psychobabble' is a form of pretend mode in which the youth treatment worker or therapist distances themself from what really makes sense in the current situation, for example, by an overly teaching or theorizing tone about 'how things are'. This must be weighed against the situations where educational interventions can also be very helpful for the client.

6.9.2.7 Parent work

Work with our young clients' parents is not a direct part of Working with your Client, but rather forms part of Working with your Network. However, given the way our method has developed, I still think the parent work is so intimately connected with the work with the client that we need to explain it, to give an understanding of our way of working. In the care plan put together by social services there is often an openly stated wish for parents to develop in their parenting role, often formulated precisely in terms of their ability to mentalize. The child is, of course, in focus. At the same time, the parents themselves are insecure and need to develop their own mentalizing skills. It is important to give time for this in the treatment.

The work involves the parent supporter meeting the parent(s) once a week or every 2 weeks. During an initial period of time, the focus of the contact with the parent is not on the child and their difficulties; instead, the parent supporter follows the parent's narrative. The focus is on the here and now, where the parent talks about their own difficulties with, for example, finances, housing, work, and relationships. The parent supporter applies a mentalizing approach here. When the parent expresses difficulties with the child, the parent supporter is first and foremost mentalizing about the *parent's* experience of the difficulties. The parent often leads the way so that we can eventually also talk about mentalizing around the child. Not infrequently, their children have diagnoses (usually ADHD and/or autism). Sometimes this becomes a difficulty in the mental understanding of the child, as the parent instead refers to the behaviour related to the diagnosis. Here, the youth treatment worker's contact with the child is crucial. The parent feels that they are no longer 'alone with the child'. This relieves the parent and opens them up to talk about their child not only as a 'problem' or in a diagnosis-oriented way. The parent may also receive positive signals from the child about the relationship with the youth treatment worker, and this can lead to competition and, at worst, splitting between the parent and youth treatment worker. To avoid this, the youth treatment worker also participates in conversations with the parent, with a frequency based on what the need looks like in each individual parental contact. In these conversations, it becomes important to strike a balance between, on the one hand, validating the parent in the difficulties they are experiencing with their child, while on the other hand, through the youth treatment worker's experience and story about the child, bringing the child to life as a subject in their own right.

We feel that many of the parents we work with are at the extremes on a scale between proximity and distance. From an attachment theoretical perspective, one could say that many are *preoccupied/ambivalent* and worried, which means they often end up in *psychic equivalence*. Others are *avoidant* and distanced, which means they often end up in *pretend mode*. In both cases, the parent supporter's first goal is to create enough security in the relationship to make mentalizing possible.

Example 1

Lisa, a 15-year-old girl we work with, has a father named Kalle. Her mother's name is Siv and her parents are long divorced. The atmosphere between them is very difficult, and Kalle wants to participate only in conversations about the treatment for Lisa. He wants no support for himself. E (the parent supporter) meets the two parents together with Jessica (the youth treatment worker). Initially, Kalle is very energetic and almost aggressive in his criticism of Siv, whom he believes is responsible for Lisa not wanting to see him. It is almost impossible to talk about Lisa. It goes so far that it becomes necessary to limit Kalle's participation in the conversation and he is instead offered individual conversations with E, to give him the opportunity to talk about the relationship with Siv. Kalle declines, however, and we agree to continue the conversations as a group together with Jessica, with a focus on monitoring our work with Lisa. After this, Kalle largely refrains from criticizing Siv as he did initially. After some time, Kalle expresses a desire for an individual conversation with E and wants to talk about his 'approach' to Lisa. In this conversation, Kalle describes problematic situations with Lisa, and E invites him to mentalize around himself and Lisa. Kalle, however, dismisses this as speculation. He declines further individual conversations with E but wants to continue the conversations about our work with Lisa.

During the conversations Kalle speaks more or less continuously in a 'teaching' and sometimes domineering way. He moves in his monologues from incomprehensible reasoning and thinking about events with Lisa, to world politics and its consequences, as well as philosophical reasoning about how people should live their lives (pretend mode). E and Jessica listen and ask questions and are eventually able to pick up a 'thread' from his monologues and bring back the focus to Lisa. This process has to be repeated during the conversations, because Kalle is quick to return to his incomprehensible reasoning and thinking. The structure of the conversations is to initially give Kalle space to talk about his own interests. Sometimes E can reconnect with the previous conversation by saying that she has thought about what he was talking about then, and gives examples and asks questions. After listening to him for a while, and when she feels it is possible, she directs the focus back to Lisa and turns to Jessica (the youth treatment worker) and talks to her about Lisa and how she is doing. Jessica develops this thread further and then turns to Kalle. This structure is repeated during the conversations.

Over time, Kalle can focus on Lisa more and more often in the conversations, and at times it is possible to have a dialogue with him. E and Jessica feel that Kalle is softening in his attitude when they talk about Lisa. At the beginning of their meetings, Kalle described a situation with Lisa, which he claimed was the reason why she now does not want to see him. From Lisa, Jessica receives information about completely different, more serious situations, where Kalle has acted out against Lisa, and the discrepancy between their stories feels unreal and strange. Kalle often returns to the situation in question, but he becomes more and more exploratory and reflective when he talks about it compared with the initial conversations, when he was dismissive and almost arrogant in his approach to Lisa and her reactions. In the beginning he was categorical and conditional when he talked about meeting Lisa again. He meant that when she came to her senses and wanted to meet him, he was ready for it, but he wasn't going to accept any anger or scolding from her. Later, he no longer made any conditions for their contact but merely expressed a desire for them to meet, and he wanted to hear what she had to say. He also expressed sadness about having no contact with her.

Example 2

Ali is a teenager who has been diagnosed with autism and ADHD. We are asked to help because there are violent conflicts in the home. Ali shows no respect for boundaries and behaves in a provocative and invading manner towards other family members, above all, towards his mother. In addition, he completely stopped going to school a long while ago. E (the parent supporter) has been meeting Ali's mother, Fawsya, once a week for a little bit longer than a year, and then every 2 weeks for a further 3 months.

Fawsya attributes all Ali's reactions and behaviours to his ADHD and autism, and she gives the impression that nothing can be done about it. She is frustrated and angry with Ali, as he invades and provokes her in different ways. One focus in the meetings is to help Fawsya find strategies and approaches to Ali in order to calm the situation at home. The meetings are often characterized by 'fire-fighting'. In parallel with E's meetings with Fawsya, Jessica (the youth treatment worker) has extensive contact with Fawsya. When Jessica makes home visits and tries to establish contact with Ali, there is room for Fawsya to talk about her problems with Ali and vent her anger and frustration. Jessica also joins Fawsya in school meetings and helps her in other contacts with different community bodies. Fawsya experiences extensive support from Jessica and is no longer 'alone' with Ali, which facilitates E's meetings with her.

The overriding problem for Fawsya is that Ali does not go to school, and many conflicts at home are about this issue. Fawsya is angry at the school, which she feels has let Ali down for a long time, and she acts out her anger at school meetings and in contact with school staff. Jessica's effort here is to have her own contact with the school staff and attend school meetings to relieve Fawsya and avoid open conflicts. Jessica can also, by virtue of meeting and getting to know Ali, help Fawsya to increase her understanding of his limitations in school and what is realistic to expect from him. The conflicts at home reduce as Fawsya changes her approach to Ali. She no longer nags him and demands that he goes to school. She also does not ask for contact and meetings with Jessica as much as before.

In E's meetings with Fawsya, she can now focus more on Fawsya and her own difficulties, where her inability to express her feelings becomes a focus. This difficulty causes problems in her dealings with her immediate surroundings, and not least in relation to her husband. In the meetings, she 'wrestles' with how to interpret her husband's reactions and signals adequately and bring herself to express her own feelings, instead of either shying away or being attacking and accusing.

At one point, Fawsya texts E and asks her to call her as soon as possible. When E calls, Fawsya is sad and heartbroken. She tells E that she called her husband and confronted him with the fact that he doesn't love her anymore and that he wants a divorce (psychic equivalence). Fawsya feels that she has expressed a question, but she hasn't received a reply from her husband. E validates Fawsya, but she also makes clear that Fawsya's question may be seen as an accusation, and E mentalizes about how her husband may have experienced and received this. Fawsya sends a new text message the next day, in which she writes that she has thought a lot about E saying that her question became an accusation. Her husband had met her lovingly when he came home, and she wrote in an upset tone that 'I am preventing myself from enjoying my marriage!' In the conversations that follow, Fawsya describes a turbulent inner state where she fantasies about the intentions of those around her, which turns out to have no basis in reality. Together, they can explore a pattern in which Fawsya attacks and where the recipient's reactions become a confirmation of her abandonment.

Fawsya now starts to talk about her own childhood. She describes how her mother never understood or validated her but instead questioned and accused her. E and Fawsya talk about how this has affected her throughout her life and not least how it has now become obvious in the relationship with her husband. Fawsya also expresses that she realizes that Ali's provocative and invading behaviour is linked to her own state of mind, as he becomes anxious and frightened when she feels unwell.

Depending on the client's needs and the contexts they are part of, we also meet in different constellations than those described above. However, the initiative for such conversations is usually based on one of the above-mentioned constellations. For example, the youth treatment worker, psychotherapist, and young client may conclude that it is necessary to meet a parent or other important person together. Another example might be that the parent and parent supporter invite others to participate in conversations.

6.9.2.8 Psychological assessment

Within the frame of our contact with clients, we sometimes pay attention to problems that we do not experience as changeable, for example, an undiagnosed intellectual disability or severe autism. Through M, our psychologist, we can then take the initiative to do a psychological assessment. We never accept assignments asking only for an assessment but are careful to assess only the clients we work with, and then only in cases where we genuinely believe there is a problem and that an assessment would benefit the client. We then make this clear with the client, social services, and parents before we start the assessment process.

Example

A 12-year-old girl, Agnes, has not gone to school in years. Instead, her mother tries to provide home schooling. She lives with her mother and an older sister. The father, who for many years regularly abused Agnes's mother, was convicted and is in prison when we are contacted by social services. The information we are given is that Agnes is traumatized and that the school thinks that this is impairing her ability to learn and making it difficult for her to attend school. Both social services and the school believe that trauma is the reason she does not come to school. Agnes is very difficult to connect with, and at first, she does not want to talk to any of us. Both M (the psychologist and psychotherapist) and J (the youth treatment worker) who work with Agnes feel pained by the rejections and by their inability to make any contact at all with her. The mother also participates, but the meetings with her often become difficult because she only wants to talk about the things she thinks Agnes does wrong. She can also be openly condescending to Agnes.

Eventually, however, M and J manage to make some contact with Agnes, and she meets them alone, without her mother. It becomes increasingly clear that she has major linguistic problems and a very strange way of understanding things. After some time, we discuss and agree with Agnes's mother and social services to conduct an assessment of her intellectual capacity. The assessment shows that she has a severe intellectual disability. With this new knowledge, we can now understand that a big reason why she does not want to go to school is that she understands neither the teaching nor the social interactions that take place between the pupils. J and M have also managed to establish a relationship with Agnes and can help her feel brave enough to go to a school adapted to her needs. Today she walks with pleasure to school every day and sends text messages to J about the things she is doing.

6.10 Evaluation

When we started our work 10 years ago, we used two evaluation instruments, FIT (Feedback-Informed Treatment) and KASAM (sense of context). FIT, developed by Duncan and Miller (2000), consists of two parts, an outcome rating scale and a session rating scale. Both parts are used for each meeting. The outcome rating scale is estimated at the beginning of the meeting and measures, in four areas, how the client feels things are going in their life. The session rating scale is estimated at the end of the meeting and measures, in four areas, how the client experienced today's conversation. Using the feedback given through the session rating scale, the therapist adapts the therapy, and the idea is that the curve of the outcome rating scale should follow that of the session rating scale. We believed that the FIT was an instrument that both measured results and meant respect for the client's experience. However, our experience with the young people with whom we work showed that the instrument somehow came between us and sometimes felt irrelevant to what was going on in their lives. Given that our work is so much more than just the meetings, it did not measure the right things, either. However, we have continued to pay attention to clients' feedback on our meetings.

KASAM intends to measure the client's experience in life based on three aspects: intelligibility, manageability, and meaningfulness. It is based on the theory of salutogenesis created by Aaron Antonovsky (1987) and is based on the notion that feeling involved in a context that is understandable and meaningful is crucial to a person's health. The instrument consists of 29 questions where the client estimates themself on a scale from 1 to 7. We make two estimates, one at the beginning and one at the end of the treatment.

In recent months, we have started to use the AMBIT Integrative Measure (AIM), developed at the Anna Freud Centre as a means to evaluate AMBIT-influenced work (see also Chapter 2). In the AIM, the client's problems are estimated in 40 areas. Six of these are selected, around which the work is built. For our part, the result of the AIM assessment needs to be linked to the client's care plan, so that they are consistent with each other and can be formulated in an implementation plan together with the client and possibly the network. In this process, it is of course essential that the client and network participate as much as possible (Active Planning). At the end of the treatment, the six areas in which they have chosen to work are re-estimated, and this gives a picture of how well the problems in the different areas have been tackled. Even though we feel that this process is very important, it has, for various reasons, been difficult to maintain the continuity of evaluations. The team has discussed how to maintain this continuity and we have made some changes to simplify the procedure. We believe that the AIM Excel sheet, which can be accessed from the AMBIT wiki manual (https://manuals.annafreud.org/ambit), can be very helpful in this. We also believe that our use of the AIM in a wider context is important, but we still need to develop a structure and routine for how we deal with the evaluations.

6.11   Final reflection

A friend of mine who read this text told me that she was emotionally touched by it. When I asked how, she said there was something about everyone being listened to. I think she put her finger on what really speaks to me with the form that AMBIT represents. The mental perspective of everyone involved is about humanity and in some sense about genuineness and maybe even love. AMBIT has for me become a structure that helps us to remain human under sometimes very stressful circumstances.

6.12   Implications

The work of the Malmö team has shown that the important knowledge and skills of highly specialist psychotherapists can be connected with and can enrich the help that young people may receive. They have developed a hugely creative method of integrating practical support with therapeutic work by beginning with creating relationships with young people, contingent to the young person's wishes, needs, and desires—that is, they respond to what is requested and needed. Contingent help is how initial secure attachment is formed, and the method used by the Malmö team recreates the mechanisms of establishing epistemic trust that have been so well documented for children in their early years. They also model a process of learning for the young person by making the relationships between themselves as a team visible to the young person through the tripartite meetings that are at the core of their work with clients.

The parent work described here is a crucial aspect of the work, but there could be an argument here that having different workers for a family (from one team alone) is excessive. However, for the reasons described in this chapter, it is critical to the success of their model. For the parent and young person, having their own worker each helps them to engage and is less overwhelming for the workers (compared with a situation in which there is one worker for the whole family) because each worker is clear about who their 'mentalizing priority' is. We suggest that this helps them to hold on to their own mentalizing capacity and in turn helps the client feel mentalized. The workers need not feel so conflicted or anxious about following the parent's lead as they describe it and mentalizing them, because they know that this will not be at the expense of the young person; someone else (the youth treatment worker) is engaging and mentalizing them, and ultimately the team will bring these strands of work together as part of their method. However, this way of working requires continuous connection between the respective workers, as the risk of dis-integration is high. Done well, it promotes integration, as workers can bring together a good understanding of each person's perspective and help the client to understand others. All too often, work with the parents is split off from teams like this, or the work is just about 'parenting' and not understanding the parent as a starting point, or sometimes involves trying to get the parent to mentalize their child too prematurely from the outset, which we know does not really work in these contexts.

References

Alexander, F., & French, T. (1946). *Psychoanalytic theory: Principles and application.* Ronald Press.

Andersen, T. (1991). *The reflecting team: Dialogues and dialogues about the dialogues.* W. W. Norton.

Antonovsky, A. (1987). *Unraveling the mystery of health: How people manage stress and stay well.* Jossey-Bass.

Bateman, A., & Fonagy, P. (Eds.). (2019). *Handbook of mentalizing in mental health practice* (2nd ed.). American Psychiatric Publishing.

Bevington, D., Fuggle, P., Cracknell, L., & Fonagy, P. (2017). *Adaptive mentalization-based integrative treatment: A guide for teams to develop systems of care.* Oxford University Press.

Bevington, D., Fuggle, P., Fonagy, P., Target, M., & Asen, E. (2013). Innovations in practice: Adolescent Mentalization-Based Integrative Therapy (AMBIT)—a new integrated approach to working with the most hard to reach adolescents with severe complex mental health needs. *Child and Adolescent Mental Health, 18*(1), 46–51. https://doi.org/10.1111/j.1475-3588.2012.00666.x

Duncan, B., & Miller, S. (2000). *The heroic client: Doing client-directed, outcome-informed therapy.* Jossey-Bass.

Fonagy, P., Gergely, G., Jurist, E., & Target, M. (2002). *Affect regulation, mentalization, and the development of the self.* Other Press.

Luborsky, L., Rosenthal, R., Diguer, L., Andrusyna, T. P., Berman, J. S., Levitt, J. T., Seligman, D. A., & Krause, E. D. (2002). The dodo bird verdict is alive and well—mostly. *Clinical Psychology: Science and Practice, 9*(1), 2–12. https://doi.org/10.1093/clipsy.9.1.2

Stern, D. N. (2004). *The present moment in psychotherapy and everyday life.* W. W. Norton.

Wilson, J. (1998). *Child-focused practice: A collaborative systemic approach.* Karnac Books.

7
AMBIT for adults with severe personality disorders

Experience from Utrecht, the Netherlands

Saskia Knapen and Rozemarijn van Duursen

7.1 Setting the scene

Although AMBIT was originally developed as a method of working with young people with multiple needs, the basic framework of AMBIT has been adopted by teams working with other client populations, such as adults with learning difficulties, chronic physical health needs, or severe mental health needs. This chapter will describe the application of the AMBIT approach to work with adults with personality disorders and will illustrate how the methods and framework can be effectively adapted to this group of clients. Despite using the same overall framework, there are important differences in some of the core themes and common situations that are typical in this often highly stressful area of work. For example, AMBIT work often involves working with young people who repudiate or dismiss therapeutic help; this is in stark contrast to the issues described in this chapter, as the overarching theme is how the team responds to the overwhelming requests and needs of some of their clients (referred to in this chapter as patients). The struggle is that the team cannot satisfy the highly distressing (and distressed) demands for ever more intensive treatment and care that do not in themselves result in improvement for the patients. Anxiety for the patients, for the team, and for the wider network may appear in different shapes than in work with young people, but the intensity of the anxiety and level of emotion experienced by both patients and the therapy team are in many ways the same. The interest for the reader is the degree to which the AMBIT framework is able to withstand the stresses and strains in these situations and enable the patient and team to hold a mentalizing stance amid these storms. It also illustrates how much AMBIT is an open system designed to be adapted to local contexts, cultures, and client groups, and highlights the need for continuous team learning in an explicit and contained way.

7.2 Working with adults with personality disorder

In 2017, we decided to adopt the AMBIT framework for our teams working with adults with very complex and severe problems who have received a diagnosis of personality disorder. The label 'personality disorder' attracts some controversy, since it is highly stig-matizing, as it implies that these people have disturbed personalities. Our view is more that these are people who have adapted to adverse (childhood) environments in a way that helped them survive in these environments. Early life adversities led to difficulties with how they learned to regulate emotions and, due to mistrust and the overwhelming nature of these emotions, they also have difficulties in the relationships that they now have with others. Furthermore, to protect themselves, people close off from contact with others and become rigid, mistrustful, and 'hard to reach'. Often this leads to a self-perpetuating circle of problems, where people with a diagnosis of personality disorder then experience blame from others (blaming the victim) and that their psychological difficulties are closely inter-connected with a wide range of social problems, such as unemployment, homelessness, financial difficulties, and social isolation. Sadly, they often also commonly experience ad-versities in relation to receiving help from others or from helping agencies, because others have the tendency to react in an unhelpful way to their sometimes difficult behaviour. This can lead to a distrust of receiving help and makes them even harder to reach.

Until 2017, we worked with the Functional Assertive Community Treatment (FACT) framework (van Veldhuizen et al., 2008, 2015) combined with mentalization-based treatment (MBT); at this point we had already realized that psychotherapy alone was not enough to best support and treat our patients. Who needs psychotherapy if they are at risk of losing their home or have huge debts? Although this approach was very successful, the original FACT framework did not fit properly and created inaccurate expectations of the type of care we were offering. FACT was originally developed for people with severe mental health problems, mostly psychosis, who need a rather dif-ferent approach. In psychosis it is sometimes necessary to take over the patient's respon-sibilities to protect both the patient and the people around them, but this can lead to iatrogenic damage in the case of a personality disorder, for example, leading to regres-sion and worsening of suicidality. In addition, the type of care offered in FACT is mainly supportive, and that challenged the need for psychotherapeutic change in our patients. Network partners, such as the police or housing companies, had wrong expectations of the type of care we provided and often would expect us to carry out compulsory admis-sions to the crisis unit, which we thought were damaging our patients. Learning from the AMBIT approach made us more aware of the need for mentalizing *systems*, because working with adults with severe personality disorders is very challenging—for workers, for networks, and for whole organizations. Severely destructive behaviour can be emo-tionally demanding on mental health workers and can also disrupt collaboration within a team or within the network, as we will illustrate later. We felt that AMBIT was a better fit with what we were already doing and wanted to develop even further.

7.3 The context in which we work

Altrecht is a large specialist mental health organization in the centre of the Netherlands offering services for a broad range of psychiatric disorders, including personality disorders. Utrecht is the smallest province of the Netherlands, with an area of 1560 square kilometres, but is quite densely populated, with about 1.3 million inhabitants. Altrecht provides services for about 75% of the province, including the capital city, Utrecht, where the headquarters of Altrecht are situated. Within the department for personality disorders, we have five AMBIT teams in different locations throughout the city (359,376 inhabitants) and in the province of Utrecht. These teams are closely embedded in surrounding social networks such as social municipality teams, housing corporations, police, and protected housing services. These connections enable our teams to provide a combination of social psychiatric care and psychotherapy.

The regulatory body in the Netherlands is the Health and Youth Care Inspectorate, which is part of the Dutch Ministry of Health. Mental health institutions are obliged to report serious incidents and calamities; the inspectorate then reviews the standard of care, based on investigations carried out by the mental health organization. If irregularities are found, the inspectorate can start its own investigation. The inspectorate does not review individual management plans beforehand. The legal system in the Netherlands is quite liberal and there is not such a culture of lawsuits as in some Anglophone countries. This gives us the legal backup (also by Altrecht as an organization) we need to operate in the difficult task of working with adults who present a wide range of risks both to self and to others.

Every team has a caseload of around 110–150 patients. Most of the patients are unemployed and have lost their connection with society. Alongside these problems, there is a lot of comorbidity, for example, multiple personality disorders, post-traumatic stress disorder, mood disorders, and substance misuse, and often a long trail of failed previous treatments, which has led to demoralization, commitment problems, and (epistemic) mistrust of helping agencies. Patients' challenging behaviour, including destructive behaviour, undermines the mentalizing capacities of many of those who work with them.

An AMBIT team consists of a psychiatrist and psychologists, but largely of keyworkers, mostly specialized psychiatric nurses. All team members are MBT trained and participate in the MBT treatment programme. Trying to maintain a mentalizing stance (see Chapter 2) is key in all interventions, both psychotherapeutic and social psychiatric (by this term we mean interventions that are mainly aimed at improvements in the social domain, such as living, working, and finances). In this regard we differ from the original FACT framework, for before acting we try to think and feel about the implications of certain interventions in a mentalizing way. This can be challenging, since pressure to act and fall into quick-fix interventions is sometimes hard to resist. There is also the risk of talking about our patients in pretend mode, often a sign of avoidance of difficulties. Because we work as a team, most of the time at least someone can keep a mentalizing stance and address these things, which again is challenging because giving feedback to colleagues can be daunting, especially when there are hierarchical differences: for example, it is difficult for keyworkers to give somewhat critical feedback to a team member who they feel is hierarchically above them, such as the psychiatrist or psychotherapist. Giving critical feedback is generally not easy for workers in any discipline, so we often tend to avoid this, but being able to give feedback, even if it is critical, is essential to avoid unhelpful, 'non-mentalized' interventions.

We work to build sustainable relationships, with the patient and their loved ones, within the team, and with the network, to enhance the chance for the patient to have a more positive experience within their own context so that this can catalyse enduring change. The AMBIT framework provides us with the means to sustain mentalizing networks around the patient and ourselves. It also validates constantly being slightly unbalanced (see Chapter 2) as the default stance in this work. In the following sections we will show our daily work by describing what it looks like in every domain of the AMBIT wheel.

7.4 Working with your Patient

Enhancing epistemic trust, while also managing risks and setting limits, is our biggest challenge in this domain. All our interventions are aimed at increasing epistemic trust or are at least being considered for this purpose. Aligning with the patient's needs and sincerely trying to understand the world from their perspective are essential for this, as is the recognition that distrust from the patient's perspective is understandable and has helped them survive in the past. Involving people who the patient *already trusts* in eliciting trust in us and our work is a very helpful piece of advice that AMBIT has given us, and we often make use of it. This does not necessarily need to be a spouse or family member; it could be a neighbour, a teacher, or anybody the patient trusts. It is very fruitful to search for these people in the patient's network.

Alongside this process, *scaffolding (healthy) existing relationships* is an important way to generate support so that patients can, for example, better put up with psycho-therapeutic treatment. People with personality disorders often have quite difficult and challenging relationships and some of these relationships are very dysfunctional, and it is very easy for others (including the psychiatric team) to adopt a judgemental at-titude towards them. In addition, the patients have often alienated other people so much that they have become very isolated. Still, it is as important to build new or better existing relationships as to conduct psychotherapy with the patients. Before we started using AMBIT, we would focus solely on creating safe and sound relationships with our patients, but often we became the only safe attachment relationship they had. This made ending therapy very hard, as it felt as if the patient was being abandoned without support. Furthermore, in psychotherapy, epistemic trust improves by way of improved mentalizing, restoring social learning, which is essential for generalizing what has been learned in therapy to the patient's own environment. A more benign environment (achieved by scaffolding relationships) gives them a chance to learn from new social experiences, which are essential for change—even more than psycho-therapy itself. With this scaffolding process a solid support network around a patient is built, which stays with the patient when professional help withdraws.

Both of these tasks are challenging when also *managing risks*. Restrictive interventions focused on controlling behaviour, rather than making sense of behaviour, are iatrogenic and damaging to our patients, but the pressure to use such interventions is often strong. Keyworkers or other professionals can feel anxious about losing their patient, while feeling responsible for their life, or can feel guilty or afraid of legal consequences. Setting limits, on the other hand, can hinder the development of trust, and this way a worker can feel stuck in an impossible dilemma. Eliciting trust while trust is low and destructive behaviour is profound is therefore very challenging but is the key to our work in this domain. We will illustrate this with a vignette.

7.4.1 Example: Working with your Patient

Brandi is a patient with chronic suicidal behaviour leading to repeated, sometimes compulsory, hospital admissions. She is often referred by the police or accident and emergency (A&E) department after disturbing the public order. Therefore, the mayor and safety authorities are involved. During her stay on the inpatient wards, her suicidal behaviour usually quickly escalates, leading to her cutting on the ward or pouring boiling water over her arm in front of other patients, after which she is forcibly discharged from the ward. In treatment, she misses appointments and frequently makes demands on crisis services after hours. Her close relatives are very much disturbed and worried. Her boyfriend is afraid of leaving her alone, but her demands on him exceed what he is able to offer. Her parents are disillusioned and withdraw helplessly from the relationship.

After multiple failed treatment programmes, Brandi is referred to our AMBIT team. She is quite distrusting and dismissive in contact with us. We find it difficult to manage risk and at the same time try to build a trusting relationship with her. Furthermore, we have to set limits to contain her challenging and disruptive behaviour. Because multiple admissions had not led to any improvement, but in fact to deterioration, we decided, after consultation with her relatives, to no longer carry out crisis interventions after hours and not admit her to the hospital but refer her to AMBIT workers the next day. Instead of controlling her destructive behaviour, we focused on understanding it and identifying precipitating factors.

Brandi, of course, felt very much rejected by this policy, but we patiently and repeatedly explained our intentions while trying to understand her behaviour. We made an effort to be trustworthy and available but within realistic human proportions. At the same time, we brought in her boyfriend and parents to also understand their perspectives and needs. Like Brandi, they felt scared in the beginning, but also understood that the multiple admissions were not helping Brandi and were preventing her from engaging with more effective treatment. We started to identify little interpersonal misunderstandings, which made Brandi feel rejected and often led to destructive behaviour. Her boyfriend tended to react in a quite over-concerned and controlling way, which was counterproductive, but we also learned that Brandi often felt consoled by her friendly neighbour in these instances. We worked on a crisis plan where the boyfriend would give Brandi some more space and we also involved the neighbour as an additional resource to fall back on.

While doing this, we kept broadcasting our intentions all the time—that we didn't want Brandi to die, but we really wanted to understand *why she* would want to do so. We especially and repeatedly tried to understand the world from her point of view, and we tried to be as available as possible after there had been a crisis to help Brandi understand what was happening. Often we brought her boyfriend with us. Brandi's parents learned to understand her a little bit more by joining a psychoeducation programme for relatives, and we had multiple sessions with them and Brandi to rebuild their relationship.

The biggest effort in all this was to accept and endure the distortion of our intentions, both by Brandi and by her relatives, and persevere in offering them contact and help, despite their rejections. It was important to understand Brandi's rejection of help as understandable from her own point of view. It made sense to her, however frustrating it was for the team, as she had had lengthy and bad experiences with help in the past. Furthermore, we focused on what we *can* offer instead of what we don't (i.e. crisis interventions out of hours and hospital admissions). Over time, the frequency of crisis events reduced and the backup team consisting of the parents, neighbour, and boyfriend became more confident in handling the storms that Brandi would still experience.

7.5 Working with your Team

Setting up a close working relationship is sometimes a daunting task, as dealing with mistrust, bad experiences, and hostility seem to collide with expressing good intentions and hope. Especially in the first months of treatment, all team members focus on forming a working alliance with the client. The keyworker tends to make frequent appointments, and makes a house visit to get a view of the patient's living circumstances and possibly meet their relatives, pets, or housemates, and observe their social skills. In the later stages of treatment, sustaining a working relationship can be a challenge. Clients can idealize and subsequently devalue our input or question our good intentions. It is not uncommon for clients to be ambivalent about treatment or express that despite our efforts, we are not helping them recover. 'How is this mentalizing helping me, why can't you just tell me what to do?' In order to understand these complex dynamics and deal with them, and to sustain our own mentalizing, all individual workers need a well-connected team.

As part of supporting each other in our teams, we have scheduled a *daily team briefing at 09.00*, in which crisis situations are evaluated and the team can oversee what lies ahead in the day and what needs to be done. It is also a moment for team members to share their worries and ask for advice or support. Apart from the daily briefings, *a weekly or 2-weekly hour of intervision* is scheduled, using the AMBIT

'Thinking Together' tool (see Chapter 2). The use of Thinking Together has made a big impact on our team time, as team discussions became less chaotic in form and content. We feel we are more able to diminish the risk of lapsing into a pretend-mode discussion leading to lengthy conversations but not to a purposeful plan. The framework helps us to focus and identify the point of friction in a situation, which turned out not always to be to do with the client. In particular, the step of mentalizing your colleague first during 'mentalize the moment' proved to be helpful. Even though we have all been MBT trained and recognized that reflecting on ourselves was the way forward, we found out that we felt it was a lot easier to talk about clients and their problems and interpersonal patterns than to talk about our own insecurities and anxieties. By explicitly mentalizing a colleague, we opened up the way to discussing our own interpersonal patterns and problems in working as a team. And, although we tried to tell our clients that seeking help is always an option, we were sometimes lacking in the 'show, don't tell'. We learned that team members sometimes felt awkward asking for help, feeling inadequate and unprofessional as they believed they should be able to manage on their own. It was already common practice to ask for help from the team consultant psychiatrist in complex cases, driven by the need to escalate in order to share (legal) responsibilities and feel protected in high-risk situations. Supporting each other as keyworkers was, however, not common practice before we began using the AMBIT framework.

As team leaders, we also made some changes to our own behaviour. First, we shifted to first trying to restore the mentalizing capacity of the keyworker, instead of immediately taking over. Although our intention was to support the keyworker by stepping in, this stance had possibly stimulated feelings of inadequacy in our colleagues. We realized we had often felt that as team leaders we needed to be strong and reliable, in order to provide holding to the anxiety of other team members. This has sometimes made us feel isolated and burdened by carrying the demands of not only our clients but also our colleagues. Demonstrating our own anxieties and need for help, and explicitly asking for support from the team, helped in gradually changing the help-seeking conditions in the team. In our role as team leaders, it has proved to be an ongoing process of finding the balance between being reassuring but not overly sure, and being firm but vulnerable, just as it is in the relationship with our clients.

7.5.1 Example: Working with your Team

Lisa, one of the keyworkers in our team, who is trained as a psychiatric nurse, repeatedly wanted to discuss Brandi's case. She questioned the management plan, as she felt that Brandi could seriously hurt herself or die, and she would be the one responsible. She seemed to be reassured when the team psychotherapist or psychiatrist explained the rationale of the treatment plan, and agreed with it, but the next day she would again voice her concerns during the morning briefing. She then reiterated conversations she had with Brandi and her boyfriend and brought up risky situations that the team might not have thought about. Although at first she received a lot of support during the team meetings, gradually some team members started to become annoyed by Lisa's input and tried to cut her short or would start joking about her taking up a motherly role for her client. Other team members felt that Lisa needed more support and urged the psychiatrist to get more involved. As tensions rose in the team, we decided to use a scheduled intervision hour to think together to address Brandi's case. Lisa asked Ken, a nurse colleague she felt supported by, to manage the process. In step 1 ('Mark the task') Lisa stated that she wanted the team to help her come up with a solid risk management plan. In step 2 ('State the case') Lisa elaborated on recent events: Brandi had been admitted to A&E after taking an overdose of her medication, which she had never done before, and this had worried Lisa even more. Apologetically, Ken interrupted Lisa, as he felt that the team was getting lost in the stories about Brandi. He suggested that the team members would try to mentalize Lisa's position ('Mentalize the moment') *before* trying to understand what was driving Brandi to this change in her destructive behaviour. One team member voiced that she felt that Lisa was over-anxious and that she had become too close to the case. Another team member felt that Lisa was insecure and was not able to deal with the pressure. A third team member then suggested that Lisa felt left alone. This was met by some surprise, as team members had tried to reassure her on a daily basis. However, as the team conversation moved along, several team members realized they had actually stopped listening to Lisa's concerns instead of trying to understand why she was anxious despite the team trying to back her up. Lisa then expressed that she felt she was leaving her client to die and was not providing adequate care as a psychiatric nurse, even though she understood the rationale of the treatment plan. She realized that she *had* been feeling alone, and this had been intensified by the annoyance she had sensed during team meetings. In the last step ('Return to purpose'), it was concluded that a new risk management plan was not needed, but Lisa needed more support in following up on the plan that existed. Ken suggested that he would be able to help her adhere to the risk management plan by acting as a second keyworker. Lisa and Ken scheduled joint appointments with Brandi, sharing the work and the emotional strain. Brandi was initially reluctant about Ken sitting in on appointments, as she felt she had to let a third party in on a relationship that had become important to her. She was, however, willing to give it a try after Lisa explained to Brandi that she needed help in supporting her as well as she could. Over the following weeks, Lisa still regularly expressed her concerns in team meetings, but she felt she was better able to support Brandi and felt more supported by the team. In the intervision 2 months later, Lisa suggested that Ken would join every other appointment, as she felt supported by the possibility of inviting Ken but that it was no longer necessary to have him in the room. Looking back on Lisa's feeling of isolation, other team members admitted they had also sometimes felt inadequate and anxious when dealing with suicidal behaviour. A relatively new team member said she had felt ashamed, as she thought everyone else did not seem to worry about risks and responsibility. The team then decided to regularly check in and offer the addition of a second keyworker in instances of serious and repeated suicidal behaviour, instead of waiting for the specific colleague to ask for this help.

7.6 Working with your Network

AMBIT made us realize in this domain that dis-integration is the default stance of networks in general (see Chapter 2). This recognition released us from constantly trying to strive for harmony and to accept that it is difficult to collaborate productively when many agencies are involved. This prompted us to strive to understand other agencies better rather than try to make them behave in the way we would like (which didn't work anyway). Much to our shame, we realized in our AMBIT training, we, as skilled psychotherapists and mental health workers, often felt somewhat superior to other agencies such as the police or support staff of protected housing services. With hindsight, we realized some of our network partners may have felt looked down upon and not taken seriously. This did not help them to be open to our advice. Hence, we contributed to the dis-integration in an unproductive way ourselves. We learned to put effort into trying to understand other agencies better, just as we have to better understand our patients and ourselves, to do this work properly. This can be quite a challenge sometimes, because we too often feel misunderstood or pressured by other agencies, and that does not help us to maintain a curious stance towards their intentions. It is sometimes hard to keep in mind that we are all in this with the same best intention: trying to help the patient. In the turmoil of things, we came to realize that we sometimes tended to attribute the intentions of our fellow network partners as inadequate.

If network problems arise, we now often conduct a dis-integration grid and a sculpt (an exercise from AMBIT training), and literally stand in our network partners' shoes. Frequently, we are surprised by what we learn from this exercise. Often, we feel all the pressure is on us and feel sorry for ourselves, but when we actually stand in the other shoes in the sculpt, we realize, for example, some of our partners feel isolated or left alone by us or are as anxious and overwhelmed with things as we are. This gives us a better understanding of them and contributes to connecting conversations with them, which elicit trust in each other and improves collaboration. In this way, trust in the helping system can be restored a little for the patients. In addition, by the keyworker taking over the responsibility for integration, the patient gets less overwhelmed and helps to regain perspective.

7.6.1 Example: Working with your Network

In Brandi's case, the police and A&E workers were not at all happy with the AMBIT team not hospitalizing Brandi when she engaged in severely destructive and disruptive behaviour. She kept repeatedly calling the emergency services out of hours or presenting at A&E with wounds. The AMBIT team got several requests from the police, the A&E team, and the protected housing service to 'do something'. We put effort into understanding their needs and found out that the community care worker would sometimes sit with Brandi for hours, as she feared Brandi would engage in destructive behaviour when left alone. The police struggled with all her calls to the emergency services, which they legally had to act upon but did not have the means to do so. All the network partners felt the AMBIT team was not helpful and was unwilling to collaborate. The A&E team expressed that they felt they were doing the job the AMBIT team should be doing, and proposed a lengthy involuntary admission. This put a lot of pressure on us to act (quick-fix). Although all this pressure was difficult to withstand, we did not admit Brandi to the hospital, but started connecting conversations with the network partners. Because this was too much to handle for one keyworker, we divided the work over several keyworkers, with each network partner getting a dedicated contact person in the AMBIT team. In the FACT approach, this is called a shared caseload, where you share the 'burden' over more workers, so the work becomes easier to bear. This is a good approach when a patient's needs exceed what one worker has to offer, which is often the case with patients with personality disorders. In addition, availability and therefore reliability increase for both patients and network partners. Shared caseload is an example of local practice from our past working in the FACT framework, which we gladly hold on to.

We worked with the community care worker around how to give Brandi space, notwithstanding the risk. We worked together on a crisis plan setting out how to act in difficult cases, so this was predictable both for them and for Brandi. We assured them we would take full responsibility for the outcome of our policy and would back them up. Their contact person kept in close contact with them. Alongside this, we contacted the community police officer and advised them to make an official report of Brandi's behaviour which was disrupting the public order, including her repeated calls to crisis services. This, of course, was challenging while we were also building trust with Brandi, but she also had to learn to deal with the consequences of her behaviour.

With the A&E team, we agreed they could inform our crisis service after hours if Brandi again visited the department for treatment. They could rely on us to follow it up the next (working) day and could confine themselves to only somatic treatment. We also gave them a psychoeducational explanation about personality disorders and destructive behaviour, to help them understand. As we described earlier, this also contributed to a reduction in Brandi's crisis behaviour. We made sure that we would be easily approachable for all these network partners.

7.7 Learning at Work

Implementing the Learning at Work quadrant proved to be the most challenging part. Although we recognized the importance of making explicit what often remains implicit in teams, it proved to be easier to discuss patient problems. In order to create a learning space, we established a 2-monthly meeting with representatives of the five AMBIT personality disorder teams in our organization, to discuss implementation and share local practice. In an effort to examine differences and try to create some uniformity across the five teams, we developed an internal audit, looking into all four quadrants of the AMBIT wheel and mentalizing. We asked the teams to complete questionnaires on their daily work. Two members of another team looked into five case files, recapped the findings of the questionnaires, and wrote a short report. This report was then discussed in the team, with the aim of improving coherence and sharing local practice.

An example of manualizing is the guideline we wrote about dealing with recurrent suicidal behaviour. From a mentalizing stance, it appears logical to try to stay curious and aim to understand recurrent suicidal behaviour. In practice, however, it proved to be difficult not to take over responsibilities and protect clients in order to prevent suicide or serious harm, for example, by organizing compulsory hospital admissions, as is described in guidelines for dealing with acute suicidality. The pressure clients put on out-of-hours services is sometimes difficult for individual workers to manage, as either they feel responsible for the survival of an individual patient or they feel inadequate in dealing with chronic suicidality as they have not had extensive training—for example, police officers or nurses in A&E. In addition, out-of-hours psychiatric services sometimes struggle not to proceed to protective interventions. In order to support individual workers to adhere to the management plan, we decided to manualize our risk management strategy. In cooperation with the clinical director, we wrote a protocol that explained the rationale and provided clinical considerations before applying a management plan that includes taking a weighted risk in cases of recurrent suicidal behaviour.

We then developed a 1-day training for practitioners as part of the suicide prevention training programme in our mental health organization, as other trainings were solely aimed at acute suicidality. The training includes different role plays aimed at explaining clinical considerations to patients, relatives, and network partners. After adopting the AMBIT framework, we updated the training and put more emphasis on dealing with the informal and the professional network. For example, we included a role play to practise explaining to the parents of a 21-year-old client that we accept the risk of their daughter hurting herself. It proved to be very powerful for trainees to step into the shoes of the parents and experience their anxieties.

Learning at work also includes exchanging local practice with other mental health organizations in the Netherlands. As we work with a specific client group that places a high emotional demand on teams, we sought connections with teams in different organizations with a similar client group. In a 2-yearly online meeting, we exchange local practice and think together about our local struggles. This is an example of 're-spect for local practice' and has led to improvements in our work. For example, we learned that a mental health institution in the north of the Netherlands had composed a letter for clients explaining their risk management policies, which were quite similar to ours. With their permission, we adapted the letter to our specific situation, and we now hand this letter to new clients at the beginning of their treatment with the team. By doing this, we address suicidality and dealing with suicidal behaviour at the start of treatment, allowing us to set the scene and manage expectations. By manualizing risk management policies on these different levels, we have improved our support of clients, relatives, network partners, and ourselves in dealing with highly pressured situations.

7.8 Concluding remarks

Our AMBIT journey started with the international team training at the Anna Freud Centre in 2016, after which we felt enormous energy and enthusiasm to implement the AMBIT way of working. We started out implementing the AMBIT framework in our FACT personality disorder teams in 2017. We feel we have since improved our daily work in many aspects. Explicitly mentalizing our clients, the wider network, and ourselves has opened up new conversations. The notion of giving equal attention to all four quadrants in order to keep the AMBIT wheel turning has been a valuable mantra. Previously, we were used to focusing solely on our clients and working out the best way to help them change. Discovering that sometimes the network or the team needs attention first, or needs an equal amount of attention, has given us a wider range of interventions and created more headspace when we feel stuck.

Applying the AMBIT framework helped us expand our focus from solely working with our clients towards trying to understand the wider context and trying to work with mentalizing systems. Although we still do not have a solution for everything, and we still struggle with complex and risky behaviour, AMBIT helps us to realize that imbalance is the natural state and that we can endure it together.

In the past 2 years we have started training teams in other mental health institutions in the Netherlands, to help them become AMBIT-influenced teams as well. In the training we have given so far, we have noticed that the teams were often looking for guidelines and a clear set of rules on how to do their jobs. It was sometimes unsettling for them to find out that we do not have the perfect solution and could not tell them how to act in difficult situations. This sometimes evoked insecurity in ourselves, wondering whether we had hit the right note and could deliver what was expected from us. Up until now, we have experienced in the course of the training that teams become empowered to create their own framework suitable for their specific work conditions, using mentalizing as the core of their activities. Training has turned out to be different every time, urging us to stay flexible and able to adapt to what each team needs. We learned that our job as trainers is to create a learning space, and that we have to keep tuning in to the needs of the team that is receiving training, by staying curious and keeping a 'not-knowing' stance. Active planning helps us in the training process, as it does when we are working with our clients.

7.9 Implications

Often, mental health treatment approaches can be described as somehow detached from the stress, the muddles, and the triumphs of how they are implemented in practice by therapists and frontline practitioners. AMBIT proposes that without including a full recognition of what it is like to implement a treatment approach, it may be hard to make sense of, both for practitioners and for their clients. This chapter has powerfully conveyed the connection between the theory and the implementation of the AMBIT approach. It has also described how the approach needs to adapt to the specific risks and contextual relationships of working with adults with personality disorder. As we noted at the beginning of the chapter, the unboundaried demand for help, rather than the avoidance of help, is a striking contrast to the descriptions of work with young people in several other chapters in this book (see Chapters 5, 6, and 8).

This chapter has suggested that there is a highly promising fit between the AMBIT approach and working with adults with personality disorder. This perhaps indicates that there are several key features that are shared across different client groups. Perhaps the most obvious of these is that the young people who we originally worked with were at an earlier stage of their lives but heading towards the difficulties so powerfully described in this chapter. They often had the same difficulties, but not the diagnosis of personality disorder. So, the degree of fit may be less of a surprise than it might appear. Second, the patients described in this chapter have psychological and psychiatric needs that are entwined in multiple social and life difficulties, and the involvement of multiple agencies increases rather than decreases the challenge of providing effective help (see Chapter 1). The difficulties experienced by workers from different agencies in trying to create a shared and collaborative approach to the needs of clients is profound. How a situation looks from the position of a police officer, an A&E nurse, and a worker at the housing department are not minor differences that can be addressed by simply considering that people need to be more 'flexible' or 'not keep being so difficult'. So often these difficulties become understood in terms of the personal characteristics of those we need to collaborate with. What the case of Brandi and Lisa has illustrated in this chapter is that these problems require larger respect, a method of addressing them, and the preparedness to think creatively when faced with the conundrums that this work presents.

References

van Veldhuizen, R., Bähler, M., & Polhuis, D. (2008). *Handboek FACT*. de Tijdstroom.
van Veldhuizen, R., Polhuis, D., Bähler, M., & Mulder, N. (2015). *Handboek (Flexible) ACT*. de Tijdstroom.

8

Enhancing multiprofessional cooperation in a child and youth social service institution

Vorarlberger Kinderdorf, Austria

Beate Huter and Michael Hollenstein

8.1 Setting the scene

In the previous chapters, we have read about the implementation of AMBIT predominantly in outreach teams. In this chapter, we turn to learning about the application of AMBIT to a service that has residential, educational, and outreach provision all within the same organization. For readers of this book, it will come as no surprise that this complexity of service provision, although hugely exciting and potentially creative, also produces major challenges in establishing well-connected teams and network collaboration. This chapter will describe how AMBIT was used to try to address these types of challenges in Vorarlberger Kinderdorf in Austria. Despite the scale of the task, we are in very good hands. We first met the authors, Bea and Michael, in 2016 and have had ongoing contact with them since then. With disarming humility, they have harnessed their enormous professional expertise to the AMBIT programme and have taken many of the core ideas to new levels of practice and understanding.

Their description of the implementation of AMBIT in their organization is supported by many case vignettes, which richly convey the complexity of the work and their humanity in how they perceive the tasks of those around them. In our view, it is a brilliant, multilayered description of implementing AMBIT. They also describe the application of AMBIT to leadership roles and how the application of a mentalizing stance in leadership tasks may enable others to make connections with the direction of travel that an organization may wish to embark on. As with other chapters in this book, this chapter richly illustrates how the development of the AMBIT model is deeply dependent on whether it can be effectively adapted to the real-world contexts in which services work. Most of all, it conveys with honesty and feeling the human process that this involves.

8.2 Introduction

8.2.1 Who we are and what we did: the story in a nutshell

The two authors are clinical and health psychologists, supervisors, and coaches who lead a team of 12 clinical psychologists, psychotherapists, and social workers who are responsible for assessment, psychotherapy, and parent counselling at the Paedakoop, a subdepartment of Vorarlberger Kinderdorf in Bregenz, Austria. Vorarlberger Kinderdorf is a privately run child and youth social service institution that cares for about 3,000 children of all ages and provides a range of services for children, young people, and families. As a subdepartment within this larger organization, Paedakoop cares for 65 young people aged from 6 to 16 years with multiple social and mental health problems. One-third of these young people are resident at the institution, while the others sleep at home and receive outreach care. Nearly all of them go to the Paedakoop School. Every family is accompanied by three professionals: a teacher, a social pedagogue, and a parent counsellor, and they often also have a child psychotherapist. Together, this 'triangle of professionals' works with the whole family system.

Paedakoop (formerly known as 'Jagdberg') has not always been what it is now. It is an institution with a dark history. Until the mid-1980s, violence and abuse were part of the pedagogy in many institutions with residential care. 'If you don't behave well, we'll take you to Jagdberg!' was a sentence that many children in Vorarlberg heard from their parents. The number of people who had been looked after at Jagdberg and reported their experiences of abuse to the Victim Protection Commission was exceptionally high, and the state of Vorarlberg granted compensation payments to them. Pedagogy and violence appear in the history of the institution as siblings.

By 1999, the institution was privatized and integrated into the Vorarlberger Kinderdorf, Austria's largest provider of services and support for children and families. Since then, the wind shifted and sails were hoisted in another direction; pedagogy set out to improve itself, but this was not easy. The social pedagogical care in the residential groups and the pedagogy in the school were often in strong competition with each other. Different styles, interests, educational methods, and attitudes collided with each other, resulting in numerous conflicts between the employees and the management. Finally, in 2003, a new school was founded, the *social pedagogical school Jagdberg*. Vorarlberger Kinderdorf took on the task of maintaining the school and, from this point on, two departments were put in place: the social pedagogical residential care and the social pedagogical school.

Now, Paedakoop's self-image is that of a complex all-inclusive offer, an 'educational intensive care unit': the boys and girls can live in one of our residential groups, or they can live with their families at home and we provide intensive outreach care. They can go to our private school and take advantage of its special teaching approach, since many of the children and adolescents we work with have histories of failure in regular schools. However, they can also go to external schools and still be cared for by us either through outreach work or as a resident. Paedakoop operates 24 hours a day, 365 days a year, and provides emergency accommodation when needed for those who have nowhere else to go. This department has carried out extensive organizational development over the past two decades, which was oriented towards professionalization, regionalization, service adaptation, diversification, expansion, and service improvement.

We adopted the name Paedakoop—an abbreviation for PAEDAgogical COOPeration—in 2013. So, cooperation was there from the beginning. The new name highlights the collaboration between school and social pedagogy, parent counselling, and therapy at all the locations where we work. But, even more, the new name expressed the will to cooperate and implicitly also the notion that help can lead to good results only if workers work together.

8.2.2 Initial contact with AMBIT

We first came across AMBIT in 2016. Our interest began at a day conference on adolescence at the Anna Freud Centre, where one of the authors and a colleague took part in an AMBIT workshop, not knowing what it was about. Our interest was elicited because AMBIT is a team-oriented approach within which consideration about workers' well-being was a core part. In the workshop, we had a feeling that AMBIT recognized the problems and feelings of workers. Our experience of our own work felt understood. We wanted to find out more. So, in October 2017, we participated in an AMBIT International Train the Trainer course in London.

8.2.3 What were the problems we needed help with?

What was it that we felt AMBIT could assist us in addressing more effectively? Looking back, we were aware of a number of major interconnected difficulties in our work setting that we were looking for help with, and AMBIT appeared to address these.

8.2.3.1 Staff well-being
We were concerned about the problem of worker well-being. Paedakoop has over 100 employees. A few years ago, about one-third of the employees left Paedakoop. We needed to think about what had happened. The organizational culture of caring for workers was good. There was constant support from team leaders, regular team supervision, and individual supervision on demand. There was a strong team spirit and definitely an attempt to be helpful to each other. Nevertheless, people left because they were worn out emotionally. This worried the management and elicited the urge to start thinking about what could be missing in the institution. Was it a question of deficits in vocational training or a lack of self-awareness in the workers? Was it due to

shortcomings in personnel selection? What was being missed? Tham (2006) examined reasons why social workers in child welfare leave their jobs and found that organizational interest in workers' health and well-being seem to be the most influential factors.

Thus, what emerged were the following questions. What help is there for the workers? How could we support workers in such a way that they have enough energy and enthusiasm to go on working with 'hard-to-reach' clients and complex systems? What surprised us again and again was that experts work together in teams but do not seem to devote much of their expertise and focus of attention to workers' well-being and network collaboration. Team meetings and case discussions were unsatisfactory. Collaboration with colleagues in other organizations was often exhausting, nerve-racking, and placed a strain on helpers—sometimes even more than the work with clients. Figley (1995) wrote of *compassion fatigue* to describe secondary traumatic stress and burnout in child welfare workers. This very vividly describes a phenomenon of losing the passion and energy, becoming tired and incapable of engaging enthusiastically or empathetically in one's tasks.

8.2.3.2 The need to pay attention to the workers' state of mind

We knew that the work demanded high resilience and affective competencies from our workers. They were often highly trained in their core profession, but what seemed to be needed additionally was a high capacity for self-awareness, crisis resilience, and the ability and willingness to cooperate with other workers or system partners. Workers were faced with resistance from and rejection by the clients, frustrating phases of stagnation, and also a high amount of aggression and violence against the self from young people or workers themselves. This elicited anxiety, insecurity, and feelings of isolation, insufficiency, or incompetence. Residential teams and teams of teachers in a class were at risk of emotions overrunning the team like a wave, becoming contagious and pulling the whole team down. Although outreach workers had more flexibility, they were often out there alone dealing with crises and needed strong bonds to experience support from the team.

8.2.3.3 Pedagogy and the problem of help-seeking for workers

Alongside this high level of need was the difficulty of how help-seeking was considered in our organization. The basic orientation of our facility is an educational one. Pedagogy is at the core of what Paedakoop offers, and pedagogical approaches are strongly dependent on the experiences that these professionals have had as children, and they are very much shaped by values and attitudes that are often implicit. Pedagogy pursues the aim of strengthening the resilience of children and young people and promoting their adaptation to social demands and norms. However, the need for help is strongly associated with weakness. When someone in a team seeks help, this person shows themself to be vulnerable. Some professional groups develop a strong identity of being 'solo fighters'; teachers may also belong to these professional groups. For us, it was important to contribute to a culture of cooperation, seeing it as a positive quality if someone seeks help and gets it. We learned to pay particular attention to ensuring that everyone looks for help at an early stage when they encounter a problem or risk, before it reaches excessive proportions.

8.2.3.4 Increasing case complexity

We also needed to recognize the increasing complexity of the families' needs on the one hand, and the demands of case management systems and the problems of network cooperation on the other hand. The fact that clients were being referred at a younger age required adaptation of care, and, in contrast to 10 years ago, their problems were much more likely to be related to wider and more severe difficulties. A retrospective quantitative survey conducted by the Vienna University of Economics (Schober & Wögerbauer, 2020) together with the Vorarlberger Kinderdorf has shown that, from a worker perspective, case complexity has doubled within the past 20 years. The problems of families have become increasingly diverse and serious, ranging from mental health to socioeconomic difficulties. Many children and young people were on the edge of care, which required far-reaching decisions from workers and increased effort in goal-directed parental work. This is one of the main reasons we had to invest in worker well-being. Complexity also arose due to larger networks, a lack of care services, and the resulting efforts to search for external care or treatment provision, as well as the challenges of handling new digital worlds.

8.2.3.5 The stress of working in networks

All workers in this field, regardless of whether they work with young people or their parents, must cooperate with a large network to be able to address the complexity of problems. State social welfare services, child and adolescent psychiatrists, external psychotherapists, preceding or subsequent helping systems, housing workers, probation officers, and social workers specializing in migration matters are just the most usual system partners in this field. Often, workers experience stress, devaluation, competition, jealousy, and conflicts of power in their cooperation with the network, and sometimes dealing with the network becomes more stressful than the work with the client.

So, perhaps not unexpectedly, the problems we needed help with were not just about working with clients, but included painful problems concerning working together in teams, cooperating across networks, and navigating a complicated multidisciplinary terrain. These were the sorts of problems that had been spoken about in the AMBIT training we attended.

8.3 Implementation in practice

8.3.1 The 'bones': the implementation process

After our AMBIT training, the implementation of AMBIT was supported by the Vorarlberger Kinderdorf leadership, and some of our time was protected for AMBIT development work. We visited teams from all the departments in the organization, including the management and team leaders of Paedakoop, to give them short presentations on AMBIT. About 80 employees from all areas participated in full-day workshops. Three complete teams were trained in AMBIT and can really be considered as AMBIT teams. Additionally, and much to the trainers' surprise, there was also great interest from external teams. We provided workshops at external institutions in Austria and presented AMBIT at various conferences. Thus, AMBIT moved and inspired the institution on various levels and kicked off a range of organizational developments.

While some of the implementation had its roots in our own team, the rest was distributed across the whole institution through interdisciplinary AMBIT workshops. Thus, AMBIT was experienced either directly via workers learning about it themselves, or passively by their being introduced to mentalizing techniques and AMBIT tools by co-workers. In this way, AMBIT has become a stance that has found its place in the working style of the workers, in addition to everything they knew before or have learned since. Some now might not even know that they are using AMBIT tools.

In the 5 years of our AMBIT implementation we have gone through several phases. In year 1, we concentrated on trying out AMBIT techniques ourselves and getting our own team curious while keeping it all voluntary. We tried to 'spread the news' by telling people about AMBIT, both formally and informally. 'Formally' meant that we told our CEOs and senior leaders about AMBIT in a short presentation. We did our first workshop and, to get people's interest, we decided—together with the management—to visit every team, including the school headteachers, to give them a short presentation about AMBIT before they sent their colleagues to the workshop. Informally, we would tell people about our experiences and conviction that AMBIT was an interesting approach in coffee breaks, team meetings, and so on. We translated material into German and tried out the tools.

In years 2 and 3, we agreed with our management a certain amount of money and time that we could invest in AMBIT within the organization as well as for external workshops. We adapted our approach with regard to focusing more on teaching whole teams. We started manualizing and formed an AMBIT Development Team in order to empower others to help us implement AMBIT. After we had trained quite a few teams, we deepened their knowledge by helping them to implement and adapt AMBIT to their specific needs by delivering follow-up workshops. By training teams and having single workers taking AMBIT techniques into their work groups, we got more and more people curious as they heard about AMBIT from different voices. Our internal magazines interviewed workshop participants and published two articles on AMBIT. Workers tried out different and new things. We used AMBIT techniques in team away days or leadership development teams, introducing it in all kinds of settings. In this way, even colleagues who had never been to a workshop learned from AMBIT. By running external workshops in other parts of Austria we learned from many incredible teams about how to do things better and what needs they have—and how adaptive AMBIT can be.

In the past 2 years we have joined the AMBIT Study Group and started to use the AMBIT Integrative Measure (AIM) (see Chapter 13). Our wonderfully engaged colleagues spread AMBIT ideas across our institution by experimenting and trying them out in their cases, inspiring other colleagues and improving our service immensely. They used their position as branch coordinators to bring AMBIT exercises to multiprofessional team meetings, which supported the co-production of the implementation. We owe these colleagues a huge thank you. Implementation could not have had this effect without their efforts. Already the effects were becoming observable; the mentalizing stance and tools play a role in everyday work and AMBIT is 'living'—humble and invisible under the surface of our everyday work, enriching cooperation and improving our work with clients.

8.3.2 The 'flesh': implementation in practice

We will now describe the implementation of AMBIT in greater detail in terms of the four quadrants of the AMBIT wheel. The emphasis will be on our lived experience of implementation in our complex organization.

8.3.2.1 Working with your Client
AMBIT has changed many aspects of our work with clients. The examples we provide here convey how AMBIT became understood by others, by seeing mentalizing techniques in action.

'The tribunal of death'—comparing waymarks and co-designing help
In our institution we have case meetings with the family and workers every 6 weeks to evaluate progress and to exchange views and ideas. These meetings can be very enriching and goal-directed—or very difficult and full of tension. A young boy once called it 'the tribunal of death'. We were desperately looking for ways to make these meetings more bearable and enjoyable, and, most of all, helpful to the client.

The most important stance we strengthened was to emphasize the young person's or family's capacity to be their best and foremost helping system themselves. Rather than teaching them what to do or what might be helpful, we began to focus more on their own knowledge about themselves, moving from educating or instructing them to not only asking them for their suggestions but encouraging them to co-design or co-produce help. To a greater extent than before we started working with AMBIT, we would compare waymarks with the clients and see whether we agreed on the next steps to take.

Example
A 14-year-old boy lived with his mother, who had borderline personality disorder. He had a place in our residential group, but he often did not turn up. His mother's illness became worse, leading to times when she had not paid the family's bills, taken

the rubbish out of the flat, or been able to buy food or provide clean clothes. Over a period of weeks, we had tried to convince his mother to refer herself to a psychiatric clinic, and had brought food, cleaned the flat, and provided money for electricity, always making sure the boy realized he was not alone, respecting that at the moment he said he could not leave. One day, I came to the boy's home after he had called me to report that they had no electricity again. I entered the flat and found him sitting in the dark; I had to use the light on my mobile phone to find him. We tried to convince him again and again to come with us to the residential group, but we came to understand that he could not leave home as he had to take care of his mother and he was afraid that she would lose the flat. Therefore, we had to make sure that we cared for the home he was protecting, so that he could care for himself and his life.

I knelt in front of him and said: 'I would really like to take you with me back to the group where you have food and a bed and can sleep. However, I know you can't go as you fear losing everything and because you have to take care of your mum. Help me to understand how I can help you. What could I provide here, at your home, so that at some point you feel you can leave the flat and find both of you safe in our hands?'

In retrospect, I consider this to have been a vital moment in which he felt understood, because I respected his devastating situation and concentrated on what he needed to be able to let go and get help for himself. He did not return to the residential home, but we managed to organize a special care plan together with social care, in which we allowed him to stay in his home, with his mentally ill mother, and took all the help—for his mother and himself—to where he was, rather than taking him out of the family home.

Mentalizing the other and oneself: 'You don't see the world through my eyes!'

Taking a mentalizing stance when working with our clients has transformed our work. We started to mentalize ourselves or our clients in various settings, to show interest, and to 'ask more than tell'. We used techniques of thinking aloud, talking to each other about the client, mentalizing the self, and asking questions. We moved from a stance of knowing to a stance of not-knowing, used our humour, and tried to hold the balance. We learned to show more curiosity when working with clients ('Let me learn from you!'), which suggested that not only could the client learn from us, but first we would have to learn from them. We implemented this by starting to talk about the client in front of them, with the intent that they might feel understood—a technique that often helped immensely to reduce the awkwardness of many meetings. What we realized was that clients listen very carefully, sometimes accompanied by red cheeks or ears. We also tried to show a stance of not-knowing and to express interest and curiosity in the knowledge the client already had about themself.

Example

I was caring for a young adolescent girl and her foster parents. The girl's mental health was poor and her behaviour was hard for the workers and family to cope with. Case meetings with Child and Youth Social Services (CYSS) and the family had usually been exhausting for everyone, followed by accusations by the foster father that everything was useless and being done wrong. After the AMBIT training, I mentalized the family in front of my colleague from social services: I started to share with my colleague what I thought life might feel like for the foster parents, who had so many hopes and dreams when they took over responsibility for a foster girl. I mentioned the fears and sadness, and maybe feelings of guilt that I could imagine they sometimes felt while doing everything they could to try to get things right. I also emphasized the love I felt they had for the girl, despite all the worries and stress. When the meeting was finished, I looked at the face of a surprised and maybe a little irritated social worker, who was not prepared for such an emotional speech. Afterwards, however, I got a call from the foster father, and expected the usual complaints and accusations. To my surprise, he said: 'Mr H, I have to tell you something! So nice how you spoke about us today ... no one has ever spoken so nicely about us, ever in our life. We finally really felt understood. Thank you very much.'

It was especially enriching to experience that sometimes it is the clients who initiate mentalizing in us, or to observe how mentalization-based work leads to the re-establishment of a mentalizing atmosphere in families.

Example
The family of an adolescent boy, A, was facing problems with A's puberty and also a cultural gap between two generations of family members with a migration background living in Austria. During a case meeting with the family, in which everyone was (partly in a non-mentalizing pretend mode) trying to understand and explain the problems of the boy, A suddenly spoke up: 'You simply don't see the world through my eyes!' Surprised that he had used an expression common in mentalizing theory, I asked him 'What would we see, if we looked through your eyes?', and he answered 'A lonely boy who lies in his bed and cries'. On his own initiative, he had got his parents and the workers to listen to his thoughts and feelings, and had stopped their non-mentalizing. Respecting and appreciating his effort to share his inner world, we thought together with him about how we could help him with these feelings and where we might be going wrong. Doing this made it possible afterwards to share our thoughts and feelings about him, which differed in a way that also allowed us to see more positive and lively elements of his personality.

'What did you mean when you said . . .?'—growing curiosity
One of the developmental tasks that we try to support in our families is the capacity to remain curious, and to mentalize self and other. Often, however, the complexity and dramatic dynamics of the family's problems undermine mentalizing and lead to harsh

and rigid thinking and interaction. If we manage together to revitalize the verbal and non-verbal mentalizing capacity of the family, then things become at least a little bit easier for our clients.

Example

The mother of an adolescent girl who tended to self-harm and had attempted suicide had been able to cope with the situation by acquiring a hard shell. Interactions between mother and daughter were harsh and full of misunderstandings and narcissistic insults. The daughter felt massively misunderstood, and her mother had no tolerance for her daughter's dangerous self-harm. Case meetings with them were often focused on risk management and crisis prevention. Self-harm elicited family crises and family conflicts triggered self-harm. It was a vicious cycle.

On one occasion I had made a home visit and talked to the mother. The daughter was coming in and cooking, and I seized the moment to mentalize in a playful manner with and between them. I invited them to think about each other's thoughts and share their own, and, meanwhile, I brought in what I thought might be on their minds. We talked about music, friends, cooking, the family, and everyday subjects. Both smiled and obviously enjoyed our conversation and to hear from each other what they thought and felt.

At the next case meeting, the mother, father, and daughter arrived in a good mood. The daughter had declared that she often felt that all adults tell her how she is feeling rather than being interested in how she is actually feeling. Therefore, we addressed this immediately and asked her to share her thoughts and wishes before anyone else spoke. We also tried to keep a relaxed and regulated atmosphere. She was extremely happy to be able to get some space to share her feelings and compare her waymarks with ours. Her parents were able to connect with her in a humorous and playful manner.

'I love these cards!'—goal-directed outcomes and the AIM cards

Working with the AIM cards (using the AIM cards is described in more detail in Chapter 4) has become a very useful and important part of our work. We translated them into German, and use them in work with the young person, in co-settings with the mother/father and young person, and in joint interventions with our colleagues (e.g. the social pedagogue or teacher uses the cards with the young person, the parent worker uses them with the parent, and then they are brought together again). Once we had seen the value of the cards within whole family systems, we created a parent/adult version of them by changing the language and adding topics. The AIM cards have become a widely used tool that enhances cooperation between colleagues, enables joint interventions, and helps families and young people to become clear about their goals.

8.3.2.2 Working with your Team: the role of mentalizing in supporting collaboration

The atmosphere during team visits was strikingly positive, I had the impression workers were in their power; this has positive effects for the work with the clients and families. (CEO, Vorarlberger Kinderdorf)

Creating mentalization-based joint leadership

Your joint leadership is not just like two people doing the leadership. It has become more than that. Something new was born, an energy that has pushed the whole team further. (A team colleague)

An unexpected, but in the long run perhaps the most profound, consequence of AMBIT was that the authors decided to lead their team of social workers, psychologists, and therapists jointly. It was the first ever joint leadership with equal rights in Vorarlberger Kinderdorf to date. There had been models of deputy leads, but no joint leadership had previously been practised in the institution. Nevertheless, the CEO was willing to support our joint leadership, emphasizing that this experiment was taking place due to his trust that we could do it. What had led to our CEO's trust in this respect was, apart from many years in the organization, the experience of our AMBIT implementation process. They had witnessed how working together can succeed and what power it can unleash. With our work on AMBIT and the idea of 'mentalizing always needs a partner, a second mind' taking root, we discovered how incredibly enriching it can be, not only in the sense of personal joy but also with regard to the quality of the outcome, to implement and develop services with another mind at your side. You have a second mind to help think things through, but you also develop yourself with and through the eyes of your partner.

Leaders bear a considerable strain with regard to responsibility, decision-making, 'Active Planning', and team development. Also, like parents, they lose their mentalizing capacity many times every day. There are things in leadership that have to be thought through or decided, which a team member cannot help with as it would lead to hierarchies becoming blurred. Often leaders try to solve problems as 'lone rangers', and Active Planning becomes a much less creative process when it is done alone. Why should the aspects we claim for the clients, the team, and the network not be valid for the leaders too? How could we be convinced of the necessity to mentalize together with colleagues and clients, but leave leaders out of this process?

Whereas many people are sceptical about joint leadership and emphasize its pitfalls and obstacles, we have become convinced that it can greatly improve the development of a team if it is done by applying AMBIT principles. AMBIT taught us the ingredients that are needed. Mentalizing each other, restoring each other's mind, talking about our thoughts and feelings, comparing waymarks, and learning from and with each other made joint leadership possible and, with time, noticeable effects were achieved in the team. The team became less anxious in relation to us, knowing how demanding the leadership of a large team in this complex setting is. It calmed them to know that we have each other to look after and care for. What was important was that we always included the team in this process—planning our strategies, broadcasting our intentions, and again and again asking for their feedback and their contributions in co-designing our joint leadership together with the team.

'Thinking Together'

When we first started to use Thinking Together techniques, it seemed a bit weird both to us, because we weren't feeling completely safe with the method, and also to our team colleagues, who found themselves having feelings like 'Interesting, what are they doing? It's great that someone actually asks for my feelings in this case!' and 'Hmm, this is kind of strange ... artificial ... I don't like this interrupting ... I just want to talk about my case!' The positive and negative feedback from the team was very helpful to us in adapting the style. We realized that we could not do Thinking Together in the same way with every person. Their needs were different and, in order to keep the team on board, we had to adapt. So, we realized that some cases need Thinking Together whereas others do not. Sometimes we still need just simple information or management decisions; sometimes the need of the worker is not related to their own feelings, but rather to hard facts. We took into account that we were working with individuals who had different needs. Some colleagues needed to feel heard without too much interruption; some needed more concrete suggestions and less talking about feelings. Others thrived once their thoughts and feelings had been addressed in the case. We still did the same thing, but in a more individualized way. In this way, we learned together as a team. After a while, the technique of Thinking Together became embedded and colleagues used it with each other. With our workshops within the organization, more and more colleagues from the various teams—teachers, social pedagogues, therapists, parent counsellors, and team leaders—became used to the technique and helped each other in their cases. As a result, fewer cases were brought to the team meetings, as colleagues mentioned that their co-workers from the school or the socio-pedagogical teams had already helped them by Thinking Together.

Example 1

It was a Friday morning. I was caring for a family with a very demanding and critical mother. Things had happened the previous evening in the family; the mother called me early in the morning, very aroused and in a dramatic mood; things had to be done immediately, she got into a rant that no one was doing things right, and nothing helped. From a mentalizing point of view, she was in a quick-fix (teleological) mode. I knew that it was very likely that I was at risk of being drawn into that mode of 'quick-fixing' too. I did what I could to calm the crisis down; however, by lunchtime, I still felt restless and insecure about leaving work for the weekend and whether I had done everything I could to prevent the next crisis. I called my colleague, whom

I had great epistemic trust in, and who was in her private practice between two patients. She said: 'I have 10 minutes!' I described my feelings of being unable to go home and asked her to check with me whether I had forgotten anything. She went through my Active Planning with me, acknowledged that I had done everything I could do, helped me out of the mother's contagious 'quick-fix' mode, and suggested that I could offer additional security calls to the mother if I felt it necessary but that I could also easily not suggest them and still be safe. These 10 minutes served perfectly well for me to let loose enough to go home and know the case was as safe as it could be for the moment.

Example 2
We held an AMBIT workshop in Linz, Austria. We were explaining to the group what Thinking Together meant. During the session, one of us (Michael) got a text message from a team colleague: 'I need your help with a case. Can you call me back?' We could not immediately answer because we were teaching, so the colleague had to wait. During a coffee break, Michael wanted to answer the message and help the colleague, but he had already received another message saying 'Already asked P and K, Thinking Together, all is well'. So we went back to the group, read the message to them, and said: 'Look, this is how Thinking together in a team works!' There could not have been a better live example.

Having multiple helpers: the use of 'case triangles'
We have already mentioned the history of the conflicts in the organization. With so many specialists working together, one might superficially assume that this would work and that the results of the help would be optimal. This is far from the case, because competition, conflicts of interest, and professional shame actually shaped cooperation and this, together with the strong dynamics and re-enactments deriving from the complex needs and difficulties of the children, adolescents, and families with whom we work, increased the risk that collaboration does not work. In retrospect, it may be that the will to cooperate was much more pronounced than any clear idea about how this will could be implemented in real life. We have looked for numerous ways to secure and improve collaboration in our organization, and taken many concrete steps. Here, we will take a closer look at how we implemented cooperation in casework. We decided on something that we call the *case triangle* or simply *the triangle*. Three specialists (social pedagogue, teacher, and parent counsellor) are jointly responsible and have a job that sounds simple: *do everything to change the child's development in line with the goals of the help plan.*

We had created numerous formats for cooperation over the years: time resources, meeting formats, ideas, and concepts of how and why our work should be done in cooperation. However, we also had the impression that we still had to work on the professional stance as a necessary link between the structure and the groove of cooperation. There was a will and engagement for cooperation. However, it wasn't so simple. To use an analogy, we were in danger of having a really cool bike with a high-standard chain—however, without oil on the chain, it was likely to rattle and stutter. The difficulties of cooperation between social pedagogues, teachers, and parent counsellors were strongly influenced by the attribution of status, and insecurities arose as to who had more experience or power or more to say and decide in the case.

Keith Johnstone, a drama teacher, describes in his wonderful book *Impro: Improvisation and the Theatre* (Johnstone, 1987) how relationships between people are influenced by status, which is displayed by gestures, movements, tone, and the eyes. Some people display high status; others tend to show low status. His theory derives from observations he made with three types of teachers, of whom he found that the most successful teachers were those who were able to *play* with status. Ideally, in his opinion, people flexibly vary their status between high status and low status when in contact with other people—for example, by sometimes allowing high status to the other, then playfully taking high status at another moment, just as the situation affords it—a phenomenon for which he uses the picture of a seesaw.

In our example, one worker in the professional triangle could constantly display or be attributed high status as the 'well-educated scientific professional', or as the older person, or as the leader of the triangle. On the other hand, a colleague with little professional self-esteem could constantly display low status in the cooperation, for example, to show that he would love to follow the others or to compensate for the fact that he doesn't feel experienced enough, or simply in order to resist taking responsibility. This very often happened in our triangles, without any explicit motive to do so. Johnstone argues that it is in our power to influence these positions. His theory suggests that cooperation will be most successful where it manages to flexibly *play with* and *vary* status between the workers.

Before AMBIT, this was mostly not the case in our professional triangles. Workers often wanted to state their position and convince their colleagues to agree and follow; disagreement was interpreted as 'not understanding' what is important and 'not getting it right'. Irritation and dismay were often the consequence; ignorance or incompetence were frequently attributed to the others. What was missing was the general respect for the possibility that the other might have had a good intention or good reasons why they argued for a specific intervention. Of course, the work with the client is the core of our daily business. It seems to us that the decisive factor for this change is that we found a common language with AMBIT. Self-mentalizing and enquiries returned, and curiosity about the point of view of colleagues and the request to check one's own perception took the place of fixed and sometimes rigid ideas about what kind of strategy the other worker was pursuing. Basically, assuming good intentions was a first step towards change. The next step was to ask frankly about mental states, about what we imagined was going on for others. People always talked about this, but often not *with* one another, but *about* one another. Things are different today: speaking about speaking, meta-communication, is now more consciously conducted in our department.

The question of who is responsible for what in the cooperative triangle, who from the specialist triangle sets which interventions, has always had the potential to be a cause of anger, distrust, competition, and guilt between each other. That has also changed because we now talk about it in advance and, even if sometimes this does not go well (and that is always part of this work), we give less room to accusation than to mutual respect. The 60 different triangles around the children and families had a great deal of variance in terms of the quality of their work. We have the impression that this variance has decreased and the overall quality of the results of the interventions provided by the specialist triangles has improved. What was previously missing in terms of cooperation was brought in by AMBIT. If AMBIT didn't bring the sound, it certainly changed it decisively.

AMBIT-influenced case screenings in addition to team meetings and supervision
In 2020, triggered by the need to work from home during the COVID-19 pandemic, we started to call every colleague once a week to provide leadership support and go through all their cases, as having case discussions about many of our 64 cases in remote team meetings would overwhelm everyone's capacity to mentalize and be helpful. We had previously had team meetings and team supervision, and spontaneous case discussions whenever needed. However, the implementation of these screening meetings on a regular basis, for every worker and every case, improved the quality of our Active Planning and mentalization-based work. How did this evolve?

Of course, we still discussed cases in our weekly team meetings and in team supervision; however, by starting the individual case screenings we eliminated the problem that workers sometimes felt left alone because their case was not discussed in a team meeting, and they no longer had to wait through several meetings for the discussion to happen. What was interesting was that our original intention was to use these screenings as a management tool rather than for extensive case support, so that we, as leaders, could get a picture of how each case was developing, whether the work was goal-directed, and to check how the workers were coping. Indeed, we realized that the quality of the strategic planning increased observably and workers less often experienced feelings of 'being fed up with the case'. They started to somehow enjoy every family they cared for, no matter how difficult the case might have been and including all the emotions that came along with this work. We felt they developed a more professional stance, seeing the case and their approach more from a professional meta-level rather than as 'their personal family'. The reasons this happened were that (a) we became better in preparing ourselves for these meetings, which had an impact on both the worker and the leader; and (b) the regular screening elicited a feeling of 'handling a case together' and not being left alone.

What did we want to know? We asked questions relating to all four quadrants of the AMBIT wheel:

- How is the case (what was the strategic planning; what was the worker working on)?
- How is the worker (getting a feeling of the mentalizing stance, feelings of being stuck, anger, etc.)?

- How is the cooperation (especially within the professional triangle)?
- Is there still curiosity and learning?

In these case screenings, we did not engage in elaborate case discussions but really focused on 'screening' the cases with regard to the workers' strategic planning; we also shared ideas that might be helpful or reflections, resonances, or questions that we asked ourselves when listening. What happened, to our surprise, was that workers powerfully improved their approaches to their clients. We think that they improved not because they followed our ideas or suggestions, but because they became clearer and more strategic in their own ideas and strategic planning with their clients. One colleague explained: 'You know, by having to tell you about my cases I already sort them in my head. And with your additional thoughts and questions I become clearer on what I want to do next.' The meetings used mentalizing techniques (e.g. noticing and naming positive mentalizing; stopping non-mentalizing modes). What also came into use very often was the Active Planning triangle, to check whether the worker had a plan, whether they had actually shared their intentions, or where their sensitive attunement tended to lead them. Wherever cooperation was the problem, we used the dis-integration grid, and when there were complex helping systems and clients who seemed to get lost in the flock of professionals around them, the Pro-Gram was introduced as a possible means of clarifying things.

Individual risk support—insisting on stopping

One challenge for us as leaders has always been to take good care of our team colleagues when they are dealing with high-risk situations. Our experience is that the more a worker gets involved and entangled in a case (to use an AMBIT metaphor, the more the worker moves towards the middle of the pond), the harder they grab hold of the case and the more difficult it becomes to help them out of the entanglement. We often used the picture of a dog who freezes and does not want to let go of his stick even though he wants to play with you. When you invite him to give you the stick or try to grab it, he might run away or growl.

The four-step CUSS (Concern, Uncertainty, Safety, Stop) model for graded assertiveness (outlined in Bevington et al., 2017), adapted from the airline industry, is very helpful for us when it comes to individual risk support in these cases. This model is based on the notion that you shift your focus from offering help directly to someone to asking them to help *you* with *your irritation about them*. We used it as leaders in our own team and also trained multiprofessional teams (teachers, social pedagogues, psychologists, social workers) in our institution to be more vigilant to cues that a co-worker might have become entangled with a case and address the person according to the model.

Example

In a multiprofessional meeting of teachers, parent counsellors, therapists, and social pedagogues, we talked about risk support between colleagues. In pairs, they did a role play in which one worker tried to stop their colleague and share their worry about them. We realized that colleagues found it extremely hard to be insistent and get their fellow worker to stop, as they were afraid that it might be considered as impolite, bossy, or encroaching. We discussed whether this is something only a leader can do, with our strong opinion being that this is not the case, and that this way of insisting and using graded assertiveness is necessary when a colleague is really strongly entangled with a case. Despite their hesitancy and fear of being intrusive, the participants found it very helpful to talk about this matter, to diminish shame and discover that they shared this difficulty. Additionally, by discussing it, they together built the foundation for this process being less awkward when they used it in the future.

In our experience, it is difficult to address worry about a fellow worker, as the more entangled they get, the less they can take it. Without grading up your assertiveness, you might be unable to help them. In our opinion, it is vital to talk about these situations and also try out and role play such stops, however awkward it may be, as this will make it easier to do in real life, and workers become more vigilant to the risks faced by others. Once we had talked about the process and tried it out, we had a mutual understanding of our responsibility for the well-being or risk of fellow workers.

Team and leadership risk support: managing the case together

In cases with a high level of risk, the role of the leader becomes especially important, as well as factors such as co-location of staff, pre-referral discussions, or joint visits to the client. Helping systems work best between colleagues who know each other and work together. We started to adapt these thoughts to our work, with special emphasis on worker well-being—not because the worker is more important than the client, but because we realized that if we cared well for our workers' well-being, they would care well for their clients' well-being. We decided to check all the cases periodically and decide which cases would become 'team cases'. This could be elicited by the leaders, or in a case discussion, or when we or someone from the team realized that a colleague was consistently becoming tense, agitated, or worried about a case. We did some Active Planning with regard to these team cases and decided that the following aspects made a case legitimate for becoming a team case, depending on whether these aspects also led to a felt burden for the worker:

- The case involves a large amount of time or energy.
- A case name is coming up again and again.
- Parents are in high conflict and cannot be cared for by a single professional.
- Emotional stress is constantly very high in the worker.
- Fellow workers constantly experience irritation in case discussions when listening to the worker.
- The dynamics of the case are not calming down.

Once a case has been chosen as a 'team case', the following options arise, taking the stance that 'from here on, everything is "team"':

- The case has to be discussed in every team meeting.
- Additional face-to-face case discussion with the team leaders and the worker involved.
- Supervision support by a colleague or leader for the professional triangle.
- Additional leadership focus on worker well-being (e.g. mental and physical health, days off).
- Optional reduction of caseload for the worker.
- Optional supervision in a single setting by an external supervisor.
- Optional co-worker in the case (joint visits).

Example
A colleague in our team generally has a high workload with a large number of cases. At one point, four of her ten cases were highly demanding. We had heard about the cases in many team meetings, and realized the team was becoming annoyed by the amount of time the colleague was taking up in the meetings. We also felt that the worker was getting entangled in her cases and was in quick-fix or pretend mode very often, talking a lot, and hardly breathing in between sentences. At one point in a meeting, she started crying, and it was clear that everything was getting too much for her. We started the 'team case' process: we took time to talk about her cases outside the team meeting, explore the issues in each case, and thought about case reduction and the possible introduction of co-workers. The colleague said she found it extremely helpful that both leaders took the time to really look at all her cases in depth and this felt like a huge appreciation of all the work she had been doing. We realized she was actually doing brilliant work, but the emotional overload that belonged to the cases had become overwhelming. The worker then dealt with one topic at a time. We held a second meeting in which we talked about her well-being. It was becoming obvious that private matters and work matters were intertwined, and it was time to sort them out. We decided on additional supervision provided by an external supervisor.

Adapting THRIVE: getting an overview of the risky cases and team workload
We started to use the THRIVE model (Wolpert et al., 2019) to get an overall picture of all our cases by, twice a year, allocating all our families to the relevant sector of the model to gain information on:

- How many families from each sector we were caring for
- Which families need what types of help
- Which families receive what types of care from our workers
- How troublesome the cases are for the workers
- Which families should become 'team cases'.

The procedure we used for allocating families was as follows: workers first choose a coloured presentation card (red, orange, yellow, or green) for each family and then write their name on the card. Red means high workload (with regard to time or emotional stress or complexity); green indicates 'easy to cope with/running well'. Then, each worker allocates the card to the sector of the THRIVE model that best represents the kind of help the family needs. This gives a picture on a meta-level: the whole team can look at their workload and see the distribution of cases to all areas of need; workers listen to their colleagues and can see that everyone else also struggles at times; and it is possible to see who has a suboptimal balance of cases (i.e. too many in the risk sector and no easier ones to balance this out). As Johannes Rauch, our former team supervisor, put it: 'A worker should be challenged, can sometimes be overwhelmed, but should always have something where they are underchallenged, in order to have a balance. If they are always in the red area of overload or too much strain, their mental health is at risk.'

The results of this THRIVE screening helped in many ways: directly for the work with the clients, but also for our managers and CEOs, who could get a picture of the distribution of clients with regard to the help they needed. Results could also be taken to the professional triangles to check how the fellow workers in each triangle would have allocated their cases and also to communicate how demanding a case was for a particular worker, thereby eliciting attention from the network partners.

Additionally, inspired by the Choice and Partnership Approach (CAPA; http://www.capa.co.uk/) model of service improvement, we adapted our parent work with the aim of efficiently and conscientiously allocating cases to the 'best fitting' workers out of our (personally and professionally) diverse team, rather than simply allocating cases according to workers' capacity or free time slots. In the course of this change, the team developed a stance of being able to talk about the allocation of cases with regard to the 'best fit' of the clients' needs to the competences, professional background, personality, or relationship to the workers. Although this process was difficult in the beginning, with workers having notions of 'being insufficient', 'being taken away from a case', or 'having to prove that the case fits', with our broadcasting of our intentions and sensitive attunement, the team got used to the change and broadened its thinking. The team members have come to see the cases less as their 'personal' cases but as something we are collectively responsible for, and the prospect of being able to talk about a possible fit as a positive thing rather than as a personal failure.

Teachers as keyworkers
The idea of the keyworker became very influential in many of our cases as a way in which we tried to establish the person who had the strongest bond to the young person in order to reach out to them. During the COVID-19 pandemic, it was the teachers who turned out to often serve as keyworkers. During home-schooling, teachers phoned their students every day to check on their tasks, teach them new topics, and ask them how they were getting on with their assignments. While parent workers or social pedagogues sometimes did not manage to get through to the young

people, because they either did not want to see them or were afraid of getting infected with the coronavirus, suddenly the teachers became the closest to the young people. By calling them and asking about their schoolwork, they got into chats about how the young people were feeling in general. Sometimes the teacher was the only person a young person wanted to have contact with, and therefore the only professional able to provide help.

Example
We were helping an adolescent girl who was self-harming and suicidal. The parent worker and the social pedagogue were concerned that the COVID-19 lockdown would increase the girl's depression and anxiety and her emotional isolation. However, the only contact the girl would accept was the teacher's calls, as school achievement was very important for her. Therefore, the other professionals started to support the teacher by, for example, providing knowledge about self-harm and suicidal symptoms, and asked the teacher to keep an eye on such indicators, with the teacher having them as supporters in the background. Thus, the teacher became the keyworker and the link between the other professional helpers and the girl, providing the best support possible in the circumstances.

8.3.2.3 Working with your Network
Mentalizing the professional triangle and multiprofessional networks
Frequently, our professional triangles, consisting of a teacher, a social pedagogue, and a parent worker, face situations in which the case dynamics influence either cooperation or conflicting ideas or priorities. In these situations, AMBIT has taught us to change our focus, especially as leaders when we supervise our colleagues, but also as workers with our own cases. Before AMBIT, we would have tried to convince our colleagues of our personal idea or plan, or put our effort into developing a shared vision. AMBIT directed our attention to sharing out thoughts and feelings *first*, to get a mutual understanding of what was happening between us or in the case. This has had an effect that we can still see is one of the most decisive changes that occurred when we brought in AMBIT. We do not have complaints about colleagues any more in our team meetings. This is not because conflicts of interest do not occur any more, but because our workers have adopted an integrative stance with which they themselves address their professional partners to solve conflicts or share irritations. In this way, conflicts are more easily resolved. It is the stance that matters, as it leads to workers spending less energy on complaining and instead accepting dis-integration as a natural resting state of cooperation and focusing on sharing their thoughts, as well as being curious about their colleagues' intentions.

Example
A parent worker, a teacher, and a social pedagogue became very agitated with a case in which a mother was very entangled with her son, unconsciously forcing him into

an emotional bond that made it difficult for him to leave her to go to school. He had an important role for her own emotional stability. The teacher saw this with increased concern and became more and more pushy towards the parent worker and started to advise the team leaders of the need for various additional interventions as a way of communicating his concern for the boy's risk. The parent worker saw the problem but felt that the teacher was going too fast and that a change in the mother's behaviour would take more time. During a case screening, we tried to look at the case from every person's perspective. We realized that the mother might have a strong transference towards the teacher, who symbolized someone (e.g. her father) who had pushed her to perform academically in her past, eliciting stress and pressure. At the same time, the teacher might have felt unheard in his concern and the perceived slowness of the parent worker might have put him into a state of even greater arousal, which in turn led to him becoming more pushy and thereby eliciting stress and pressure himself. We got the impression that the mother was somehow pulling the parent worker to be understanding and being 'on her side', perhaps like some validating person she might have wished to have had in her past. This dynamic led to the triangle becoming dis-integrated, splitting the parent worker and teacher. The perspective-taking process enabled the parent worker to see how the dynamics of the case had affected cooperation within the triangle, and that the teacher had been forced into a position as if the boy's school performance was his concern alone. The parent worker decided to talk to her colleagues and share her new insights and take responsibility to integrate some of the concerns the teacher had into her interventions and make it their joint goal. This enabled the teacher to slow down and respect the parent worker's feeling that it would take a little longer for the mother to be able to change.

Mentalization-based team development of multiprofessional networks
In our institution we have strong cooperation between teachers, social pedagogues, and parent workers, as well as therapists. Although all of these workers felt connected and were willing to cooperate, what was sometimes missing was something to make sure everything ran smoothly—the 'oil on the bike chain'. One very powerful aspect of the AMBIT implementation process was using our regional multiprofessional team meetings to enhance the quality of cooperation and client work. As every branch is led by a leader of each team (social pedagogue/teacher/parent worker), it was already a fundamental part of team development to use the meetings of the branch leaders to introduce the AMBIT stance and techniques in order to compare waymarks and get a shared vision of how we want our teams to work together. We used various interventions, between us but also within the teams, that were related to all aspects of AMBIT: addressing dis-integration, sharing minds, speaking about what we thought and felt about each other, sharing irritations and worries, talking about structures or our well-being, helping each other out, or speaking about the risk faced by workers. All these AMBIT-based interventions have led to probably one of the most profound

changes: a culture of learning with each other, respect for each other's ideas and priorities, joint interventions, talking about conflicting approaches, and willingness to solve conflicts directly and with humility.

Mentalizing in complex professional networks

In our setting, we work together with a vast variety of workers from many fields, as our clients are usually at the edge of care and have multiple problems, meaning that different services are needed to help them. We have different professions within our own institution, but we also work with various other systems, such as CYSS, child and adolescent psychiatry, housing workers, external psychotherapists, and external schools. Dis-integration is not the exception, but the natural resting state of complex professional networks like these. We are therefore responsible for contributing everything we can to improve understanding. In our work, of course we encounter dis-integration and conflicting ideas or plans between colleagues and beyond our internal network.

Colleagues might be irritated by colleagues in their triangle or by workers from, for example, the CYSS or the psychiatric unit. As AMBIT-influenced workers and leaders, we have a responsibility to invite our fellow workers in such situations to stay curious, get back in contact with the person who might have elicited the irritation, and mentalize themselves as well as asking the other about their intentions. This was an important step towards a different approach in situations where there was irritation. For example, previously workers might have complained about someone in front of a colleague, and this fellow worker might have added to the irritation and anger (e.g. 'Yeah, I know this person, she really is annoying!'), thereby creating shared arousal and getting carried away with blaming the other. AMBIT led to a stance in which colleagues would stop each other when they were being non-mentalizing and invite them to stay curious or to mentalize themself to the person in question.

Example

I needed family support for a family I was working with. As I had never used the family support service before, I called the service and asked the colleague whether she could explain to me how the service worked. She did so but, unfortunately, I did not understand, as her explanation was confusing and incoherent. So, I asked whether she might be so kind as to tell me again, as I hadn't understood some aspects of what she had said. She became annoyed, and I could feel her tension when she ranted on about the CYSS who did not get the funding straight, and that she couldn't help me as my case was wrong and did not fit, and anyway why don't I understand what she had explained? I realized I was getting slightly tense. I decided to mentalize myself and said in a friendly tone: 'Listen, I just called you because I am in need of help for a family. I have never used your service before, and I kindly asked you to explain to me how it works so that I can see if you would be the right one to help. Unfortunately, I still don't understand how you are organized. I also do not understand why I am confronted with all this anger—I just asked you for information—and I must admit I did not find this helpful at all.'

We said goodbye and I put down the phone. Two minutes later, my phone rang. 'I am very sorry and want to apologize,' she said, 'you faced an anger that wasn't about you. It is all the tension we have with the CYSS and their funding, and my tone expressed my pressure to be helpful when I am getting all these referrals and not knowing how to deal with it all. Please let me explain again to you what you wanted to know and see whether I can be of help this time.' It was a very good conversation, and she was really very helpful, which I thanked her for. This example shows that mentalizing the self or expressing irritation can sometimes elicit self-mentalizing in the other and make cooperation easier. It also shows that mentalizing myself restored her mentalizing in the brief period between the two calls.

Pro-Gram

As we often find ourselves working with large networks, we, or our clients, can lose sight and understanding of who is responsible for what, or about what relationships the young person has with all the workers around them. This is especially important in the work with 'hard-to-reach' clients, when you intend to establish who the keyworker is who could be supported to strengthen a relationship of trust with the client. The Pro-Gram can be of help here, and we used it in various ways.

Example

A 14-year-old boy often mentioned that no help from anyone was ever actually helpful. We wanted to help him explore who in his network might yet be a helpful resource for him. We decided to hold a case meeting with the workers (teacher, social worker, parent counsellor) and family to address the boy's network, and made plans for how we would do this (Active Planning). I (the parent counsellor) told the boy what we planned to do (broadcasting intentions) and that I needed his help. I said I would like to explore his network with his social pedagogue and his teacher, and that I would ask him to listen carefully and give us feedback at the end on whether we had got the picture of his network right. I asked the workers to talk aloud about the professionals the boy was working with, and to discuss what relationships they felt the boy had with each of them. I drew the Pro-Gram on a flipchart as they talked. The boy concentrated fully while the colleagues shared their thoughts, and his family was also listening curiously. At the end, I invited the boy to share his views and tell us whether we had got it kind of right. He stood up, took a felt-tip pen, and corrected the diagram, explaining to us how the relationships were from his point of view. It was obvious how seriously he took the task and how important it was for him that we were thinking about him and trying to get it right. At the end I asked the mother what she thought, and what her picture of her son's network was. The father was forgotten by mistake, because he usually never said anything in these meetings, but suddenly he reminded us indignantly: 'Don't you want to know what I think?!' This was a wonderful side effect of our task, because the father actively asked to be invited to share his thoughts, and the boy got a chance to understand what we all thought about him.

8.3.2.4 Learning at Work

The learning from difficult cases and the openness to speak about it improved with AMBIT. (Team leader)

Manualizing

Difficult topics are discussed in more depth and with more serenity from the leaders; more time is invested. (Team member)

The AMBIT International Train the Trainer course had introduced us to manualizing (see Chapter 2 for a description of manualizing). However, this was not enough for us to feel ready to really use manualizing, so we created a special AMBIT Development Team, which involved the workers in our team who were willing to take an active part in the implementation. We taught them how to use the manual, how to chair a manualization meeting, the purpose of manualizing, and how to actually write in the manual. Thus, we had a number of workers who were able to be scribes and chairs. From then on, the sub-teams met every 4 weeks and chose subjects to manualize— and they loved it! What we experienced was that the quality of the work of our team improved observably as we realized how everything that had been manualized had become 'team knowledge' rather than individual knowledge; for example, if you were working with a client who had made suicide attempts, you could rely on the fact that the team had referred to their shared experiences and wisdom and manualized them.

We could see how team development in these separate sub-teams sped up and thrived. It was a pleasure to see how they developed their own ideas, shared their knowledge, and referred to manualized expertise, which enhanced their work with their clients. We also started to use manualizing in multiprofessional meetings beyond our own team. While we had implemented manualizing on a regular basis in our own team, we used it in various other multiprofessional settings, however occasionally. In this way, we introduced the technique to our child protection team, and the team leaders used it in multiprofessional teams at our different branches— always with the aim of enabling the development of a 'team mind' and building joint learning. Speaking about topics together meant learning from each other, sharing our experiences, anxieties, successes, thoughts, and knowledge. The way in which the chair created a mentalizing atmosphere was crucial to support a culture of listening, being curious, asking, and showing respect for colleagues' thoughts and feelings. Without understanding this aspect, manualizing is just writing down team expertise, but this is not what it is supposed to be, namely learning at work in a mentalizing atmosphere, showing interest in and respect for the mind of the other. Manualizing has given the workers more power to develop their own expertise, guided and trusted by their leaders.

Example

We ran a workshop for a very experienced team that worked with adolescents in acute crises, which often led to confrontations and high levels of aggression in their work. It was obvious that the aggression they faced in their daily work had also infected their style of interacting with each other, despite their great expertise. We did a short demonstration of manualizing, and they then chose the topic of 'being confronted with a violent parent'. We manualized this topic, and after the session they expressed, with great relief, how much they had enjoyed the style of the chairing of the session with regard to the mentalizing atmosphere. They said they often talked about these types of topics in their team but mostly the style was one of interrupting each other, telling the others what to do, suggesting interventions, and so on. They enjoyed the way that in this session the chair had let everyone speak, invited workers to share their own thoughts and feelings, and respected every view. And they were puzzled that after just 20 minutes they had all their knowledge on the topic in the manual, ready to read and use.

Learning from cases

We decided to have one intensive case discussion in every team meeting. However, instead of a presentation (as we had used before), we introduced a new approach to our case discussions. Colleagues could decide whether it was a case they needed help with or a case they wanted to learn from. In the first case, they chose a fellow worker as chair for their case discussion. Together, they chose a method and clarified what question the worker would like to address. In the latter case, the worker could decide to also have someone else chair their case or do it themself. However, they had to include two aspects in the learning case discussion: first, what they had learned themselves from the case, and second, what the team could learn from the case that might generalize to other cases. We also included the invitation to share the learning with the families they had been talking about and to tell them what we had learned from them. In addition to this process, after a case had ended, the professional triangle of workers would come together and discuss what they had learned from the case process and from the family.

8.4 Evaluation

8.4.1 The clients' perspective: using the AIM outcome evaluation

As a result of the AMBIT Evaluation Day in 2018 we joined the then newly established AMBIT Study Group (see Chapter 13). The group has two aims: (a) offering the opportunity to share experiences and develop AMBIT further, and (b) evaluating outcomes to gain evidence that AMBIT does have an immediate effect for the clients. This was done by evaluating outcomes with the AIM form. Between 2019 and 2020, a first trial was launched within the team, with every team member being asked to rate at least one client at two times during their work with the client. Some cases were also evaluated by using the AIM cards with the client. The AIM measure was rated by the clinician. In this way, 15 cases were rated within the year, with new cases being started after this period. The first results showed, taking into account the small sample, very good results for our clients. Average ratings for all aspects of the AIM were significantly better at the second evaluation time.

We also evaluate all of our cases using EVAS, Germany's largest evaluation system for CYSS (https://ikj-online.de/). EVAS evaluates change in symptoms or diagnoses, and the development of resources around the goal-directed outcome. It is used every 6 months and is rated by the parent counsellor and the social pedagogue together. This outcome measure provides the major proportion of our outcome data. In addition, quality of care in general, as seen by the client, is evaluated at the beginning and the end of care by using a version of the Inventory of Life Quality in Children (ILK; Mattejat & Remschmidt, 2006) adapted for use within Vorarlberger Kinderdorf. At present we do not have empirical evidence from the client's perspective whether AMBIT has made any change, although we can see from the EVAS and other outcome measures that cases have mostly developed positively for the young people. However, we cannot yet make an empirical conclusion on the impact of AMBIT. What we do have, however, is verbal feedback from the clients and our clinical impression of what changed in the handling of a case or within the family dynamics since we have been trained in AMBIT.

8.4.2 The stakeholders' perspective: implementation process evaluation

> After all these years, we finally speak the same language in the network!
> **(A social worker from Paedakoop)**

We have also done a formal evaluation of the implementation of AMBIT. A selection of 12 stakeholders in the organization took part, comprising all members of the top management team (three CEOs), the quality manager, the manager of Paedakoop, three team leaders, and four workers trained in AMBIT. Data were collected via an online survey consisting of open (qualitative) and closed (Likert-scale) questions. The survey questions covered knowledge about AMBIT and perceptions regarding the implementation strategies, observed changes, and expectations of where the process could lead to in the future.

Based on the results of the survey, the implementation was perceived as successful. Three important factors were related to this: first, the personality, conviction, and vision of the local facilitators (AMBIT trainers) and their ability to elicit curiosity;

second, that the model was applicable in daily work and addressed issues relevant to workers so that they felt understood in their own needs; and third, that the strategic planning and methods of communication played a vital role in the implementation process. The participants also rated specific aspects of change on a scale from 1 to 10, as far as they perceived the observable outcomes of the AMBIT implementation process; the results are shown in Figure 8.1.

The majority of the stakeholders perceived that AMBIT had positive effects on the quality of work with the clients, learning at work, and the quality of cooperation and communication both internally and externally. Furthermore, AMBIT had changed the personal professional stance of the stakeholders, as far as they described it. As an unexpected side effect, the interest of other institutions in the work and expertise of the organization was raised through AMBIT. What seems to have been underestimated by the stakeholders is the effect on leadership, which we would rate higher with regard to how AMBIT had influenced change. This might be due to the fact that the stakeholders were from different departments and hierarchies, and therefore leadership outcomes were not observable for all of them.

The evaluation set out to gather impressions of whether AMBIT effects can be observed by relevant people in the organization. The findings suggested that substantial changes had occurred with AMBIT. This now gave us permission to explore further how these changes had come about. We also realized that these findings were incredibly important for teams who were becoming interested in AMBIT training. It was not primarily the data or empirical evidence that was of importance to them; it was the conviction of our stakeholders, especially leaders and managers, that enabled them to trust that AMBIT can be useful to elicit change and better quality in client work.

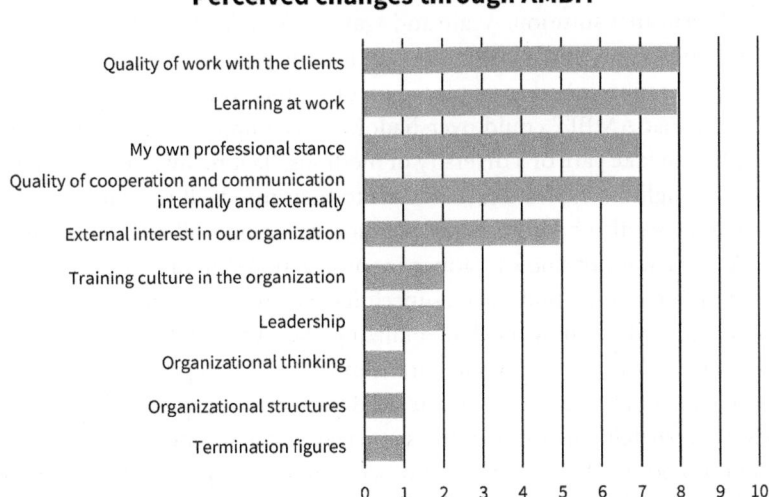

Figure 8.1 What changed through AMBIT, as perceived by relevant stakeholders.

8.4.3   What we learned about AMBIT implementation

8.4.3.1   Bumpy roads: what did not work so well

The most difficult part was the beginning, when we were introducing something new that we had not even fully grasped ourselves. We were trying to convince other people and trying out the techniques and tools while it was still bumpy and clumsy. Everything became much easier after a while, when we were much less engaged in inspiring people and more confident with mentalizing and AMBIT, when more colleagues had become familiar with it and the language and techniques were no longer so new. It would have been better if we had self-mentalized more often in front of the team, in the sense of 'We don't know how it will feel but we would like to try it out; maybe it seems awkward, but let's learn together'. We were faced with openness in most colleagues, but also resistance in others. We needed many supervision calls with the team in London to encourage us to mentalize our team, stay curious and humble, and take the team with us on our journey, step by step and patiently.

While we think our enthusiasm and inspiration were vital for the successful implementation, we know that we also sometimes got on the nerves of some of our colleagues. Our happiness to learn something new, our joint work, the travel to different locations to learn and spread AMBIT, and the joy we had in working together were inspiring but also sometimes elicited envy, provoked scepticism about our motives, and might have been hard to follow at times. 'Why do they get to have fun while we are doing the hard work?' was one of the feelings elicited in other teams, even though we were doing exactly the same hard work as them. Looking back, we would still be authentic with regard to our energy and excitement, but we would be more careful to keep a good balance between displaying our passion for AMBIT and at the same time showing restraint and humility.

Another bumpy road was respecting that AMBIT is just one approach among many others circling in an institution. Again and again, we were faced with leaders and managers who reminded us that AMBIT was not the only programme that was important, and that equal emphasis had to be placed on other methods. What we perceived was a certain fear that AMBIT could overshadow other important approaches and that managers had to take care of a diversity of methods. 'Is it really nothing that we have done so far?' might be a question that came to their minds. It was vital, therefore, to emphasize that we also had the same intention to support all relevant programmes and that AMBIT was not a new treatment approach that should replace existing paradigms, but rather a stance that can be superimposed on any existing method.

What we realized was how much mentalizing played a vital role in AMBIT. We had understood what AMBIT was about, but the most important part and the heart of the whole model, mentalizing itself, was the hardest part to grasp. After our workshops, we found that participants were, in the same way, quick to understand the tools and model, but did not really have any idea of what mentalizing capacity is and how you actually do it. For this reason, we started to learn more about mentalization-based treatment (MBT), do additional training courses, read articles and watch videos on the different versions of MBT (e.g. MBT for families, or MBT for children and adolescents) to get a grasp of how you actually go about stopping non-mentalizing, noticing and naming positive mentalizing, or chairing a mentalization-based family meeting, and what non-mentalizing modes look like in clients and workers. As a consequence, we embedded other mentalizing techniques into our AMBIT workshops. This made a huge difference, for us as well as the participants, in terms of the competence they gained after the course.

8.4.3.2 The little and big successes: what worked

> There's a fire in my head, there's a fire in my chest/Can't you see it burning? It is never gonna rest. ('Riot', song by Steiner & Madlaina)

When we are asked by other teams, 'What are the basic ingredients for successful implementation; what do you recommend?', we come up with the following elements that we think are essential.

Start small, dream big—have strategic plans and a guiding vision

1. Don't make overambitious plans. Have a vision, but start small. Start with yourself, slowly influence others, and let curiosity do its thing.
2. Don't expect everyone to be excited about AMBIT. Be kind and patient. There will be some who are immediately interested, while others might be sceptical or even resistant. Accept this, stay curious about their reservations, and tell them it is OK if they cannot see any advantages in AMBIT right now.
3. Go on doing it yourself, trying things out, and invite them to watch the effects and develop a stance about AMBIT. It might take a week for some, 2 years for others, and some might never come be convinced that AMBIT can be useful. That is OK. Trust in the other multiplicators. Maybe they won't be convinced by it from you, but they might be impressed if they watch someone else using AMBIT techniques.
4. It is equally important to have a vision—'What do we want to have in the end?'— and never let go of this idea, even if it is vague. As a team of local facilitators, we find it vital to always make strategic plans—for the near future, the next steps, and for the longer-term future.

One step forward, one step back
AMBIT implementation is not a linear process. As we speak of 'comparing waymarks', broadcasting intentions, and sensitive attunement in the work with our clients, we also need to always check where we are in the process, adapt, change plans, listen to feedback, and see where we are and what we might have to change.

Choose the right people

Don't just send any worker to the training. We consider it vital—as shown in our evaluation—that careful thought is put into the wise choice of local facilitators. Who has epistemic trust from the workers and management? Who is already influential in the organization in a positive way? It also seemed very helpful for at least one of the trainers to be a team leader or, even better, a manager. The hierarchical power makes it much easier for decisions to implement elements from AMBIT to make it through. It also seemed helpful if the selected people already had a positive experience of working with each other.

Enthusiasm, humour, and curiosity

When we got to know different teams who work with AMBIT and MBT, we found that they seemed to have a natural liveliness, a bit of fun, a light-heartedness and creative energy, and they gave the impression that they were happily experimenting with AMBIT and having fun in succeeding, as well as failing and trying again. These were the teams who served as role models for us, who we wanted to learn from. So, although AMBIT is a serious matter, it can settle down in a playful manner. Like a dance or play on stage looks like simple joy, but behind the scenes requires training, patience, and ... practice, practice, and practice.

Don't forget the purpose

When implementing a new approach or programme, it is important to always remind oneself and others of the purpose and intention—that is, why we consider it vital or helpful to our clients. AMBIT carries the risk that it might be seen just as a model that simply serves to enhance team functioning. The purpose behind it, however, is to help clients to be better able to adapt to their life, to improve family functioning, and to enable access to education. Therefore, considering the complex nature of our clients' problems, we need well-connected teams, high-quality risk support, and a flexible learning culture. These are the reasons why we think AMBIT is helpful.

Communication and involvement

While in the beginning it will be the local facilitators who push AMBIT forward in the institution, it is important after a while to let others play a role in the process. Establish the individuals who show interest in AMBIT and its development. Encourage their attempts to implement it in their cases and to tell colleagues about what they are doing. We were helped by having an AMBIT Development Group that included those who showed ambition to design an adapted version of AMBIT for their team or institution. We not only wanted to educate and engage them in AMBIT, we wanted to co-design it with our colleagues and finally reach a level of co-production (in line with the model of Arnstein, 1969).

8.5 Where are we now?

Of course, we sometimes fail. We still have competition, conflicts, shaming, and blaming. We are human beings. We come from different backgrounds and professions. We are emotional when it comes to our emotional work. But, first, these conflicts occur much less than they used to, and blaming has almost vanished from team meetings. Second, what has changed immensely is how we handle these situations, and how willing we are to talk about them and solve conflicts without causing damage to individuals and teams. What has changed is the amount of space and energy that was absorbed by such conflicts. Today, they are mostly solved without leader involvement, directly and easily. We see great differences in the general stance that multiprofessional colleagues encounter, and we observe the curiosity and respect that we generally show for each other. Cooperation is not a structural thing any more; it is a lively organism, which is developing and thriving.

AMBIT has improved our leadership skills. Recently, we had a huge restructuring of our residential and outreach care, which meant that some of our colleagues moved into different teams. We noticed that AMBIT-influenced leaders showed a very thoughtful approach to handling this situation. They hadn't just taken in the new people into their team. They had done Active Planning, mentalized the needs of the new colleagues as well as the existing team, invited the new workers to the team, shared their own thoughts and feelings, and asked the team to share their 'team mind'; they had also invited the new colleagues to self-mentalize who they are, what they need, and how the leader and the new team could help them. We could see that mentalizing had played a vital role in their planning and the steps they took.

AMBIT is not magic; it cannot solve the problems we face and make life easy. However, it can improve our multiprofessional cooperation, help empower our clients, and enable them to adapt to life, and it simply helps us to do better work with each other, not against each other, and for the clients.

8.6 Looking back: the AMBIT implementation wheel

We have had many different experiences in the past 4 years and now we are surprised by how many of the suggestions, approaches, content, theories, methods, and tools from AMBIT we have been able to implement in our team and our organization. 'Life can only be understood backwards; but it must be lived forwards': this quote is attributed to Søren Kierkegaard. We feel the same way with the implementation of AMBIT. Today we try to understand what we did, how we acted, and what happened. So, what can be said about the implementation of AMBIT in general? To cut a long story short, we basically applied AMBIT to the implementation of AMBIT. Analogous to the AMBIT wheel, we have developed an *AMBIT implementation wheel*, which is intended to summarize and illustrate which segments the implementation of AMBIT is dedicated to and what challenges the implementation will face (Figure 8.2). We hope this may be a useful tool for others involved in the implementation process.

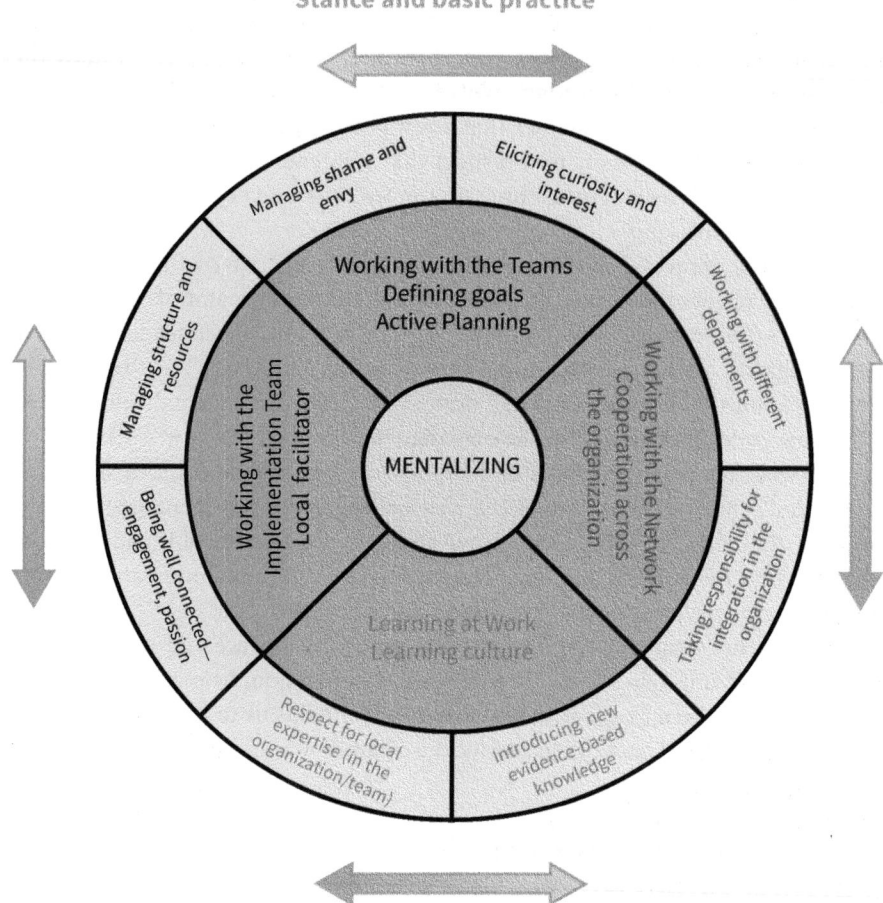

Figure 8.2 The AMBIT implementation wheel: holding the balance between conflicting interests.

8.6.1 Core element: mentalizing

As in AMBIT, mentalizing is also at the core of the implementation processes. Taking a mentalizing attitude towards all the people relevant in an implementation process, from team to management, at the same time recognizing and avoiding non-mentalizing processes, appears to us, in retrospect, to be of the greatest importance.

8.6.2 Working with the Implementation Team (local facilitators)

The responsibility for the implementation should be carried by an implementation team. This team will need to balance being well connected through shared enthusiasm with also ensuring that it is supported by good management of its own structure and resources. The enthusiasm will disappear if the structures and resources are missing, so it is important to involve the management of the organization from the start. As implementation takes time and interests might vary or change, the facilitators are required to repeatedly reflect on their cooperation and work towards a shared goal.

8.6.3 Working with the Teams (defining goals, Active Planning)

The implementation of AMBIT will inevitably involve working with teams. The first step is to arouse curiosity and interest. Often this is best evoked by sharing with colleagues what experiences you have personally had with AMBIT. You have to be prepared for negative feedback, as competition, professional shame, and envy are omnipresent in human cooperation. Communicating your intentions very transparently is an effective way to reduce these dis-integrative forces and arouse curiosity.

8.6.4 Working with the Network (cooperation across the organization)

Teams are often part of departments and these in turn are part of an overall organization. Each professional team has its own story and culture. In working with the network, the implementation needs to balance working with different departments and taking responsibility for wider integration in the organization. This involves respecting different interests and boundaries.

8.6.5 Learning at Work (learning culture)

Creating a culture of active learning in an organization and in teams is a particularly challenging task. It requires a similar emphasis on learning and talking about our work and cooperation as we already use in the client work itself. On the one hand, it is about respecting, maintaining, cultivating, and sharing all the knowledge and experiences that workers have acquired in an organization. On the other hand, it is about strengthening a culture that is open to seeking and integrating new knowledge. The same goes for the implementation itself: there is a need to frequently rest and reflect on what has been learned and what has to be adapted to the local situation, and how this can be integrated into the further Active Planning of the implementation process.

8.7 Implications

In its beginnings, AMBIT was designed as a mentalizing approach to community outreach work. It particularly focused on the potential isolation of workers and the problems of establishing helping relationships with clients who did not immediately see the value of what was being offered. In this chapter, Bea and Michael have illustrated how AMBIT can be applied to more complex service settings, which include residential, educational, and outreach services. Their positive and enthusiastic observations and experience of the utility of AMBIT in this setting are consistent with other chapters of this book, in that the core of the AMBIT approach is not confined to any specific service context but is defined by its relational and mentalizing principles applied to complex processes of help. When we started thinking about AMBIT, a decade ago, we did not know this. We thought that we were working out a specific treatment approach to a specific service context.

We are hugely indebted to the authors for the insights and observations that they have brought in helping us change our point of reference. They have demonstrated a real attention to the state of mind of both young people and workers, and recognize the individuality in the helping process in terms of what different clients and families need. This helps the workers with their work, this being the primary source of stress and therefore the thing to focus on. The best approach is to treat not just the symptoms of their stress but the source, in varied and layered ways. As the authors comment, this can be easily missed in the ways organizations approach supporting their workers' well-being.

References

Arnstein, S. R. (1969). A ladder of citizen participation. *Journal of the American Institute of Planners, 35*(4), 216–224. https://doi.org/10.1080/01944366908977225

Bevington, D., Fuggle, P., Cracknell, L., & Fonagy, P. (2017). Working with your team. In *Adaptive mentalization-based integrative treatment: A guide for teams to develop systems of care* (pp. 170–209). Oxford University Press.

Figley, C. R. (1995). Compassion fatigue: Toward a new understanding of the costs of caring. In B. H. Stamm (Ed.), *Secondary traumatic stress: Self-care issues for clinicians, researchers, and educators* (pp. 3–28). Sidran Press.

Johnstone, K. (1987). *Impro: Improvisation and the theatre.* Routledge/Theatre Arts Books.

Mattejat, F., & Remschmidt, H. (2006). *Das Inventar zur Erfassung der Lebensqualität bei Kindern und Jugendlichen (ILK) [The inventory of life quality in children and adolescents (ILC)].* Huber.

Schober, C., & Wögerbauer, J. (2020). *Studie zur Entwicklung der Betreuungskomplexität von Kindern und Jugendlichen.* Kompetenzzentrum für Nonprofit-Organisationen und Social Entrepreneurship, Wirtschafts Universität Wien. https://www.wu.ac.at/fileadmin/wu/d/cc/npocompetence/09_NPO_Abgeschlossene_Projekte/NPO___SE_Kompetenzzentrum_Forschungsbericht_Entwicklung_der_Betreuungskomplexit%C3%A4t_von_Kindern_und_Jugendlichen_Langversion.pdf

Tham, P. (2006). Why are they leaving? Factors affecting intention to leave among social workers in child welfare. *British Journal of Social Work, 37*(7), 1225–1246. https://doi.org/10.1093/bjsw/bcl054

Wolpert, M., Harris, R., Hodges, S., Fuggle, P., James, R., Wiener, A., McKenna, C., Law, D., York, A., Jones, M., Fonagy, P., Fleming, I., & Munk, S. (2019). *THRIVE framework for system change.* CAMHS Press. http://implementingthrive.org/wp-content/uploads/2019/03/THRIVE-Framework-for-system-change-2019.pdf

9
Creating and supporting a Team around the Worker

Laura Talbot

9.1 Setting the scene

In Chapter 1, we emphasized that AMBIT was designed to work with clients with multiple needs who often have multiple workers and have to deal with many systems all at once. By this stage of the book, these are now familiar themes: that the multiplicity of workers often adds to the difficulties the family or client may be experiencing. The involvement of multiple agencies and teams is not only a problem for the client but creates difficulties for the frontline workers in all agencies with regard to how best to link up with other forms of support, or at least not inadvertently undermine the work of other agencies. We do not believe that there are simple solutions to these problems, but AMBIT has proposed one method for trying to address this, which is called creating a *Team around the Worker*.

When this idea was first developed, we had no idea what major challenges it would present to implement. So, this chapter will look at this in two ways. In the first part, following our deployment-focused approach (see Chapter 1), the chapter will focus on what the AMBIT programme has learned from the experience of training practitioners in the 'Team around the Worker' idea. We have learned a lot in terms of the changes of attitude and behaviour needed for practitioners, and the barriers that may arise in trying to implement this approach. In the second part, the chapter will describe a specific service example where this aspect of AMBIT has been successfully placed at the centre of the service design. This involves an edge-of-care team called the Adolescent Multi-Agency Support Service (AMASS), which adopted the principle of the Team around the Worker as axiomatic to their whole approach. This team has been in operation for over 10 years and is presented as a good example of how the idea works in practice.

9.2 Introduction

The Team around the Worker is one of the aspects of the AMBIT approach that often captures the interest of teams during training. It can be an idea that makes a lot of sense to workers but generates a number of questions and feelings about how it might actually look and work in practice. We see some great examples of teams implementing the idea of Team around the Worker in their work. For some, this has required what has felt like quite radical adjustments to their working methods; for others, it has affirmed and clarified the rationale for existing ways of working. We discovered that we needed to attend more closely to the experience of workers and teams who were considering the idea of a Team around the Worker. Mentalizing some of the ambivalence that can be experienced by workers has enabled us to better understand complex aspects of multiagency working. We are aware that what seemed simple in theory has proved to be not so in practice, but the potential benefits of this approach seem to us to remain substantial. Our hope is that by the end of this chapter the reader will feel clearer about the radical nature of this idea and encouraged by some of the benefits that implementing it could bring for both clients and workers.

9.3 What is a Team around the Worker?

In Chapter 1, we described traditional approaches to multiagency work, where a client with a number of needs usually has direct contact with professionals from different teams, each offering help with a specific need. This is commonly known as a 'Team around the Child' (or a 'Team around the Client' in adult services). When clients are able to manage the task of forming relationships with multiple workers and are actively help-seeking (i.e. they share ideas with the workers about what their problems are and how they might be best addressed), this arrangement can be experienced as helpful by clients and can be effective in creating change. When this works less well, these networks around the client can increase in size and complexity as more professionals are brought in to address areas of need that are not being met. This may result in the client being faced with a myriad of helping relationships and approaches, where it is not clear whether any of the workers in the network have a real working relationship with the client. In these congested networks, workers can struggle, finding themselves unable to sufficiently engage the client in the piece of work they have been referred to them for, or feeling that they are duplicating another worker's current or previous efforts.

The AMBIT principle of a Team around the Worker is designed to address some of these difficulties by suggesting that helping efforts might be more successful if we consider two issues, namely (a) that we apply principles of epistemic trust and (b) that we aim to reduce the complexity of helping relationships for the client. This approach requires workers to reflect on where epistemic trust (see Chapter 3) might already exist within the relationships around the client or, better still, might involve asking the client 'Who do you already trust?' to help decide who might be best placed to contribute to the work. Similarly, it may be valuable to ask whether it may be possible to delegate some roles to those who know the client best, to reduce the demands of workers on the client. In practice, applying these principles results in many different ways of creating a working network for both workers and clients alike, which depends on the specifics of the case, the opportunities for involving trusted others, the views of the client, and the demands of case coordination (i.e. where there are greater risks, the requirements for tighter case coordination may be greater). There is no single set of arrangements that applies in all cases for how to apply the idea of a Team around the Worker. The key principle is that attention is given to the quality of the helping relationships, the role of trust, and the wish to avoid duplication and repetition across different teams.

In AMBIT terms, a person with a high degree of trust may be called the 'keyworker', referring to the fact that this worker is 'key' to the client because the client trusts them. Often, this keyworker will work very closely with a worker from a core agency, such as social care or mental health services. This idea is distinct from the role of 'keyworker' that is sometimes assigned to a worker by the professional system to take on a specific set of responsibilities and tasks in relation to the client. For example, a parent may say that their daughter gets on best with her football coach, who she has known since childhood and really respects. Despite all her problems at school, she always goes to football training. For the football coach, the idea of being a keyworker to a young person may be a very long way from how they see their role as a sports coach. But this idea of a keyworker is not like a case coordinator. This person may well not have a role in coordinating others, but they are *key* because they open up the possibility of the client developing other trusting helping relationships. How this may happen is the focus of this chapter.

In our experience, being guided by those whom the client trusts represents a radically different way of identifying who is important to include within a helping network, a process that is usually dominated by system-driven decisions about which team or worker(s) and professional expertise most closely aligns with the perceived solutions to the client's presenting needs. If you place the need for trust in the helping process at the centre of the work, then status and professional background may have a more limited role in the early stages of establishing help. Once trust is more established, it is 'infectious' and others can be perceived as becoming trustworthy too.

Given that clients with multiple needs often require help in multiple domains, the expectation that one keyworker (e.g. a football coach) will be able to meet their needs on their own is unrealistic. To offer a comprehensive form of help to the client, this trusted adult will need to be part of a team of workers who have other specialisms and skills relevant to the client's situation. In addition, given what we know about the emotional impact of work of this nature, particularly on those whose position or relationship brings them closest to the client's experiences and circumstances, the keyworker is also likely to be vulnerable to experiencing fluctuations in their capacity to mentalize, which may compromise their ability to sustain an effective helping response. Therefore, a proactive and responsive network is needed to enable the keyworker to be supported by others to strengthen their own helping capacity (i.e. managing dilemmas and restoring their mentalizing) and to ensure, as much as possible, that the right forms of help are available to meet the client's needs. This may take the form of other workers offering their input indirectly through the keyworker by providing expert knowledge outside the keyworker's specialism. We will provide a detailed example of how this approach might look later in the chapter.

9.4   Learning from training about what supports a Team around the Worker

In the following section, we will set out what we have learned from trying to support teams to understand and implement the principle of the Team around the Worker and what this has required us to change in our approach. We have come to see that we have perhaps not been following one of our own principles when thinking about this particular aspect of practice change, which is to attend first to the worker's state of mind. On reflection, our efforts to explain, and train teams in, the Team around the Worker idea perhaps initially focused too heavily on the experience of the client, because we (implicitly) assumed that describing the benefits that clients might feel from these arrangements would be sufficient to promote uptake of the ideas into practice. In mentalizing terms, we had not adequately held the balance between the perspective of the client and the perspective of the worker when thinking about how to support these ideas to best make sense and connect with the workforce. As is so often the case in AMBIT, paying attention to the worker's state of mind first has been key for us, and we will move on to describe both what we have learned from this and how we have adapted our approach in response.

9.4.1   Mentalizing the worker: 'This Team around the Worker thing seems like a good idea, so why don't I want to do it?'

Those familiar with the motivational interviewing literature (Miller & Rollnick, 2012) will recognize the above question as being characteristic of the state of ambivalence: the experience of having contradictory thoughts or feelings about something or, as some describe it, of 'being in two minds'. We have increasingly recognized that this is a helpful idea to hold on to when beginning to make sense of what might be going on in the minds of workers in relation to first hearing about the idea of Team around the Worker.

During training, we tend to find that, when the idea is first described to them, workers can immediately see some benefits for clients of Team around the Worker arrangements. The notion of clients being supported (in the first instance) by those who they trust, rather than being expected to form and sustain relationships with lots of people, is often met with interest. However, after this initial enthusiasm, we have noticed that workers' minds begin to turn quite quickly to the question of exactly how this might all look and work in practice. More specifically, they start to imagine what it might be like to be a worker enacting these arrangements (either as the worker with the trusted relationship or as a worker in the team around them), and a different set of thoughts and feelings arises. Box 9.1 summarizes some of the responses that have commonly been expressed during training.

Box 9.1 Some initial responses to the Team around the Worker idea

Worries/concerns

- If I'm the keyworker, I'm going to be expected to do all the work, and I've already got too much to do. I'll be asked to solve problems that I don't have expertise in.
- If I'm the keyworker, I'm just going to get left to do all the work—people say that they will support me, but they are not actually going to do it when it comes down to it.
- I don't really want to start asking other people for help with my work—they are going to think that I'm not cut out for the job. I might get negatively judged by my colleagues or my manager.
- I'm going to lose my professional identity if I start doing things that are outside my training or that don't make use of all the professional study and training that I've done.
- If I share my skills with others, by working through them, it might mean that my role or skillset won't be needed any more because I'll have given all my knowledge away.
- I'm not the kind of person who needs help with their work—I can usually deal with most things on my own.
- I don't really like the idea of doing joint work with people from other teams—it will feel as if all my skills are on public display!
- I'm not that keen on having other professionals in my sessions—they might get in the way of me being able to do what I need to do.
- I'm not senior enough to support another worker with their work—people won't take me seriously, especially if they are more experienced or highly paid than me.
- I'm not sure I want to support another worker to do what I do—I'm not convinced that someone without my training can really do the tasks I'm trained to do properly or safely (e.g. a non-mental health professional helping a client with their mental health).
- If I start trying to bridge other workers into my relationship with the client, it could ruin our relationship—my client won't be happy that I'm mixing in with certain professionals, because they don't like that group of professionals.
- I don't want to step back from trying to work directly with the client—other workers won't share information properly with me about what is happening, and it might become unsafe.

System barriers

- If I'm helping indirectly through another worker, how is that work going to be reflected in my caseload? Does it count as an open case, even if I'm not seeing them? If it's an open case, I have to have face-to-face contact with them.
- I'm not allowed to offer consultation in my role, only face-to-face work.
- Our team only gets paid to see people face to face.
- In my role, I have formal/statutory responsibilities for particular types of need (e.g. a psychiatrist and medication; a social worker and child protection; a probation officer and a court order). I have to see the client directly; I can't work through another worker.
- There's no point in only our team working in this way—how are we going to get other people in other teams to work like this when they've not had this training?

The workers' responses seem to us to be a very legitimate mix of worries about some of the (imagined) implications that this change in practice might result in, and some of the anticipated or actual system barriers to working in this way. These responses make sense and are often a genuine reflection of the anxiety that can arise about how these ideas might work in practice. As one social worker asked in a training session, 'Are you suggesting that monitoring safeguarding may be delegated to an untrained professional? If this went wrong, it would be me who was sacked, not the keyworker'. These anxieties may be amplified and feel more insurmountable when only one team in an area signs up for AMBIT training. In such situations, workers frequently express feeling unsure about whether they have the authority and/or confidence to influence the practice of colleagues from different agencies: it feels to them to be outside their 'ambit' (i.e. their sphere of influence).

We have found it helpful to allow more space for workers to share the thoughts and feelings that arise when they first hear about these ideas and offer validation around these, as well as broadcasting our hopes that by the end of the training we might arrive at a place where they feel clearer about whether and how these ideas might fit best for them. It has also been helpful for the trainers to share any observations they might have about what is happening to the group's mentalizing capacity as they consider these ideas, in terms of highlighting mentalizing (e.g. people showing curiosity or playing with ideas) and terminating non-mentalizing in a supportive manner (e.g. drawing people's attention to where dialogue might have become characterized by certainty about what will and will not work) to help the group think together as productively as possible about this.

We have also come to realize that illustrating the Team around the Worker idea through a diagram (as in Figure 2.7 in Chapter 2) may have led to it being interpreted as a particular fixed, structural configuration of a network, whereas in reality there are a multitude of ways of enacting it. While it can mean a team (or network) making

---

Box 9.2 Examples of Team around the Worker implementation

- Using the AMBIT programme with clients during the engagement phase to understand more about who they already trust (i.e. the person who is the keyworker).
- Asking the keyworker for their ideas on being introduced to the client and their tips on how to best do this (if you are a new professional in the network).
- Asking the keyworker to attend sessions with the client if they need to be seen by workers who they don't yet trust.
- Talking positively about other workers in your sessions with the client in order to help build their trust in others.
- Offering to include other workers in your sessions with the client if you are the keyworker, to help scaffold their relationships with others.
- If the client has a need that could be met by your role/team but does not want to meet directly with you, thinking with the keyworker about how they could support the client to consider this.
- Offering help to the keyworker via a regular check-in or being open to being contacted by them to see how their work is going with the client.
- Thinking strategically about the mix of workers and methods in a team, to ensure that the team's approach maximizes opportunities for building epistemic trust (e.g. some ability to work flexibly on an outreach basis).

---

some structural changes to how it organizes help around a client, it can equally mean holding the *principle* of a Team around the Worker actively in mind during casework and recognizing situations in which it might be helpful to make use of it. Box 9.2 contains some examples of what this might look like; this will be further illustrated through the extended case study provided later in this chapter.

9.4.2 Trying it out: the importance of helping processes for the Team around the Worker

As well as helping teams get to grips with the idea of the Team around the Worker (the 'what' and the 'why'), we have increasingly recognized that we need to address some of the processes on which it rests, namely the challenge of help-seeking and help-offering between workers (the 'how') across agencies. Workers have described finding it hard to imagine how they might ask each other for help with their work (since this usually happens only by a process of client referral) and, relatedly, how to support each other to mentalize. Both of these dilemmas pose a challenge to the successful enactment of a Team around the Worker, but their resolution is crucial for supporting effective mentalizing in the keyworker and getting the right mix of help for the client. There can be several challenges to overcome. Being the giver rather than the receiver of help may be a core part of the identity (perhaps both professionally and personally) of those who work in helping professions, meaning that it is hard to reverse these roles. There may also be some hesitation around offering help to colleagues outside of supervisory structures; for example, how would it be to offer help to a colleague whose mentalizing appears to have gone offline? Will this help be received in the spirit in which it was intended? Will it be perceived as a criticism or generate shame, or will it simply feel like extra work for which there is no time? Exercises in training that focus on extending the idea of help-seeking in teams to thinking about how these processes might look across networks have been important in this, as has creating opportunities for discussions in mixed groups across teams in which examples can be shared of times where practice consistent with the idea of a Team around the Worker has already been possible locally. These are often useful starting points that can help with generating more ideas about how these approaches can be further embedded through the team's and network's implementation plan.

So, in starting with what seemed to us to be a simple principle of putting trust at the centre of the helping endeavour, so as to support engagement and reduce the number of helpers directly involved with the client, we inadvertently opened up huge challenges for teams and further exposed patterns of relating between teams in which mutual trust and help-seeking were not prominent. We have come to see how common it is for teams to connect with and relate to each other primarily through referral methods that can often generate feelings of resentment, distrust, and suspicion between adjacent teams. When we started developing AMBIT we were not aware of how strong these emotions can be or that there can be such a stark absence of trust between neighbouring teams of well-intentioned and highly competent professionals. Because AMBIT always evolves in dialogue with teams, in response to recognizing the extent to which we have underestimated the anxieties and conflicts that the idea of the Team around the Worker may provoke, we have adapted our stance in the ways that we have described above. We want to move on now to balance our recognition of these challenges by sharing how this key AMBIT principle can be effectively implemented in practice.

9.5 The Team around the Worker: a case example of AMASS in London

9.5.1 Building Team around the Worker into the service design

The AMASS was set up over 10 years ago as a multiagency team to support allocated social workers in addressing edge-of-care concerns. Based in a London local authority's children's social care department, AMASS has been jointly managed by a social care manager and an NHS-employed clinical psychologist. The team was set up to include a range of professionals, including two specialist social workers, a teacher, an assistant psychologist, and a sessional outreach worker. A parental mental health worker and an adult employment worker also offer sessional input to the team. The team was intentionally set up not to take referrals of young people and families, but to be a team that responds to a social worker's request for help with a family where there are edge-of-care concerns. In response to a request for help, the AMASS team forms a *team around the allocated social worker* and jointly undertakes the intervention work required with the young person and their family. The key point here is that the social worker is not referring the *family* to the AMASS team but is in effect referring *themselves* to the team to request help with their work.

In terms of how this looks in practice, not all of the workers in the team are directly involved with the family. The social worker and AMASS senior social worker join together to work with the parent(s), and the young person is offered the support of the assistant psychologist, outreach worker, or teacher, depending on how they might view their primary need (although this person's role might initially involve connecting up with another worker outside the team who is already trusted by the young person, as we will go on to explain). The other workers in the team are then brought into these relationships according to need as help-seeking develops. Throughout, the social worker is supported to develop or maintain their relationship with the young person to continue to uphold their statutory responsibilities.

This deliberate and explicit decision to build a Team around the Worker into the service design was made for several reasons. First, in contexts of such significant safeguarding concerns, it is crucial that the allocated social worker remains central to any work being undertaken with a family because they need to be able to continuously assess and address risk. Second, it is often the case in edge-of-care contexts that it is difficult to develop and maintain an effective working relationship between the social worker and the family, because the social worker and family often may be increasingly conflicted about the preferred course of action. Either the family wishes to relinquish the care of the young person to the local authority, which in turn is resisting this move because it believes that more interventions need to be tried first, or the local authority wishes to instigate legal proceedings to seek alternative care for the young person, against the family's wishes, due to significant safeguarding concerns that the family has not been able to sufficiently address. This is understandably very stressful for both the family and the social worker, which creates a very difficult context for mentalizing and the development of a trusting, collaborative, and purposeful relationship. Third, the risk of a young person coming into care is usually driven by a complex interplay of multiple risk factors (both acute and chronic) across the young person, family, school, peer, and neighbourhood systems, which are inherently connected and will benefit from being addressed by an intervention that can target the range of issues in a way that makes sense of and takes into account how these issues influence each other. As we have said repeatedly throughout this book, it is unrealistic for any worker to deliver such a set of interventions singlehandedly, but the usual alternative here is for the social worker to enlist or coordinate this help from multiple outside services to ensure that the range of needs is met. However, this approach can present additional problems. The family may not feel ready, willing, or able to make use of this increasing number of forms of help, and the social worker may be experiencing a high burden from trying to coordinate and maintain communication with a busy network, which is likely also to be characterized by significant levels of dis-integration.

To illustrate how such an approach might look in practice, we are going to return to the story of Alice and Lucas that we described in Chapter 1. We will use this imagined case to illustrate the different parts of the AMASS intervention, which connect to multiple cases seen by this team. Since Chapter 1, the situation for Alice and Lucas has deteriorated. After multiple failed attempts to establish regular attendance and improved behaviour at school, Lucas has been permanently excluded from his school and is now receiving some level of home tuition, but he does not cooperate with this. Alice is still on antidepressant medication but is not attending any therapy sessions and has begun drinking heavily. She has significant rent arrears. There have been major rows between Alice and Lucas, which have become physical and resulted in her threatening that he should go and live with his father, who is living in rented accommodation in another part of the city. His father does not agree with or support this idea and in any case is not deemed suitable due to his own current substance use difficulties. Alice has now decided that Lucas is beyond her control, that nothing is going to help with this, and that Lucas needs to 'go into care'. Lucas is staying up most nights playing on the computer and sleeping during the day, partly to avoid his mother and the demands of home tuition. Martha, his social worker, does not support the idea of placement in care but is struggling to make any positive impact on the family situation. Dominic, her manager, suggests that they ask AMASS for help.

9.5.2 Requesting help versus making a referral

The AMASS team recognizes that social workers, like most other professionals, are accustomed to getting help for families via a process of referral rather than by being joined by someone in their work, and that these are quite different processes. A referral is in effect a situation where someone (usually the client) is sent to a different place where a separate helping process will be set up. For families facing edge-of-care concerns, we have described some of the challenges to setting up an entirely separate helping process independent of the social worker at this stage of their difficulties. So, as an alternative to the client being directly referred to the AMASS team, the process of AMASS involvement is instead initiated by the social worker and their manager making a request to the AMASS team for help with their work.

Rather like the first meeting that might take place between a client and a worker, one of the AMASS managers then meets with the allocated social worker and their team manager for an eligibility meeting. The purpose of this meeting is to clarify what kind of help is wanted, whether AMASS is best placed to help, and to check for shared understanding about how this help might be provided. This includes the AMASS team manager broadcasting the intention that the team's approach has an equal emphasis on helping the social worker and helping the family; this means that the social worker commits (and is supported by their manager) to undertake the work jointly with members of the AMASS team and to attend a weekly 20-minute slot in the team's group supervision meeting. In general, this approach has become both familiar and acceptable to the social work teams over time, as illustrated by the following quote from a social worker:

> When I refer to AMASS, it's because I'm stuck and I'm not getting anywhere at all. I know from working with you before that you guys can get results and you know, the fact you have more people in your team and you have a combination of people in your team, when I think of families and what they need, they'd have that all in one bag and I think that's brilliant if you can offer all that to a family.

So, going back to our case example, Martha and Dominic met with Adeyemi (Yemi) from the AMASS team. Yemi's task was to make sure that there was a genuine risk of Lucas coming into care and therefore that supporting the social worker by offering an intensive, multicomponent intervention to the family would make sense. It was agreed that Lucas's father could not provide an alternative home and that the situation was deteriorating markedly, with Alice increasingly contacting Martha to express that she could no longer care for Lucas. Yemi recognized that Martha felt 'rubbish' about her work with this family, emphasized to her how stressful supporting this family appeared to be, and acknowledged the risk that it would be easy for the AMASS team to inadvertently add to this stress. Yemi discussed with Martha the team's aim to be helpful to her (as well as to Lucas and Alice) and that they would regularly ask for feedback from her as to whether this is what she experienced in practice. Martha left the meeting a little reassured by this but, not having worked with AMASS before, still felt confused by exactly how this might all look in reality and had some worries that this unknown team might negatively judge her previous helping efforts with the family.

9.5.3 Seeking the family's perspective on whether working with AMASS would be helpful

The next stage is for a 'sign-up meeting' between the parent(s), the allocated social worker, and a manager from the AMASS team to be set up, within which the family's views about receiving joint help from the social worker and AMASS can be sought. The AMASS manager and the social worker meet ahead of the sign-up meeting so that the AMASS manager can explain the format that the meeting usually takes. It begins with the social worker clearly broadcasting their intentions behind inviting AMASS to help them and the family. It is important that this is only a recap of their reasons for thinking that additional involvement might be helpful at this point, rather than this meeting being the first time these reasons are being shared. To hear information about the local authority considering care proceedings, or this being the first time that the family are told that their wish for their child to be taken into care is not going to be granted (particularly in the presence of an unknown worker), is likely to lead to significant distress and emotional arousal for the family, which does not provide a conducive context for thinking about embarking upon a new form of help. Sometimes, the eligibility meeting reveals that this conversation has not yet taken place with the family, and the social work team are tasked with completing this ahead of a sign-up meeting being scheduled.

Once the social worker has shared the reasons for AMASS involvement and checked with the client that this fits with their understanding of what has previously been discussed, the AMASS manager offers to explain more about what working together with AMASS involves so that they can discuss together whether it might fit for the family. As part of the preparation for the meeting, the AMASS manager would usually seek the social worker's guidance on how best to explain the service, in terms of whether there are any parts that might particularly appeal to the parent's state of mind (e.g. that there is a worker with a particular skillset in the team who might align with the parent's priorities; that the young person is also expected to attend meetings as well as the parent). In the spirit of transparency and enabling the family to make an informed choice, other key aspects of the service are highlighted: that it is a service designed for families where there is a teenager who is struggling at home, at school, and in the community, leading to there having been some serious discussions between the social worker and family about whether the young person could carry on living at home; that the service tries to help make it safe for families to stay living together, but that they also help to make the decision about whether this is possible; and that because things are so difficult, the help is offered very intensively (twice-weekly visits for the parents and one to two visits a week for the young person, with the possibility of joint sessions as things progress). The parent(s) are invited to share how well this fits the description of their circumstances and raise any initial thoughts or questions that they have about the involvement of this additional team of support around the social worker and the family. The parent(s) are then invited to take some time after the meeting to consider their decision, before feeding this back via the social worker. A 10-year service evaluation showed that 85% of families opt in to receiving the service when they are given this choice (Talbot et al., 2020), via this initial introductory process of a joint meeting with the social worker and the team.

In our example, Martha and Yemi arranged to meet with Alice for a joint meeting. Martha explained that she felt aware that her attempts to help Alice and Lucas were not helping Alice to feel able to continue caring for Lucas at home, which is something that she wanted to support Alice to be able to do, rather than looking for Lucas to be placed in care. Yemi briefly explained how AMASS worked and offered Alice the chance to share her thoughts. Alice shared her feelings of hopelessness and anger and that she wanted someone to take authority with Lucas so that he listened to them and did what they said. She was exhausted. She thought Martha had good intentions but that all that had happened had been a lot of talking and Lucas was still the same. Lucas knew about the visit that day but was in bed, probably asleep—a sign that he didn't care what happened next. Yemi explained that he would join the work with Martha and Alice, and that Lucas would have a worker from the team, too, unless he already had a worker who he already trusted, who the team would join up with and support. He explicitly broadcast to the family the AMASS way of working: that the team had people with different areas of expertise who helped each other to help the family. Yemi then got interested in what Alice made of all of this: were there any parts that she thought might be helpful to her current situation? Her choice in whether or not to take up the offer was emphasized. This method of the AMASS worker being introduced by the social worker and taking a collaborative approach to the meeting was the first step in the family seeing the social worker and the team working together in this way. Alice said her main worry was about Lucas going to school and not getting involved with local gangs. Both Martha and Yemi gave examples of ways that they might work together to help with these needs. Alice agreed to think about it, and Martha said she would call her in a couple of days to check in. Both Martha and Yemi left the meeting pleased that they had been able to cover all they had planned, but unsure how much Alice had really grasped of what they had discussed. Yemi shared that the sense of despair and depression was powerful and that he was able to get an immediate sense of what it might be like for Martha to work with this family. Martha acknowledged that she felt the same for much of the time in her contacts with Alice and felt validated by Yemi sharing that the meeting had had a similar impact on him. Feeling mentalized by Yemi in this way felt like a bit of a relief to Martha, and she began to feel more hopeful that involvement from AMASS might be helpful to her as well as to the family.

9.5.4 Supporting the development of helping processes between the social worker and the team

As we have described earlier in this chapter, the successful enactment of a Team around the Worker cannot be guaranteed by just making a structural change to how the helping relationships are organized within a network. As such, paying attention to the *relationship* between the allocated social worker and the AMASS team was key to the social worker experiencing the support of the team as helpful rather than as overbearing or as being there only because the social worker couldn't do the job well enough, akin to having extra supervision. It was critical to recognize that the AMASS team being experienced as helpful could not necessarily be taken for granted, and that this would need to be attended to in an ongoing manner throughout the process with the social worker and equally with the family.

It was important to consider how the AMASS team might develop a relationship with the social worker grounded in epistemic trust, so that the social worker would feel able to seek help from the team. In order to do this, the team aimed to develop a mentalized understanding of what it might be like to be the social worker in relation to the family they were seeking help with, and used this understanding to guide their approach to building a trusting relationship with the social worker. The AMASS social worker took some of the lead within the team of mentalizing the social worker's position, which was aided by many of the AMASS senior social workers having previously worked in the social care department and having had an experience of working alongside AMASS with one of the families on their caseload before joining the team.

This process included directly eliciting the social worker's perspective about their experience of working with the team, how they were thinking and feeling about their work with the family, and what they felt they most needed help with. As with clients, the AMASS worker would pay attention to how help-seeking the social worker appeared to be and would attune sensitively to this so that their efforts to get to know more about the social worker's state of mind were not experienced as intrusive, overwhelming, or shaming. Usually, the AMASS worker could draw on their own experience to normalize some parts of what the social worker might be experiencing (e.g. perhaps a sense of feeling relieved to have all these people in the AMASS team on hand to help, but confused about what they were all going to do; a bit unclear what their own role was going to look like; worried about being exposed in group supervision and whether the team would think 'What have you been doing all this time with this family?'). In establishing this shared understanding with the social worker, the AMASS worker could then think with the rest of the team about how best to refine their approach to support the development of this new working relationship. The team also often thought together about ways in which they could be affirming, strengths-focused, and validating in relation to the social worker's previous and current efforts and interactions with the family, to further support the development of trust and safety. In essence, as with work with families, there was no 'one size fits all' approach, but the important thing was that the relationship with the social worker was given this conscious attention and monitored and adapted accordingly. This approach intentionally parallels the approach that the AMASS workers would take in building a trusting relationship with the family, as getting into the position of being able to offer meaningful support to another worker through a Team around the Worker approach requires a similar relational context to be established.

Trust between the social worker and the AMASS team usually continued to evolve throughout the intervention in such a way that it supported the social worker feeling able to ask for and accept help from workers in the team. Sensitive attunement to the needs of the social worker was key throughout this process. The team thought carefully about how to make themselves readily available as helpers, without overwhelming the social worker, in recognition of the fact that their joint family was usually only one of many on the social worker's caseload. Being co-located helped to improve the ease with which the team and social worker could communicate about their work, and the team members were explicit about the social worker being welcome to come over to the team's desk area to speak to them at any time. The team would carefully consider and coordinate their efforts to communicate with the social worker throughout the week outside of the family visits and group supervision (i.e. what needed to be updated in person, or where an email with reference to an updated case record would be more helpful), to balance a reduction in some of the demands on the social worker with ensuring that they felt sufficiently involved and up to date with what was going on. While this is not to say that the balance was always achieved perfectly, it was reviewed often with the social worker, and general feedback from social workers about their experience of working with the AMASS team reflected an appreciation of the team's stance:

> If a crisis had come up, then I would try my best to pop over to AMASS to get some insight—or update them first—but also get some insight into why this may have happened or what steps to take next. I found that the most useful thing. They knew the family extremely well from their visits—to be honest, better than what I knew of the family sometimes, and so they were able to provide me with additional insight in order to help me to support the family during times of crisis.
>
> I still felt like the lead professional, which I think is important. I always felt like that throughout. I know recently there was a change in worker … but no matter who I was working with, I didn't feel undermined. I always felt they had a good working knowledge of the case and if I was wanting or needing support, I could ask for that.

Let us return to our example of how the relationship between Martha and the AMASS team developed in relation to their work together with Alice and Lucas. In the early weeks, Martha hated coming to the group supervision; this was a meeting that she had to attend for a 20-minute slot every week, in which the team would review the current week's work, explore any dilemmas arising, and then plan the visits and activities for the following week. She felt vulnerable and thought that some of the support was a bit patronizing, as she felt that some members of the team did not always acknowledge that she might have already tried the things they were suggesting. A change happened when the team were discussing how to support Lucas in getting out of his daytime sleeping routine, as Martha was not sure about the approach the team were suggesting and volunteered that she had already tried some of what was being suggested. This prompted Yemi to explicitly recognize that the team were beginning to run away with their own enthusiasm and ideas about what might work and were not paying enough attention to Martha's perspective in all this. He reminded the team that their task was to support and understand Martha's way of making sense of the family, as this was the basis of creating an effective team around her as the keyworker. Using 'Thinking Together', the group set itself the task of better understanding Martha's view of the relationship between Alice and Lucas with regard to the sleeping issue and what approaches had already been tried. This process yielded new understandings about the situation for the team and also led Martha to reflect that it might be worth trying again some of what had already been attempted, with the bolstering of the support of the team. At the end of this meeting, Martha felt validated and less wary of the group, and from that point she had increasing trust in the work of the team.

9.5.5　Building relationships with the young person using the Team around the Worker

Edge-of-care work is very difficult to carry out effectively without the perspective and inclusion of the young person who is considered at risk. However, it is also often very difficult to engage a young person in doing any work jointly with their family at a point where family relationships have broken down significantly. In mentalizing a young person's typical experience in such situations, they are usually feeling blamed for the problems their family is experiencing and are getting into trouble in other contexts (e.g. in school and the local community), so have often come to expect that any new adult will also see them as 'the problem' and repeat these experiences.

To tackle these dilemmas, the AMASS team ensured that discussions with the social worker included consideration of where epistemic trust already existed (if at all) within the network around the young person. This enabled planning between the team and social worker together from the outset about who the team and social worker might best join up with to build or strengthen the relationship with the young person to give the best chance of them wanting to engage in the AMASS work. Having the young person's perspective within this work was critical to its success. Often, there already appeared to be a more trusted person in the young person's life; this could be, for example, a member of the extended family, someone at a youth hub, a learning mentor, a mental health nurse, a youth offending worker, a gangs worker, a head of year at school, a careers advisor, or a substance use worker. In the team's experience, the person with whom the young person formed a trusting relationship was not predicted by professional background but by how much they felt understood by this person.

Enormous care was taken over the initial contacts between the AMASS team and the young person, to avoid old patterns of intrusive and non-collaborative helping processes being repeated. If there was a trusted person already on the scene, the team would seek this person's advice as soon as possible about how best they thought they could connect up with the young person about the work that they were going to be starting with the family, and to think about how they might want to be involved. Sometimes the trusted person might feel that the young person would be quite open to meeting someone from the team and would just give the AMASS worker tips about how best to go about it. On other occasions, they might suggest an initial meeting that included them as someone who could introduce the AMASS worker to the young person. Other times they might feel that getting the young person's agreement to meet someone from AMASS might take longer, in which case the team would ask for their help in brokering this by talking about AMASS to the young person, or sharing a note or message the team had written to help the young person understand more about them or seek the young person's ideas about something that could be fed back to the team via the trusted person. The focus of these initial contacts with the young person would always be to help the young person understand the work of the team, what they had been asked to do to support the young person, and to ask for their help to make sure they were helping in the best way. Sometimes the young person would be gradually able to build a relationship with someone in the AMASS team and work with them independently, but at other times the team invited the trusted person into the group supervisions for the duration of the work, to support them and to feed some of the work that the team hoped to undertake with the young person through this relationship.

After some discussions with the outreach worker from the AMASS team about how to approach this, Martha managed to get Lucas to agree that she could come into his room for 10 minutes one day and talk to him while he was in bed. Martha explained that she felt as if she was not being that helpful to Lucas and wanted to find out whether there was anyone he already knew who he might prefer to come and talk to him to help Martha get to know him. From under the covers, Lucas was able to help make a list of people he knew, and he selected those who he felt OK with. Two people stood out. He had always liked his paternal uncle, Matt, and he had stayed in contact with Matt after his parents' relationship had ended. Lucas also got on with one of the youth workers from the youth club near his flat, George, who had shared interests in a number of computer games and was 'not that serious'. Lucas agreed that Martha could speak to Matt to see whether he would be up for coming over to meet Lucas and Martha together. Although Matt was not enthusiastic about statutory services, he did care about Lucas and could see he needed help to get out of his current situation. He was surprised that Martha was asking for his advice, as this did not fit with his experience of how social workers operated when he was younger, but he agreed to come over when Martha was next due to visit Lucas. In this meeting, Lucas sat up in bed and, with Matt's help, they had a useful conversation about whether Lucas might be open to having a visit from George one day if Martha could arrange it. Even though Alice was sceptical about this working and worried about wasting George's time, she agreed to the suggestion as well, but agreed with Lucas that now was not the right time. Martha suggested that they could revisit this idea in a few weeks. This is the beginning of creating a team who might be able to work together to support Martha in what she is trying to achieve with Lucas and his family, composed of people who might also be present in Lucas's life beyond the involvement of AMASS and the social work department.

9.5.6 Bridging other professionals into relationships where epistemic trust already exists

As the 'keyworker' in a team working with a client and/or family, part of the task is to introduce the client to others who have expertise that could be useful for helping them with their life problems. This process needs to pay careful attention to the role of trust and is very different from the usual processes of 'making referrals'. It is more a process of showing the client that you (as the keyworker) trust the other person yourself, so the process has more of a flavour of a social introduction to an individual person rather than a message to an anonymous team. This may need to be a gradual process, as the client's/family's level of distrust and disappointment resulting from previous experiences (or from strongly held attitudes) may be very high.

As Martha's work with AMASS and the family progresses, they decide that it would be useful for Lucas and Alice to receive some advice about options for getting back into school. Martha is not knowledgeable about this area, so suggests to Alice that they could ask for help from the education worker in the AMASS team, Kelly, to begin thinking about this. Martha mentions this worker by name and talks about how she has been helpful to Martha for another young person in the past. Alice is not sure, but reluctantly agrees that Kelly can come to the next meeting, which Martha is able to arrange for the next day. However, while they are on their way to the visit the next morning, Alice texts Martha to cancel, following an argument with Lucas, although Martha and Kelly suspect that Alice might also have been feeling wary about the appointment. Because the education worker is part of the AMASS team and has knowledge of the work with the family, the cancellation was not entirely a surprise to her, but it also means that there is not any pressure for the family to engage with her immediately; she is not going anywhere! Instead, Kelly is able to support Martha to think about how her involvement might happen in a meaningful way, at a pace that suits the family. Kelly suggests to Martha that rather than pushing Alice to reschedule, she takes some time to explore Alice's thoughts and feelings about meeting her in more detail in their next meeting. She gives Martha some information about different educational options that she can share with Alice instead and says that Martha can always call her from the meeting if needed. When Martha shows Alice the leaflets, she has a question, which Alice agrees she can call Kelly about; they do this with Martha's phone on speakerphone, so they can all hear the conversation. A few weeks later, a conversation comes up in which Alice expresses some worries about Lucas's future. Martha again suggests calling Kelly for help, in front of Alice. Martha models help-seeking, showing vulnerability and respect to Kelly for the advice she gets. Afterwards, Alice agrees to meet Kelly to talk further, as long as Martha is there too. Alice also insists that Lucas has to come to the meeting too. Martha really welcomes Alice's suggestion that Lucas comes too and enlists the help of Lucas's uncle Matt in supporting this to happen.

The above example illustrates several important aspects of the Team around the Worker. First, it shows how helpful it can be for workers to be able to approach their involvement through a more relational process, rather than through traditional referral routes, which are not usually contingent on the windows of opportunity that might open (and close just as quickly) in the client's help-seeking. The education worker could work flexibly with Martha in a way that both she and Alice might experience as being attuned to their state of mind about receiving her help. This sequence illustrates what we mean by attending to the place of trust in the process of enabling Alice and Lucas to access additional help. The process also rests on Martha mentalizing Alice, with respect to monitoring what is wanted and needed and being proactive in mobilizing the network in response to this. With Alice's increasing trust in Martha, this process is facilitated by Martha modelling help-seeking in reaching out to Kelly for her help. Alice sees Martha take a vulnerable position by asking for help, which we could understand as giving her permission to do the same, and this is facilitated because some of the trust that Martha shows in Kelly has generalized to Alice. In this process, Martha is drawing on the support of the team of workers around her to support the creation of a team of workers around Alice who she is more able to trust and thus benefit from their specialist areas of expertise.

Another process of creating a Team around the Worker can be the value of reconnecting a client or family with someone who had offered help previously. In this example, we return to thinking about Lucas's relationship with George the youth worker, who Martha had discovered was previously helpful to him. About 6 months previously, Lucas had been referred to the youth service and had had some sessions with George, but this had been for only a brief intervention before George had been signed off sick from work, after which Lucas did not return. As a result of Alice's sessions with Kelly, they have been thinking about ways in which Lucas could get some practice leaving the house to go and do something, before he returns to school. As part of this, Alice and Lucas agree to Martha arranging for George to join her for a visit to see whether Lucas would like to come back to the youth club. Martha and George had some preparatory conversations before the visit to mentalize how Lucas might be feeling about reconnecting with George. They thought that it would be important to recognize that Lucas may have been disappointed when his sessions with George stopped suddenly and that he might find it helpful to know that George had still been thinking about him and wondered about how Lucas was getting on now. They hoped that it might help Alice and Lucas to see that George was still interested in how Lucas was getting on and that he could share positive memories of his previous contact and maybe encourage Lucas to meet up with some of the other young people at the youth club. We acknowledge that this sort of transparent dialogue and time dedicated to planning joint work between workers in different teams may appear very different from what goes on—or feels possible—in routine practice. This type of activity takes place only when attention is given to the process of trust and is actively supported by managers and leaders across a range of teams working with similar clients.

9.5.7 Team processes that support the Team around the Worker

9.5.7.1 Having the right mix of people who can work flexibly in the team

In AMASS, the principle of Team around the Worker was integral to the design of the team, as the team had a mix of professionals within it that included most of the specialisms that might be required to help clients with multiple needs in relation to education, mental health, parenting, adult mental health, employment, and so on. As we saw in the example of Kelly the education worker, the availability of different forms of help within the team was key because it meant that families did not experience any delay in receiving a form of help in relation to a need (whether they were directly asking for help, or a worker was asking on their behalf). The matter was not 'referred' to another agency, where service entry barriers or waiting lists might be encountered, by which time the conditions that enabled the family to ask for or accept help might have changed. Expressions of help-seeking by clients with multiple needs may be tentative and fragile, and the state of mind associated with them may not be sustained if help is not provided more or less immediately. Expressed another way, the containment of the range of help within the team was important because families were not necessarily equally help-seeking in relation to all aspects of their circumstances. In edge-of-care work, there is often a balance to be struck between working on factors that are necessary to promote safety and working on those the family feels willing, able, and ready to address—these factors do not necessarily overlap.

Addressing this by nurturing clients' capacity to seek out and make use of help may open the door to them being able to make use of help for other aspects of their situation. Families may wish to prioritize a different issue from the one the worker may wish to start with, but when different forms of help are readily available within a team, it is not necessarily a problem to start with the client's focus, as the trust in the helping process that may be generated from this experience may pave the way for conversations about what other forms of help the client might want. This worker has the flexibility to be introduced at a pace that suits the family and to come in and out of contact with the family as needed. The experience of having to fill in referral forms, sit on waiting lists, and be discharged for not attending does not often match clients' help-seeking patterns. When teams are composed of workers whose remits are the different specialisms relevant to the multiple needs of the client group with whom the team works, there is no waiting list, the referral is not closed if the client changes their mind, they are not discharged, and the door remains open for the next time when the family is in a position to try again to address a particular issue. We recognize that many teams will not have the range of expertise that was designed for AMASS but feel that this could be given greater consideration when setting up services working with clients with multiple needs. Even where this is not possible, we hope that we have illustrated how the process can be successful when the team members incorporate a willingness to work in this way into their approach and make efforts to think about their role in 'bridging' in workers from other agencies who might also play a valuable role in supporting their clients, as was the case with George in helping Alice and Lucas.

9.5.7.2 Establishing and sustaining help-seeking in the team: make it part of the work

The degree of coordination and trust required to work as a team in this way does not establish and sustain itself without conscious and explicit efforts by the team. It rests on a team of workers who are comfortable to move in and out of the position of being a keyworker for some clients and a member of the team that forms around another worker for other clients. These processes require mutual help seeking, help offering, and help accepting between team members. To maintain this culture in the team, the AMASS team has regularly discussed and manualized its ideas about what supports this way of working. There is a sense of shared values and a shared approach in relation to the task; that supporting the family is a team effort, requiring people in the team to help each other out in the work. When people join the team, there is an explicit focus on supporting them to build relationships with other team members. Any new worker is encouraged to meet with each member of the team in order to understand their role and also to join them to shadow something that they are doing. If you observed the team 'at work', you would notice that people talk to each other about their work. People are encouraged to talk and plan together about what they are going to do in visits/meetings and to enquire/share how these things have gone afterwards. This is not done in a procedural way, but it is made explicit that it is the responsibility of team members to actively share their work as well as to check in with colleagues (rather than waiting to be invited to do so). Team members routinely ask each other for help with planning sessions; asking if there's anything useful that they need to be aware of to feed into a session that they might be planning with another family member or asking another member of the team to pick up on something that might be helpful to their piece of the work. Team members talk to each other about how they might join with each other to support each other with particular aspects of the work. The things that make this 'OK' relate to shared ideas about this work not being possible for one person to do alone; that it is positive to ask for help and that's what is needed because the work is challenging and causes difficult feelings that need to be talked about and shared, rather than solved alone.

9.5.7.3 Applying 'Team around the Worker' to group supervision

As we have mentioned, the AMASS team had a weekly group meeting where all the cases were discussed. This was a long meeting; each case was scheduled for a specific time and the social worker for each case was invited to join the team discussion of their particular case. For each case, the actions and goals for the week were reviewed and impressions about the family were shared. The risk in relation to this meeting was that the social worker could easily feel that the team had taken over the case and that they were an outsider to the team, as was Martha's experience at the beginning of her work with the AMASS team. Explicit attention needed to be paid in these meetings to ensure that the plans for the coming week took account of the views of each social worker and how they were feeling about their case overall. Often, where there were safeguarding concerns, the level of concern would fluctuate, and it was essential that the social worker experienced the team as validating their current level of concern, that is, that they felt understood by the team. Sometimes this was nurtured by having a prior conversation with the social worker before the meeting about what their principal concerns were and making sure these were covered in the discussion. Most essential was attention to ensuring that the social worker did not feel isolated with their concerns and was able to reflect openly with the team about them. This underlies the importance of the development of epistemic trust between the social worker and the AMASS team to contain the anxieties that such work inevitably brings.

We shall finish by returning to the example of creating a team around Martha, who was the keyworker in work with Alice and Lucas. In this case Martha was the keyworker not because Lucas had the most trust in her but because, in this service context, there was the possibility of the local authority taking a decision for Lucas to come into care. So, this was a local adaptation that was needed because this task would require the social worker to be central if the situation with Lucas and the family reached this point. There was a need to build a team around Martha that took into account the family's existing trusting relationships (e.g. Matt and George) but also included members of the AMASS team, who paid attention to Martha's state of mind. In particular, Yemi needed to ensure that the team supported Martha's understanding of her client and attended to Martha's own state of mind, acknowledging disappointments, frustration, and the need to notice small improvements. For Lucas, the important steps were to begin to talk with Martha and his uncle Matt about his relationship with his mother and about how they could spend more time together without this leading to arguments. It also involved Lucas being able to share some of his worries about his mum's drinking and for Alice to commit to getting some help with this. Following these steps, Lucas began to engage more with his home tutor, as he felt more comfortable being around Alice in the house during the day. He remained out of school, but Kelly had lined up a place at a college that would accept him when he felt ready to return. Because Alice felt less worried about Lucas's future, there was less stress between Alice and Lucas. At the end of the AMASS intervention, they agreed to a referral to a return-to-school programme run by a specialist education team, provided that Martha remained involved in the early stages to support them to attend.

9.6 Implications

This chapter has explored the implementation of a Team around the Worker approach to working with clients with multiple problems. As with all aspects of the AMBIT approach, it relies on a foundation of very strong team working based on mentalizing and supporting the vulnerabilities and states of mind of everyone in the team. The chapter has highlighted that the practice of creating a Team around the Worker cannot be seen as separate from the culture of team working that AMBIT advocates. There is no simple formula for creating such a culture, but we have learned that it needs to be given explicit priority and supported by those in positions of authority and leadership. It also recognizes that having many professionals directly involved with the client is not always helpful to the client. There needs to be support for trying new methods to provide help when this is the case. Most crucially, there needs to be an explicit recognition of the vulnerabilities of workers and teams and that recognizing states of mind, feeling validated, and being trusted are not 'luxury add-ons' but the building blocks of effective practice. The role of leaders and managers in making this possible is crucial. Without this, workers can be left feeling vulnerable and that help-seeking indicates weakness rather than strength. The service culture needs to extend to establishing trust between teams, and this will be the focus of Chapter 10.

This chapter has described in detail some of the early meetings that take place when creating a Team around the Worker as a way of paying attention to processes of help. Some readers may have found the degree of consideration of the fragility of the helping process surprising and perhaps excessive. We recognize this and acknowledge that we have come to see that creating effective multiagency helping systems requires this level of attention to detail about the process of beginning helping relationships, attention to the beliefs and attitudes of both clients and workers, and recognition of the vulnerabilities that clients and workers may experience in this process. We have come to see that the apparently simple principle of organizing help around those whom the client trusts is far from being simple in reality. It relies on investment in the relationships between helpers, which we believe is one of the most neglected areas of effective joint agency care. It emphasizes more than anything that AMBIT is fundamentally a relational system of help.

AMASS is an example of a service that was set up and designed around the principle of the Team around the Worker—in this case, the social worker for a family. The approach followed AMBIT principles and fitted them to the local context, service culture, and priorities of local leadership and needs. This service design was significantly different from the design of other services that you will read about in this book. The reader will recognize many similarities between the teams, and the underlying principles are the same, but local context is important too. AMBIT proposes no uniformity of service design and hence cannot be rolled out through a top-down initiative, even if this were desirable. As is fundamental to AMBIT principles, the service must be shaped by the relationships of those who bring together such services and through an obligation to take seriously the need to be curious about the states of mind of all those involved.

We also have much more to learn about how teams can work effectively together in networks, and it is to this problem that we now turn in Chapter 10, which describes the enormous creativity of the team in Roskilde in Denmark in their development of the AMBIT network approach.

References

Miller, W. R., & Rollnick, S. (2012). *Motivational interviewing: Helping people change* (3rd ed.). Guilford Press.

Talbot, L., Fuggle, P., Foyston, Z., & Lawson, K. (2020). Delivering an integrated adolescent multi-agency specialist service to families with adolescents at risk of care: Outcomes and learning from the first ten years. *British Journal of Social Work, 50*(5), 1531–1550. https://doi.org/10.1093/bjsw/bcz148

10
Working with networks

Implementing AMBIT in disrupted healthcare systems

Janne Walløe Vilmar and Stefan Lock Jensen

10.1 Setting the scene

One of the enormous pleasures of the AMBIT programme is the people we have met who are interested in AMBIT. We have found it fascinating to learn how they have taken the basic AMBIT model and have developed it further within their own work context. In this chapter, we will learn about the work of the team in Roskilde, Denmark, in terms of how they have taken forward ideas about how to work in networks. A large part of this chapter will describe the work they did around a particular case, which required enormous creativity and professional courage across the network of services working with the same young person. The authors will also invite us to step back from the details of practice and to locate the problems of their work in a wider philosophical frame, to zoom out before we focus in and explore how networks are constructed around shared meanings that may be highly elusive and intangible.

Working with networks involves developing skills and understandings that are rarely covered in professional trainings. Readers may be surprised by the strength of feeling that may be involved in this aspect of the work. The way professional responsibilities are demarcated through these trainings leads to profound challenges when a team is faced with needs that do not fit easily within these categories. Very easily, these distinct responsibilities between health, mental health, social care, and education become weapons or accusations between agencies rather than enabling a collective process of help. This chapter deliberately not only includes a description about the needs of a young person but also explores what it felt like for practitioners in such a network.

To support this type of work requires a team. At different times, Peter (Fuggle) and Laura (Talbot) have had the pleasure of visiting the team in Roskilde, a beautiful town by the shiny grey northern sea. There, we met a team that was establishing the sort of team culture advocated by the AMBIT approach. This was no better illustrated than by being welcomed to the wonderful team breakfast they had together once a week. They understood the old wisdom that to create a team one must 'break bread' together.

10.2 Introduction

In this chapter, we will describe how AMBIT, to us, enabled a new form of knowledge, integration, and purpose necessary to help young people and their families in times when their lives are disrupted, distressed, and disconnected from the world at large. It is a newly named genre especially suitable for our field of work, namely child and adolescent psychiatry, at the present time. We have, in our professional lives and our lives in general, and in our network of people, lots of knowledge about how to offer psychiatric help to children and adolescents, but we have lacked a model that organizes the complexity necessary to offer adequate help. We have searched for a common stance in assisting knowledgeably in distressed young people's lives. We are motivated by trying to understand and help families struggling with mental illness, and to help young people back on to developmentally functioning tracks in their lives. However, the uncoordinated helping system and our lack of understanding of the helping systems discouraged us.

We will begin this chapter by sharing a case example of a lost young person and her family, in need of help. We call it 'The Case of the Teenager Behind a Closed Door':

A general practitioner (GP) contacted our child and adolescent psychiatric clinic to refer a teenage girl whom he had not been able to evaluate. According to the GP, the matter was urgent and the teenager, who had not been eating regularly for 6 months, was possibly so underweight that she was in a serious condition and needed acute admission to hospital. The hospital would not admit the teenager until the GP had evaluated her. Her mother was not able to get to her behind the locked bedroom door. She was now having only very rare contact with her daughter and served her food through the half-opened door. According to the mother, the girl was starved, pale, short of breath, and talked slowly and incoherently. The GP tried to respond to the mother's cry for help and suggested involving the police in order for a doctor to be able to examine the teenager. However, the mother did not want the 'mess' that could potentially arise. The girl's school had notified the Family Services, which in turn had sent a social worker to visit the family. The social worker talked with the mother and had progressed in connecting with the teenager—at first through the locked door and later when the teenager sat on her bed with a blanket over her head.

The referral to the child and adolescent psychiatric unit looked straightforward, and it stated that the GP was referring the teenager for evaluation and treatment of an eating disorder. Upon contact with the GP, however, it turned out that there had been no objective evaluation of the severity of the possible eating disorder. It appeared that there was an urge to place responsibility for the teenager somewhere else. Certainly, the mother could not carry the heavy burden of looking after her daughter alone; the family worker was not medically trained; the school had no idea what problems the teenager was facing, as she had not attended school for 6 months; the GP claimed no responsibility as he had not been able to examine the teenager and had passed his knowledge of the case on to the hospital; the hospital staff said they could not be responsible for patients they had not seen; and the police did not have the necessary information to coerce the teenager to accept medical help. Quickly, all these parts of the helping systems united in naming 'the mess' as a psychiatric problem—regardless of whether or not the cause of the general sense of helplessness was psychiatric. It seemed that everyone had predefined the psychiatric unit as the correct 'pigeonhole' for the referral.

This left us in a position where we recognized the cry for help but had no idea what it was really about, and realized that the teenager might die and that the entirety of the helping systems around her could agree only on the situation being our problem. We could all agree on the delicacy and lack of clarity of the whole situation. We ended up agreeing that we should all (rather than the psychiatric clinic alone) try to help, and we started wondering what existential problems could force a teenager into isolation in her bedroom and to the verge of starvation, and what could lead a mother to somehow accept and tolerate this situation. What kind of help did the teenager need? What would be of value to her? How could we reach her? How could we get her to eat? Whose problem was it if we did not succeed and she died? What was going through her mind? And how were we to figure this out? One thing was certain: no one would figure it out without reaching out.

We will return to the case later in this chapter, but before we do so we will describe the helping system in Denmark and then explain our process of implementing AMBIT as a common stance in our psychiatric unit, sparked by the obstacles of integrating the different organizations in the networks in which we operate. Next, we will narrow our focus on to integrating networks in practice and circle back to finding new knowledge in the theories of the broader healthcare system. We integrate an understanding of the very complex cases we are faced with by looking to other theories and introduce the concept of the 'mentalizing case manager' (MCM). We try to connect with a broader understanding of the current society, and finally we intend to share how we handled the case according to the theories, processes, and practices described.

10.3 The value of values: AMBIT in the age of disruptive dynamics

Denmark is well known for its Flexicurity system, a social welfare system financed by one of the world's highest tax rates. The Flexicurity system provides citizens with free education at all levels, free access to the public health system, and a relative freedom to change jobs as the tendencies of the markets change. This system makes Danish society socially robust and dynamic in its essence, and it works as a protection against otherwise disruptive changes in market demands and changing paradigms of under-standing, as opposed to the low social mobility that exists in the more plutocratic[1] systems that prevail elsewhere in the world.

The system of mental healthcare in Denmark is, as a consequence of the way in which it is funded and organized, a topic of great interest for the public and political spheres nationally and internationally. Ongoing dynamic transformations are regu-larly made to optimize resources and maintain the Flexicurity system. This type of so-cial process is complex, as Rittel and Webber (1973, p. 155) described almost 50 years ago in their description of 'wicked problems':

> The search for scientific bases for confronting problems of social policy is bound to fail, because of the nature of these problems ... Policy problems cannot be definitively described. Moreover, in a pluralistic society there is nothing like the undisputable public good; there is no objective definition of equity; policies that respond to social problems cannot be meaningfully correct or false; and it makes no sense to talk about 'optimal solutions' to these problems ... Even worse, there are no 'solutions' in the sense of definitive and objective answers.

Rittel and Webber (1973) formally described the concept of 'wicked problems', con-trasting such 'wicked' problems with relatively 'tame', solvable problems in mathem-atics, chess, or puzzle solving. Conklin (2006, pp. 14–15) defined the characteristics of wicked problems thus: (a) the problem is not understood until after a solution has been formulated; (b) they have no end (what Conklin termed no 'stopping rule'); (c) they have no 'right' or 'wrong' solutions; (d) each wicked problem is essentially novel and unique; (e) every solution is a 'one-shot operation' (you can never go back and do it over, as any solution you attempt will have consequences); and (f) they have no given alternative solutions.

The Danish professor of philosophy Finn Thorbjørn Hansen (2018) has worked with 'creative innovation' in exciting ways and he has coined the term 'delicate prob-lems'. He is inspired by the discourse of wickedness of problems but claims that we have missed another dimension of human growth—the existential aspects of life and their role in shaping behaviour and meaning. Up until now, the primary focus has been on technologically focused problem-solving. What is needed in his opinion is the creation of 'meaning- and wonder driven innovation', or 'existential innovation'. Hansen quotes D. H. Lawrence in *The Plumed Serpent* (1926): 'Give me the mystery and let the world live again for me ... and deliver me from man's automatism!' The organizational theorist Russell L. Ackoff (1974) also thought about complex social problems and called them by what is perhaps their true name, 'social messes'. He wrote: 'Every problem interacts with other problems and is therefore part of a set of interrelated problems, a *system of problems* ... I choose to call such a system a *mess*' (Ackoff, 1974, p. 21).

---

[1] *Plutocracy*: a society that is ruled or controlled by people of great wealth or income.

Many organizations experience the burden of wicked problems in a world of increasing stress and optimization of processes, and many individuals will carry that burden in their hearts, in a world that moves ever faster and where disruption of facts is a given. Do we have the time, and the contexts, for asking the bigger questions about what we are doing? Can we just 'be' and not 'act' all the time in our life, or in the lives of others? We are often, as individual health system workers, more than welcome to innovate and wonder, but more often than not, we can do this only in our spare time. Most of us know that it is this 'wondering' that is often required to help the client, and that provides the innovation and creativity to actually solve complex problems. However, our system is not creative and flexible on a day-to-day basis, and in trying to do 'the right thing' for the patient, the worker at the same time probably crosses the lines of at least a couple of guidelines and rigid systems. This means that the help we are contracted to offer and the work we are paid to do (by the population, as citizens and taxpayers) in these wicked situations more often than not requires the worker to carry the responsibility alone. This calls for a well-connected team and psychiatrically competent and robust leaders—otherwise the burden of helping others may end up causing helplessness for the worker who is offering to help.

Alongside 'wicked problems', we also conceptualize the 'delicate problems' experienced by our clients. These are not just wicked and messy, they are also the 'living mysteries' of our clients that need to be released or revived in their complicated and distressed everyday lives. The delicacy of such problems is threefold: they are *fragile*, *private*, and *essential*. A focus on the 'wickedness' of problems mostly highlights the view of the hard-to-solve issues seen from the perspective of helping systems, whereas a focus on the 'delicacy' of problems is a shift to the existential and subjective perspectives of the life of the client: the why and how of lives worth living. We desperately need that perspective if we are to reach out and try to help our clients.

Can you solve loneliness? Should you? Is there a model of action that can eliminate inner turmoil? What is life all about, and how do you value peace of heart—and should you? With very little time to reflect on these matters as a team and very little room to secure common ground, how are we to help at all? In Denmark, the land of the existential philosopher Søren Kierkegaard, we are inspired to look for windows of opportunity to bring back the 'wonder of life'. We try to reinstil in ourselves the view of the young child, who thinks that the world is full of magic. We try to find a way to keep wondering about what gives meaning to the life of our clients. We try to keep 'the wonder' at the forefront of our way of reflecting when we approach AMBIT cases in our quest to ignite the spark of wonder needed in these cases—and in the co-workers trying to establish a complex helping system around each of our young clients.

We believe that the solution to wicked problems, and the service muddles that surround AMBIT clients such as the planning of treatment and the allocation of resources, depends on how the problem is framed—and that the definition of the problems depends on the solution. Different stakeholders might have different frames for understanding a given problem, and different interests might be at stake. Since the economic crisis of the new millennium, and amid growing awareness that medical treatments are becoming more expensive and the workforce is ageing, increasing political emphasis in Denmark has been placed on optimizing economic value through the 'New Public Management' approach, which has meant more focus on giving the right treatment/support to the right problems. 'Economic value' has been an increasing preoccupation, somewhat to the neglect of 'mental health value'. The focus on identifying the right problems and providing the right treatment, as well as the imperative to keep the helping system intact in the fact of economic pressures, has called for countless descriptions of visitation rules and social and clinical guidelines, along with directives about which part of the helping system is to help in what way. Despite the fact that the whole idea of a public helping system is to serve the population and that the money to do so comes from the population itself, the minute management of the helping system leaves different parts of it fighting over whose money is to pay for what. This dis-integrated health system does not serve its workers or patients/clients as intended, and the arousal this social climate creates tends to undermine mentalizing; to put it plainly, common sense, humility, humanity, empathy, knowledge, and development—the necessary building blocks for integration and the ability to help at all—are threatened. Integration is crucial in the AMBIT model and crucial for the everyday worker, if that worker is to be able to help their clients as intended. The New Public Management movement has not delivered the promised results, and a new discourse has come to light. 'Value-based management' (VBM) (Porter & Lee, 2013) provides new hope for organizing healthcare systems in ways that combine high clinical standards with a more modern, person-centred approach, and network-based intervention. The 'value of values' as a way of guiding healthcare for the public promises a broader and more relatable way of providing help across different helping systems.

The region of Zealand in Denmark has chosen to focus ambitiously on VBM, in part on the basis of a published McKinsey report (Menon et al., 2019) outlining the components of a 'value-based healthcare system'. Porter and Lee (2013) summarize the standards for the paradigm shift—a shift that might as well have been a description of the AMBIT approach:

- Treatment should be organized into integrated helping systems, as opposed to highly specialized units with restricted functions.
- Treatment outcome should be focused primarily on patient-related outcome measures.
- Budgets should be planned for the 'whole treatment course' for the patient/client.
- All treatments for the patient/client should be coordinated and integrated.
- Locality and geography should not restrict the treatments offered.
- Relevant IT systems should be developed to organize and support the above aspects.

VBM was, of course, also developed to optimize the healthcare system financially, but it is a paradigm that sets out to do so by optimizing the integration of treatment across different helping systems (reducing costly dis-integration) and by tailoring treatment to the individual client (reducing costly and often redundant standard treatment packages) and making treatment more focused on 'real-life functioning' (as opposed to blindly applying best-practice treatments based on categorical diagnosis). This is an almost verbatim description of the intentions of the AMBIT model. ·

10.4 AMBIT as outpatient milieu therapy in the real world

When we first stumbled upon AMBIT, we were not looking for it. We had been working for more than a decade with inpatient psychiatric adolescents but had now taken on a new challenge of managing and rebuilding an outpatient child and adolescent psychiatric clinic.

Inpatient treatment is a complex type of treatment, and the central point of focus in our previous work centred on building up a unit around the young people that re-establishes a sort of 'miniature real-life situation' that on an everyday basis tries to elicit and develop the symptoms and attachment patterns of the young people and, over time, reintegrate new and more constructive patterns through their new attachments to the staff of the unit. Central to this type of treatment was a highly constructed and controlled differentiation of roles, such that each worker in the helping system had a different psychological and social function, with the different roles together forming an 'integrative treatment circle'—like the spokes in a wheel. This type of treatment is called milieu therapy and has a long tradition in Scandinavia—and it has a mentalization-based form as well (Skårderud & Sommerfeldt, 2013).

At the core of milieu therapy is the understanding that the milieu in which healing can take place is a healthy and robust one, one that can tolerate and handle irrationality and intense affect—that is, non-mentalizing states. To create healthy attachment patterns, you need authentic and trustworthy people, as well as time and knowledge. No one gets real knowledge without authentic curiosity. Once insecure expectations about the world, and the value of living, emerge, it is not easy to trust people to be able to help, and you ultimately need a trustworthy and robust helping system. We set out to search for ways to create just that in our outpatient unit, equipped with the baggage of knowing the current disrupted state of the healthcare system. We saw a lot of similarities between AMBIT and milieu therapy: a focus on the necessity of different roles in the treatment process, a focus on the integration of treatment across sectors and modalities, and a key focus on attachment and mentalizing in well-functioning networks. To this day, we think and talk about AMBIT as 'outpatient milieu therapy'. Our interest in the importance of well-integrated networks and a well-functioning healthcare system may well lead back to the understanding of how crucial a safe and well-integrated milieu is for developing mental health. Building a safe relationship is one thing, facilitating a network of safe relationships is another, and supporting a whole helping system, such as the healthcare system, is a third—but all three may well rely on the same basic understanding of human dynamics.

When we started managing the new outpatient clinic, we were inspired by milieu therapy's insistence on having 'a common language' as a starting point for the creation of a well-connected team. In AMBIT we found that common language and a way of working that we were already very familiar with. We trusted that way of working and thinking, had seen it work and create results, and we felt that we were on safe ground, which gave us a feeling of freedom and confidence. In other words, we felt that we could more easily mentalize in that context, and hopefully use that capacity as we set out to build the new clinic.

It has been common in the past decade to suggest that organizational culture is like the operating system of a computer (e.g. Dykstra, 2019). If you want to create new networks of help and well-connected teams, you have to start to focus on your own milieu—your own team. Having a common language for describing the work, a common 'operating system', is the starting point. The language defines (explains), directs, unites, and is the gateway for reaching out. If you do not speak the same language as the rest of your team, dis-integration will quickly emerge. To use an analogy, according to the legend the Tower of Babel never reached the heavens, even though the 'apps' (the instructions and techniques of the people doing the work of building) were working correctly. The Gods invented different languages to stop the process, meaning that communication was hindered, and the coordination disintegrated (Bevington & Fuggle, 2012).

Transformation into a value-based healthcare system is, above all, a journey of culture change. Hopefully it is a curative one that authentically offers help to the helping system, or at least leaves room for empathy, humanity, curiosity, knowledge, and, most importantly, the 'wickedness' of human problems. On the day we first presented the new AMBIT project to our new clinic, we were excited, and a bit proud that we had managed to persuade our senior managers to send us to the Anna Freud Centre for training. When we announced the project to the staff, one started crying and one person walked out in protest. We were, looking back, naïvely optimistic and inexperienced in the art of transforming a culture. One could argue that we started a top-down process and got the response one would expect. In a way, we did an overnight reboot of the operating system of the clinic—and anxiety and uncertainty resulted. The old 'apps' would not work, and people felt alienated and were afraid that they were no longer agents in their work life. We were unaware of the state of our colleagues and of their insecurity. We learned some lessons the hard way!

10.5 Nothing unites people like a common enemy . . . but an enemy could become a friend

We wanted to build the foundation of our new clinic on an AMBIT approach, and as managers we would commit to the journey. We wanted to instil the value of good clinical practice and the integration of different types of treatment, not only in our own team, but also across the different helping systems that inhabit our working landscape—and the AMBIT approach was the mortar to hold the bricks together.

However, AMBIT is not a fixed package of tools and processes. AMBIT is a framework that has to be integrated with different teams' specific tasks, history, culture, and way of working. We learned better ways of framing and nurturing these processes through the 'Train the Trainer' course at the Anna Freud Centre; gradually, our team began adopting the language and practices of AMBIT, the team increased its well-connectedness, and the 'operating system' seemed to function without the need for too many disruptive updates from the outside. One specific problem united us as a team and started the process whereby AMBIT found its real use and integration in our new clinic. When we started managing the new clinic there was a very problematic, almost non-existent, collaboration with one of the municipalities that the clinic served. Former managers of our clinic were said to have established a very asymmetrical relationship with this municipality, which meant that there was no integration of treatment or exchange of perspectives, but rather one-way communication from both sides. This had been going on for a couple of years, resulting in the municipality hiring external psychiatric consultants who were more 'anti-system', and the two different paradigms drew both parties further away from each other. Neither the psychiatric system nor the municipality carried the heaviest consequence of this—the young people and their families did.

For the sake of the clients, we all wanted to improve the external relationship between leaders and staff alike. We reached out to the municipalities affiliated with our clinic in different ways, held mediating meetings with their senior managers, and managed to restart the connection, but it was a delicate beginning, mostly upheld by individual relationships and necessity. What really ignited the dis-integrative fire and kept it burning seemed to be a non-mentalizing stance and way of communicating with each other in different relationships. Non-mentalizing is most often brought about by emotional arousal. We would never know what emotions sparked this non-mentalizing if we were not curious, and one will not succeed in getting answers in an aroused system without authenticity and real curiosity. Even though the managers on both sides of the fence seemed by now to be getting along, we realized that we needed to change the problematic behaviour at its roots—and in that process, we saw a way to put the AMBIT approach to the test in our new clinic by focusing in on the part of the AMBIT wheel that encourages evaluating the work done.

10.6 Can you establish mentalizing network meetings? The NET-Aim-Questionnaire

We chose to focus on the one setting where we could not avoid working together with the municipalities—the obligatory 'network meetings'. When a young person has been examined and treated in our clinic, we most often inform the school, the social worker, the family worker, and other relevant parties by having a meeting where we talk about our understanding of the young person. The purpose of the meeting is for the network to agree on a joint approach to treatment across the different sectors and agree on responsibilities and optimally coordinate the work in a way that enhances the functioning of the young person in their everyday life.

These network meetings have a complicated nature due to the complexity of their group dynamics and the ambitious aim of finding common ground; they tended to be very difficult for the staff to host due to the way each of the parties involved reacted negatively to the others because of prior history. The arousal caused by the fact that two (or more) parties had to meet left well-intentioned workers in non-mentalizing states on both sides. This is not the most promising way to start a meeting in which a young person's mental health is the focus. Helping young people with mental health issues is hard enough without further obstacles.

Inspired by the AMBIT focus on networks, and in gathering and using data to learn, we set ourselves the task of improving the network meetings by trying to evaluate the meetings after they had been held. By broadcasting our intentions to improve our own mentalizing abilities and host more constructive meetings, we set a standard for ourselves by which we would ask the municipalities to evaluate us—and in the process perhaps themselves. We wanted to start a new culture of working with and understanding the network around the young person, but we needed to create an 'app' to achieve this. We had to commit to doing something different, or else we would just fall back into old habits.

If the municipalities, the schools, the social workers, and so on seem 'wickedly problematic' to us, could we learn to maintain our curiosity about their intentions and the world they inhabit? Could we try to mentalize why they might feel stuck and frustrated? Could we reframe the messiness of the experience of hosting network meetings? Might we even create a culture where we can understand the delicacy of their roles and their work in the life of the young person? Could we perhaps start to see the wonder of our common task at hand—the wonder of how we create a team spirit as a common united network, starting today, at this specific meeting?

We developed the NET-Aim-Questionnaire (NET-Aim-Q).[2] This was the 'app', the tool we wanted to guide us towards a new way of hosting network meetings—and in turn we hoped for a broader transformation and the integration of mentalizing as a core dynamic in our clinic. The name is an abbreviated combination of the words *network* (meeting), *aim* (goal), and *questionnaire* (the 'Q')—and it pays homage to the AMBIT tradition of using evaluation tools that focus on aims and coordination, like the AMBIT Integrative Measure (described in Chapters 2 and 13). We searched the literature for suitable tools but did not find one that had the specific focus that we needed, and so we set about creating and developing a tool of our own in the hope of it being useful for us and for others with a similar interest in network functioning.

---

[2] We wish to give a special acknowledgement to the psychologist Sune Bo, PhD, who was a central part of validating the NET-Aim-Q.

The past decade has seen growing research into feedback-informed approaches to therapy, and we were broadly inspired by this way of putting ourselves 'out there' for evaluation, because psychotherapy research has shown that greater effects can be achieved when you dare to let evaluation inform clinical practice (Prescott et al., 2017). By giving the participants the possibility of evaluating the network meeting in the here and now, we thought we would get the most unedited and authentic response and give ourselves the most information about how the network is functioning right now.

Research into the common factors of psychotherapy (Wampold, 2015) has focused on the effect of concepts such as warmth, empathy, and a model of the psyche/psychoeducation as the most important factors in treatment. This, as well as Fonagy and colleagues' focus on epistemic trust and its effects on social factors outside the therapy setting (Luyten et al., 2020), all seemed to us to be central to the task we had set ourselves. We could in some regards summarize this under the concept of mentalizing, and by framing statements about trying to see each other's perspectives and nurturing this capacity during the meeting (by the host of the meeting—a specific role taken up by one person) we hoped to elicit information about the joined network's general ability to mentalize, through evaluating the specific meeting.

We drew some inspiration from measures of 'group climate' in group therapy; research has shown that the concept of the emotional and social climate of the group has a large impact on the effectiveness of, and adherence to, therapy (MacKenzie, 1983). From AMBIT and from milieu therapy we knew that group dynamics play an essential role in the integration and well-connectedness of teams, and therefore we tried to create statements relating to the emotional quality of the meeting (Bevington et al., 2017). The NET-Aim-Q became a 12-item self-rating measure using a Likert scale to evaluate statements about the climate and quality of the network meeting that had just taken place. Participants answer whether they 'agree', 'agree very much', or 'do not agree' (and so on) with statements about the meeting they have just attended. Each participant at the meeting completes a questionnaire (if they consent), so in a given meeting you might get the view of, for example, the father, the mother, the young person, the social worker, the schoolteacher, and the leader of the meeting. The questions contained in the NET-Aim-Q focus on the meeting as a whole; no one participant is singled out or asked other than the host of the meeting (i.e. ourselves). We focus specifically on the host of the meeting to highlight that the host has a special role in trying to nurture and facilitate the sort of mentalizing and coordinated atmosphere we strive for.

The host of the meeting has a central role in the process and execution of the meeting, just as a therapist has the overall responsibility of therapy. The host cannot control the dynamics and outcome of a meeting, but a large part of doing the NET-Aim-Q is to ensure that the host has tried to live up to and guide the meeting according to expectations (i.e. creating a relatively safe/trusting atmosphere, perspective-taking (mentalizing), and coordination (integration) of the network and planning the intervention in the life of the young person). Factor analysis was performed on more than

250 questionnaires and a three-factor model emerged showing the internal reliability of the test; the 12 questions seemed to cluster in groups of four questions each that seemed to measure some of the same aspects of the network meeting. When we asked experienced clinicians, there seemed to be consensus about the validity of the three factors, which we identified as trust, perspective-taking (mentalizing), and integration/coordination of treatment.

When the participants in a meeting complete the NET-Aim-Q you get different scores: there is one total score for the summarized quality of the network meeting (for each participant), and subscale scores for each of the three factors listed above (for each participant). The host also evaluates the meeting in the same way. It is therefore possible to analyse the general and/or subscale scores from the perspective of, for example, the mother of the young person. Does she feel that the network meeting had an atmosphere of trust (which we aim for, since trust enhances connectedness) or not? Could it be improved? Similarly, how does the social worker rate the factor of trust? Are there differences in the scores that could point to aspects of difficulty in the relationship between the mother and the network, or between the mother and the social worker? You get a range of perspectives on the meeting that has just taken place, and relational dynamics emerge out of the scores, which could surprise the team or confirm what the team already knows. One of the most interesting things to look for is discrepancies between the scores assigned by the host of the meeting and the other participants from the network. In some ways the questionnaire can reveal dis-integration or even the degree of dis-integration in the helping network.

The questionnaire is introduced at the start of the network meeting, and we broadcast the intention of getting evaluations on our ability to host and nurture a network meeting characterized by collaboration, coordination, and trust. Our staff were at first reluctant to do this, as they were afraid their abilities in the very difficult setting would be exposed to leaders and other members of their own team and, at worst, the broader helping system. Workers in the system of psychiatry are often very experienced in evaluating others and in discussing clients, but they are not as experienced in evaluating and discussing their own efforts. We argued that such openness is required to establish a safe and healthy environment, and that our staff members would only develop and enhance their own mentalizing abilities in a healthy milieu and therefore would be able to support the development of a healthy helping system only if they themselves succeeded in meeting the requirements they demanded of their clients. In addition, how could we expect families to expose their insecurities to us if we did not grant them the same courtesy? The team agreed to support each other in this and agreed on the very vulnerable position they were putting themselves in. A benefit of this process was experiencing the very real parallel to the exposed position of the families at the network meetings.

On implementing the use of the questionnaire in network meetings, we learned more about aspects of people's and networks' real functioning—and also about responses to the measure itself. Some team members easily introduced the questionnaire while others did not until months later, even though we had all agreed to use it in these meetings. Wondering what this was all about, we learned that some members were anxious about not having understood the intention and therefore were anxious about implementing the questionnaire in a meeting. Would they know how to? What would happen? Would they be able to handle the responses? Others were still anxious about their abilities to host a meeting being compared with those of their colleagues.

As mentioned above, we chose to inform participants about the questionnaire at the start of a meeting and thereby broadcast our intentions, and just the fact that attendees knew they could evaluate the meeting after it had finished seemed to change the way they engaged in the meeting. At the beginning of the process, some workers from the municipality would object to completing the questionnaire—they said they did not see the point or did not have the time, or would openly say they would not participate in wasting the family's time, had plenty of important work themselves so would not engage in our quality assessment work, and so forth. We accepted this, of course, but sought to be curious about it and sometimes phoned them afterwards to try to explain our intentions and understand their resistance. When we began to share the results of evaluations of specific cases, some workers regretted not having completed the questionnaire and started to join in. All in all, the pretty good evaluations, and the fact that we used them in our conferences and at meetings, engaged the clinicians in our own team. Clinicians did not seem as insecure about their own abilities as before when they found out that the families and municipalities had shared that they found the meetings to be mentalizing and purposeful. When we asked our staff members before introducing the questionnaire, they said that they expected low scores on the evaluation and felt they were not as good as they could be at hosting network meetings, but when they realized this was not the opinion of the attendees, they grew more confident, and with it more curious and mentalizing.

From early on in the process, results (in the form of the NET-Aim-Q total score) seemed to show an objectively positive evaluation of the meetings held in the clinic. It seemed that the process of evaluating the meetings in itself had a positive effect. We know from research into mentalization-based treatment that a mentalizing stance seems to improve mentalizing in relationships (Luyten et al., 2020). Maybe the task of improving our own mentalizing stance and signalling that intention in itself initiated a process and improved mentalizing, by reducing non-mentalizing. Mentalizing is an interactive and common process that people use for regulating themselves; strong affect will often trigger non-mentalizing states of mind, but a marked effort to re-establish mentalizing (via mentalization-based treatment techniques or via a mentalizing stance in a meeting) can bring trust and coordination back again.

10.6.1 What will mentalizing network meetings improve?

One very clear consequence of developing and integrating the NET-Aim-Q into our clinical practice was that the AMBIT stance became more accepted and began to catch the interest of the staff at the clinic. We could all feel the change in the way we collaborated with the municipalities: there was simply better treatment coordination, integration, and collaboration between the different helping systems. This improved job satisfaction and team integration and the internal ability to mentalize each other within the team. We did an internal team AMBIT baseline measure (the AMBIT Service Evaluation Questionnaire) before we started and after 1 year, and we saw an improvement that clearly indicated that the efforts we had made in trying to integrate the AMBIT approach were progressing—and, we would argue, that our use of the NET-Aim-Q played a big part in that.

The meetings were easier to attend, and the climate was simply better; as a result, parents and young people received the required focus and their situations were directly addressed. They were often part of the network meetings and they, too, felt that all parties (including themselves, quite often) seemed to convey a more collaborative style. In some instances, a person attending one of the meetings would be obviously different from the others in their evaluation of the meeting—for example, if they gave a negative evaluation even though most attendees evaluated the meeting positively. It might be, for instance, that the father of the young person was quiet during the meeting, and no one really noticed it, or interpreted it as a sign of agreement. However, the NET-Aim-Q showed us a different picture, which gave us the possibility of addressing the issue after the meeting, or at the next consultation if we deemed it to be clinically and dynamically relevant. In this way, the father would not have to feel alienated for a longer period of time or be left feeling angry or disappointed with us, the treatment of his child, or himself. We came to appreciate the clinical opportunities the NET-Aim-Q gave us in this respect, and it sometimes gave us a second chance to mentalize otherwise mistaken conclusions we may have jumped to in inferring intentions or motives of important agents in the treatment planning of the children.

10.6.2 Will using the NET-Aim-Q improve patient-related outcome measures?

Our clinical experience suggested that use of the NET-Aim-Q would improve patient-related outcome measures, as intended in AMBIT and in the VBM approach. Common sense would argue for a positive outcome as well. We have many cases that demonstrate a positive outcome, but we are very motivated to document an effect even more clearly, and we think we are making progress in coming up with clinically relevant and easy-to-apply models of gathering data in this area. Collaboration with the AMBIT Study Group established at the Anna Freud Centre in 2019 has created a forum on this matter, and progress is being made in Denmark and in other teams to implement the NET-Aim-Q. One of the areas for potential further development of the tool is to try to create an online evaluation that could be used via a smartphone app (Mentimeter) so that the network could get instant feedback to the whole meeting/

team. This could create a new possibility to engage the participants/team in the process of working with the themes of the feedback, such as a lack of trust, or a lack of mentalizing. By contrast, such instant feedback could potentially start a group process that the time frame cannot contain and therefore could destabilize the network rather than integrate it, if the process of feedback is started but not completed at the time.

Another effect of the NET-Aim-Q process has been a deepening of our curiosity about what role the network, and especially integration/dis-integration of treatment across sectors and helping systems, plays in the daily functioning of the patient. We are currently developing another questionnaire, the NET-Stat-Q, to measure trust, mentalizing, and treatment integration over time as the treatment evolves. The items of the NET-Stat-Q are quite similar to the items of the NET-Aim-Q but aim to disclose subjective experiences over time in relation to whether or not an integrated and healthy helping system is helping the case, which we would expect to be an even more valid influence on the outcomes for the young person, that is, their quality of functioning in everyday life. The broader question remains: how do you best measure network integration? By measuring the 'temperature' at specific meetings where team functioning has stood its test (NET-Aim-Q) or by asking network members about functioning outside the direct confrontation of experiencing functioning (or lack of functioning), for example, at a network meeting (NET-Stat-Q)? We hope to move closer to an answer in the future.

10.7 The mentalizing case manager: the new specialist-generalist

If there is an AMBIT case manager, is there an AMBIT case as well? We have argued against the concept of AMBIT as a specialized model narrowing in on treating a specific problem or group of clients. AMBIT is a stance, an understanding, a common language, or even an attempt to 'cure' a helping system that has become 'ill', but it requires authenticity, time, security, knowledge, experience, and courage—all resources that are scarce and mostly upheld by brave individuals locally organized within the broader helping system.

There are certainly many clients who do receive appropriate help within the current organization of the system. There is no need to secure more core AMBIT approaches for such cases, especially as these are needed for the more wicked problems or complex cases that do not get the necessary help from the system as is, and resources are not plentiful. So, how does one differ one's approach without defining cases that are in need of the AMBIT approach? We have also argued for individualization and a value-based approach with a proposed economic gain, which is definitely in support of an AMBIT understanding and approach, guided by patient-related outcome measures. But how does one measure the outcomes of employing the AMBIT understanding to cases without defining the cases? And how does one learn from the cases without having defined them in some way?

When people are referred to our service, what seems to make the biggest difference is if we take on a leading and coordinating role for the helping system. We are more likely to take on this role in the more complex cases and with clients who services have found difficult to engage. We have talked about this role as that of the MCM. What the NET-Aim-Q tries to convey and measure is a trusting, coordinated, and mentalizing treatment network. What often seems to be most indirectly asked of us, other than assessing the possibility of psychiatric problems in the complex cases, is to coordinate and to reinstil hope and direction into the broader helping network. The network has tried to help as best as it can, but the complexity of the case has obstructed the process. The MCM works to reinstil trust and mentalizing.

We are not experts in all types of the multifaceted problems we encounter in such complex cases; we are at best experts in psychiatry, but many cases are not stuck on account of a lack of psychiatric knowledge or psychological insight, but because of confusion, lack of clarity, anxiety, group dis-integration, or lack of novel ideas to open up the case. Such problems do not draw on a specific psychiatric competency but, nonetheless, this is what we are often faced with: the psychiatric system in Denmark often handles the most difficult cases, so we are often the last party to enter the helping system, when it is most likely to have got stuck in this way. Often by this point there is certain amount of pessimism and/or helplessness in the network, and it sometimes feels that we are being asked to produce miracles. This is a hard task, which can sometimes undermine our own mentalizing capabilities and requires a well-connected team and a shared collaborative stance.

The MCM, as a concept, is our way of highlighting the function we often have to adopt (for a period of time), acknowledging as we go that we may be part of the helping system only for the short period of time it takes to reinstil hope for change—we have taken on this much-asked-for role and seen the effect it can have! The MCM takes on the role (via a process of delegated authentic agency) of case leadership from the network. The MCM is delegated the role of coordinating the case, the assessment, the understanding, and the way forward—a bird's eye view of the case. The MCM is a practical *and* an emotional manager of the case (the mentalizing aspect of the concept). The MCM is at the forefront of the case when needed but drops back when not needed in that capacity.

The MCM is in dire need of a well-connected team and a well-connected keyworker, to ensure that a real relationship with the client can unfold. The MCM needs to be humble and learn from the inevitable unsuccessful attempts at establishing mentalizing in the helping system, and the MCM needs to be acutely aware of their role as MCM within the helping system. Additionally, the MCM needs to be well trained in the AMBIT model and provided with the direct support of leadership and supervisors, to further back up the role.

The MCM role requires groundedness, knowing when to respond to a crisis, and knowing oneself and one's reactions emotionally and by action; it demands knowing when to be authoritative and when to be curious and humble. Our role as leaders/supervisors is often to help ensure that the MCM balances experience, authority, and relational support effectively. It is a role we discuss and reflect upon in AMBIT meetings within our AMBIT team. We often need a person to take on the role of MCM in the most complex cases.

We suspect that the role may differ according to the nature of the AMBIT team in question, but our experience in a child and adolescent psychiatry clinic is that it is not a role that 'just anyone' can easily carry, and (certainly in the most messy and delicate cases) it demands a rare combination of experience, courage, and humility. It is evident that one cannot be the MCM of many cases at the same time, so in our clinic the role changes. The role calls for time to reflect rather than to take action, but at the same time it is crucial that the MCM knows when to act—either in relation to the case or in seeking help for themselves or others.

The reward of being the MCM in our setting is getting to work with very complex systems and learning along the way. The job is not paid or rewarded differently. Often the experienced workers who engage in this type of case are motivated by learning, knowledge, and personal development, and are given an opportunity to join a team with a theoretical stance they can learn from, supervision, and colleagues engaged in the same kind of wicked problems. Sometimes the opportunity to work more intensely with fewer cases can be a reward in itself for an experienced worker in the current systems.

The idea of the MCM is consistent with the work of Kenneth Mikkelsen and Richard Martin in their book *The Neo-Generalist* (Mikkelsen & Martin, 2016), which describes a new type of worker in high demand for companies across different sectors. A neo-generalist is both a specialist and a generalist. They master multiple disciplines and will not be constrained by just one area of expertise. They combine a deep insight into several disciplines with the ability to act and coordinate across these disciplines and to cross-pollinate them. The concept of cross-pollination is central because creativity and innovative ideas will not come from specialists who know every detail of their area (the 'hyper-specialist') but from people who are able to combine different ideas in new ways, because they master several areas and know how to travel across these, like bees looking for nectar. Neo-generalists are the ones who see 'the whole', instead of the details. They are the explorers, who are comfortable with not having all the answers in advance but have the ability to navigate in an ever-changing world without a fixed manual or a clear map.

The MCM has to be a generalist who is able to cross-pollinate the client, the network, and the helping system, to travel in social, psychological, and somatic seas, to try to find and reinstil hope and meaning, and to succeed in coordinating the network around the client and the helping system. We see the MCM as a function that is essential in AMBIT cases because they are complex, wicked, and messy—but they are also delicate. They are existential cases with no clear answers; they are handled in much the same way as they are understood, and the answers have to be created in coordination with the person around which everything revolves—the client (the AMBIT case)—and the network. This is a very complex task, but it is done one step at a time—and it should be done within a team integrated into a mentalizing network. Above all, being able to mentalize is the central requirement of the role.

Not everyone can take on the role. We would love to say otherwise, but there is little room for pseudo-mentalizing, pseudo-coordinating, or pseudo-hoping in such rough seas. The person who takes on the role of MCM should be experienced enough in coordinating/managing ways to keep themselves calm enough to mentalize and see the bigger picture, and/or well educated in the AMBIT model.

10.8 The resonance of young people and their helping systems

In our attempt to conceptualize and expand upon the role of the MCM we have drawn inspiration from the German sociologist Hartmut Rosa (2019), who is at the forefront of theorizing about the challenges faced by late modern societies. His concept of 'resonance' in relationship to the world is an impressive formulation and integration of psychological and sociological research and concepts that in many ways create a model that encompasses and engulfs the principles and challenges that the AMBIT model tries to address.

Rosa seeks to highlight, at a sociological level, the way that late modernity (and especially its institutions) often alienates its inhabitants and diminishes the opportunities for being connected to the world in resonant ways. He draws upon developmental psychology and modern research into theory of mind, to create a model of human social–psychological development that in many ways resembles mentalization-based theories. He states:

> Resonance is a kind of relationship to the world, formed through 'af←fect' and 'e→motion',[3] intrinsic interest, and perceived self-efficacy, in which subject and world are mutually affected and transformed. Resonance is not an echo, but a responsive relationship, requiring that both sides speak with their own voice ... This is only possible where strong evaluations are affected ... Resonant relationships require that both subject and the world be sufficiently 'closed' or self-consistent so as to speak in their own voice, while also remaining open enough to be affected or reached by each other. (Rosa, 2019, p. 174)

Rosa's overall project is to create a theoretical model that can join the social and the psychological into a model that describes the specific challenges faced by individuals and systems under the accelerated development of late modernity. People feel alienated from themselves, the world they live in, and the social contexts and relationships that they long to become members of. Rosa claims that human beings are

---

[3] af←fect'—inward; 'e→motion'—outward.

most basically motivated by connectedness—that is, the experience of being part of relationships to the world of people and things that provide a sense of resonance, or of being in the world. Daniel N. Stern (2010) echoes this by talking about 'vitality moments and feelings' as the means by which development unfolds. When we meet children and adolescents in our psychiatric clinic, they are all struggling with some kind of problem connecting to the world, suffering from being alone, or feeling depressed or anxious—being alienated from the world they inhabit, not being in a resonant relationship to the world or the network trying to help them. The candle of vitality has gone out; they experience negative affect, and the motion of their emotions is often self-destructive (acting out) or non-mentalizing, resulting in the creation of a negative self-fulfilling dynamic of feelings of hopelessness and negative affect in the helping system. The network is often in a non-mentalizing loop of systems, and their efforts to break this chain are drowned.

As a parallel, members of modern helping systems also long for resonance and connectedness, in the same manner as the keyworker of an AMBIT case needs to be well connected to their team. The difference, though, is that the AMBIT-inspired team has the same reference and stance—AMBIT—whereas the helping system has a plurality of references. Our healthcare system is more often than not a 'sick-care' system, focusing on restoring members of society who have already been hurt instead of focusing on improving care and reducing cost. Treating problems after they have set in is itself likely to cause some harm in the course of treatment. We treat hurt individuals instead of promoting good health, and promoting good health demands a totally different helping system—one that is populated with healthy, authentic, and curious workers who are not afraid to make mistakes and learn from them within the boundaries of safety. Without safety in the system, these workers may suffer from compassion fatigue, and in the context of the current rigorous governance expectations and threats of litigation, curiosity, and eagerness to learn from mistakes are scarce.

We could also call the task of reaching out to the network, which the MCM tries to succeed in, a delicate task. It is delicate in its attempt to try to re-establish the resonance of the system, that is, scaffolding and igniting in the whole network a new resonant relationship that will bring healthy development to the client. Finn Thorbjørn Hansen (2018) has created a 'Four Voices' model that gives us a way of conceptualizing and connecting the experience of the helping systems with the different approaches to understanding and intervening, from which the MCM can try to (re)build the integration and the resonance of the network. The four voices are Acting, Knowing, Being, and Existing. The problems that to us, as a helping system, are 'hard to solve' (acting) and very difficult to understand (knowing) might begin to get a more practical voice if we nurture authentic curiosity about the subjective experience of the child/young person (being) and open up the way of seeing and experiencing the wonder of the case, by connecting to the resonant existing aspects of the world of the client—thereby creating small islands (experiences) of connectedness in the life of the client, or even moments of resonance between the client and the network. Perhaps this spark of hope can start as an experience of resonance between the otherwise dis-integrated network partners—it may be kicked off by experiencing a resonant mentalizing net-work meeting, which instils a new sense of coordination, which in turn sparks a vital new experience of being reconnected to the client, and so forth. This is clearly not a linear process but rather a circular and ongoing process, but we often have to talk about it as if it were linear, to simplify the otherwise complex dynamics. We think that one of the key aspects of the MCM is to be able to shift focus and integrate these fo-cuses. We have used Hansen's model to analyse where there is a lack of coordination between the voices and where there is an alienated voice that might contribute to the dis-integration of the system.

Sometimes a problem might be 'stuck' primarily in a practical (acting) and delicate way, because we know what to do in theory and we have overcome the dis-integration of the helping system, but we have to reach out to the young person, who is existen-tially stuck and lacks ways of reconnecting to the world. How can we, for example, (re)introduce a caseworker who can resonate with the lost existential themes of the young person, thereby creating novel flashes of resonant experiences for the young person that ignite hope of a more lasting connection to the world? Establishing these flashes of resonant experiences is essential for 'reaching' the AMBIT cases, as they are the building blocks that might establish more continuing experiences of resonance, in what Rosa (2019) calls 'stable axes of resonance'—that is, a stable relationship to a caseworker, or a parent, or a system/institution such as the school or the youth foot-ball club.

10.9 'The Case of the Teenager Behind a Closed Door'

To return to purpose, what we are trying to do is to inspire the reader and perhaps expand upon the concepts inherent in the AMBIT approach to the difficult cases that we see in our child and adolescent psychiatric unit. By integrating different practical and theoretical concepts, we aim in this chapter to exemplify the challenge of the MCM, and the challenge of working with AMBIT cases in general, namely, keeping up the ability to mentalize, innovate, motivate, coordinate, and integrate—in essence, to resonate—when confronted with the complex and delicate problems of the young people referred to our clinic, in the current understanding and state of our helping systems. This task requires being creative in the face of the complex, messy, and deli-cate lives of young people and their families, and an effort to keep up hope and act as a 'lighthouse', showing the way to re-establishing the coordination and integration of the helping system, and thereby reaching out to distressed and stranded clients who need to experience relationships to the world and others that resonate with the emo-tional and existential aspects of their lives. To demonstrate these aspects in action, we now return to the case we introduced at the start of this chapter.

In 'The Case of the Teenager Behind a Closed Door', we decided to offer our help but emphasized our 'not knowing' what to do exactly and that our experience was in child and adolescent psychiatry, not in the specific case or in other problems unrelated to mental health. We could reasonably have argued that the case was not 'ours' for now (as the rest of the network had done at the time of referral) but, knowing from experience that the case would keep knocking on the door to child and adolescent psychiatry and agreeing that it was more important to try to offer help to the girl than argue whose responsibility it was, we engaged ourselves. We needed everyone to pitch in and help this girl, and we offered ourselves in the role of what we have named in this chapter the MCM. Specifically, this meant that an experienced specialist psychologist trained in child and adolescent psychiatry took the role as MCM, and a senior child and adolescent psychiatrist agreed to take responsibility for the well-being of the girl and, in addition to this role, for 'supervising' the MCM. This supervisory role entailed a responsibility to offer oneself as a 'Thinking Together' partner (see Chapter 2). Both the psychologist and psychiatrist were well connected to the AMBIT team at the clinic. The case was frequently shared in meetings and by Thinking Together with team members who did not have an active role in the case. We offered to take charge based on our knowledge of the AMBIT model and the balances within the model. We dared to offer our professional help because we felt safe that our knowledge had international resonance and because we had a professional framework to refer to. We dared to offer our help because of the social flexibility still left in our Flexicurity system. Finally, we dared to take the case because we did not feel bold enough to refuse it; we knew from earlier work that doing nothing might be much worse personally than taking on a potential responsibility for life or death. We will stretch this a little further by adding that we dared to take the case because others did not, and this left the girl alone and unfairly vulnerable in a country with a healthcare system like the one in Denmark.

We shared our intentions and invited relevant parties to join in the network. The municipality involved in the case reported that it had almost used the budget it could devote to the case, and it was more than willing to get 'expert help' (which is free for the municipality). The people involved from the municipality had lost hope, and when presented with ideas to progress the case often told us it would not work and that they had tried this before. The MCM spent some time educating them about the AMBIT model, and the municipality hired a previous employee as a social worker, who they regarded as an expert in this field. They agreed that this attempt would be the 'last shot', which put pressure on the helping network—we had to succeed. Our MCM argued that we needed some safe haven of security and hope before we could let that pressure be felt too much by the broader network, and the municipality agreed to not limit the case by a set time (which was an important teleological sign of trust and cooperation). The GP was more than happy not to have to take responsibility for the girl's life and totally withdrew from the case, arguing that it was not his business until the girl's condition was again in a state that demanded only his care. He was not able to join the network meetings, which is a common situation in Denmark.

We held meetings with the municipality to define roles and discussed the environment we had to create for the teenager, as in milieu therapy. We tried to establish who was actually welcome in the room with the teenager—who would resonate with her? We chose the social worker, who we all agreed to support in being the keyworker with regard to creating a relationship, and who we were beginning to trust to be able to connect and mentalize and be open, so that we could work through him. We had no way of getting to the girl without forcing our way in and decided this was not the right approach. The psychiatrist in charge decided to be brave and use a creative approach to reach the girl, which would be based on knowledge gathered from the mother, the keyworker, and the MCM and not only following guidelines. The psychiatrist accepted responsibility for this approach (while also realizing the existential fact that no one can ever truly be responsible for other people's lives, despite the system's eagerness to place responsibility), despite knowing that if things went wrong and the teenager died, it was likely that the system/authorities would hold her to blame.

The MCM coordinated all of this, well aware of the fact that these matters were messy, complicated, and delicate; aware of the responsibility; aware of the fact that he did not know the answers and had to map them out as he went along; and aware of the fact that he had to support his own mentalizing (by using his experience, his personal qualities, his team, and the psychiatrist) to contain arousal, projections, and non-mentalizing around the case. He only once talked to (but not with) the teenager through a door and for the rest of the helping operation had to rely on other helpers' perspectives. He hosted monthly meetings with staff from the school, the social worker, doctors, and the mother. At every meeting, he distributed the NET-Aim-Q to show respect for and curiosity about their experiences of the meeting, and to raise awareness of the mentalizing within the system, the purpose, and the group climate. A good climate in the helping system was essential to support the keyworker and resonate the proposed milieu of the teenager.

After the first meetings, the MCM started to share the results of the NET-Aim-Q with the participants towards the end of each meeting; this led to another level of sharing intentions and greater mentalizing and awareness of each other in the meetings. Increasingly more focus was directed to try to engage people to understand the mother and her vulnerability. Some of her perspectives and misunderstandings, and her well-intended actions (which tended to sustain the problem), became more relatable for the team via the keyworker. In turn, the team's mentalizing stance towards the mother made her feel safer over time, and she ended up sharing important relational experiences from the past. The keyworker set up regular meetings with the mother and talked to her mainly about her own situation at first. She was anxious and she was afraid of meeting the girl's father, whom she had divorced, in public due to former domestic violence (one of the intimate themes she felt safe to share). The girl had witnessed the violence many times. The mother was relieved that the keyworker who came into their home had this knowledge, and she felt he was looking after them in this matter too. She realized that having a man in the house regularly with a well-defined role was not dangerous.

Everyone succeeded in enduring the unknown and the risks and exploring the very existence of the teenager. This took just about 1 year of intensive work with the network and involved many people around the teenager, but a relationship with her slowly developed. Only the social worker had contact with her; he talked to her mainly through her bedroom door or just sat outside the door speaking to her, and sometimes just speaking his mind aloud, trying to mentalize what she might be feeling. After a while, he insisted on the girl showing herself because the psychiatrist needed to know more about her physical state. The psychiatrist described to the social worker what he should be aware of—the colour of her skin, aspects of her appearance, and so on. The social worker was able only to stand at the door and see the girl sitting on her bed with a blanket over her head—but this was enough to make the psychiatrist feel safe enough to let the plan continue. The team was trying very hard to avoid being forced to admit the girl to the inpatient unit against her will, because they feared that would re-traumatize the girl and undermine the efforts towards having the girl 'come to us' of her own will.

When the mother left the house, she sometimes found on her return that food was missing, and the keyworker noticed that the girl was very slowly starting to look healthier when he caught a glimpse of her. The team used this knowledge to plan the mother leaving the house at certain times and making sure certain foods were available. The keyworker never confronted the teenager but enabled her own progress as planned—all in due time, and sometimes with a step backwards, but always coordinated and reflected upon with the MCM. The teenager slowly started to taste the flavours of life again and gained weight. A spark was ignited and passed on by the MCM to the keyworker, to the mother, and to the teenager.

The keyworker had a hard time enduring the slow progress and was eager to show he was worth his money. He asked for supervision himself and felt this had to be outside of the team/network around the teenager. The MCM was uncertain about adding more people to the network or more factors to the equation but, with help from his team, he decided to accept this need provided the social worker shared with the team the main themes of the individual supervisions—which he did, because he knew he needed the backing and coordination of the team. The MCM was insecure about how the external supervision could affect the management of the whole case and had often in his experience met people naming experts in other parts of the country who they claimed could definitely 'solve' a case. This insecurity was shared and, based on trust within the network, which was again frequently examined with the NET-Aim-Q, he balanced the different aspects of the matter. The MCM gained security in his team and shared the existential dilemmas apparent in the case. The team was well connected and safe enough to explore the case, in resonance and in parallel with the teenager's exploration of the world outside her bedroom. In truth, none of us is in charge of life or death, but sharing the acknowledgement of this instead of pretending to be right supported the helping system and brought about a more authentic dynamic, a humanistic outlook, and common grounds for action—we all wanted to help with whatever we had to help with. We were all connected. We were ready to step in the whole time and take appropriate action if the teenager's physical condition deteriorated further. That was an intoxicating feeling!

The girl apparently left her bedroom more and more when no one else was at home, and her mother reported that more food was disappearing. The mother met her former husband in public one day by coincidence, and the experience was not as frightening as she had expected. Somehow—none of us never really knew how—the girl started to visit her grandfather when her mother went out. He succeeded in inviting her to join a fishing trip at one point. This was revealed at a network meeting, which took place after the municipality had changed its case manager in charge. The municipality wondered why the teenager could not attend school if she could go fishing, and why they had to continue paying the freelance social worker (keyworker) when the teenager was no longer threatened in the same manner. The municipality decided to terminate the arrangement with the keyworker and instead use a social worker employed by the municipality, and they decided to plan for the girl to be enrolled in a school where this social worker worked during the day. The network became anxious about these plans, but the MCM saw the opportunity to carry this on his shoulders and hosted meetings where he, supported by his backup team and the psychiatrist, explained that the time could be right to demand something from first the mother and then the teenager. He argued that the system was secure enough and that the 'push out of the nest' was inevitable eventually, and he chose to support the municipality, despite his own worries about the timing, being very well aware of the limitations in the public healthcare system for economic reasons.

The keyworker was able to draw confidence from extensive experience in complex cases from inpatient wards, milieu therapy, and the AMBIT framework, but doubt was always there and so was the fear of things going badly wrong with the whole case. The mother luckily supported the plan because she was afraid of having no help at all, and she was probably now more psychologically and socially ready for the changes to come, both for her and for her daughter. The teenager was involved in the plan and its 'take-it-or-leave-it' character, and, after a short while, via the new social worker, agreed from one day to the next to go to the new school if the social worker promised to be there with her. The social worker went with her to and from school.

We had to creatively interpret a couple of standard treatment packages and clinical guidelines along the way in this case. We had to bend the rules of visitation to the child and adolescent psychiatric unit and the general hospital somewhat. We had to carry the insecurity of taking responsibility for a severely underweight girl, without having access to a full understanding of her physical state. We had to take more time than the current official system offered us (and fight for extensions along the way), and we had not followed procedure in evaluating the teenager in time for correct registration in our medical records. However, we used all of our professionalism. We collaborated with all parts of the helping system and integrated the different parts of it. We timed our interventions according to the teenager (as best we knew) and we took every chance we were given to find out what could be helpful to the teenager and her family. We did all this by using our experience, being curious, being professional, and referring to AMBIT as a model for understanding and entering the messy, delicate, complex thrill of a teenager's life. It was an individualized one-shot operation where we made mistakes and learned new moves along the way.

We succeeded. The teenager is now thriving and going to school, and she is healthy. To this day we may not be able to define her potential mental illness—although we can certainly think of many possible diagnoses—but by the time we got around to it, she was doing so well that there was no need. We will leave it to the reader to evaluate whether this approach is careless or in fact the very essence of care. Was there a clash of the New Public Management and the VBM paradigms? A clinician's most important task is, in our view, to be professional, regardless of whether they serve one or the other of these political systems.

The teenager's affect (hopelessness) became the tone we could try to resonate with, and we tried to make the system resonate along with us, containing this affect and trying to build up hope along the way. This was not an easy task at all, and it was impossible to undertake it without getting stuck, making mistakes, arguing about what was whose responsibility, being scared of losing the teenager, and being frustrated with the team and each other at moments. However, everyone dared to enter the unknown territory of the case, trusting that everyone in the helping system actually intended to help and that no one would leave anyone behind, and respecting the knowledge of every person contributing. The MCM supported the keyworker, the team, and the network, accepted his own lack of knowledge, and accepted learning from others as he went along. In our understanding, this was an AMBIT case. This is just one case out of many in our clinic that needed this kind of effort—which was possible only because of our ability to differentiate, individualize, and be socially mobile within the safety that is still provided by parts of the Flexicurity system.

10.10 Implications

The authors have highlighted the contexts that have shaped their thinking in the application of the AMBIT approach to their work—that of their national healthcare system and that of diverse philosophical, literary, and sociological discourses relevant to making sense of the needs and life experiences of clients who stand in the gaps between existing parts of our social world. In our original descriptions of AMBIT we simply called this the 'Tower of Babel', reflecting what some of the complexity of discourses between different parts of the mental health and care system might be like for clients. In this chapter, Janne and Stefan have insisted that the process of moving towards greater collective and network care must address both pragmatic care issues and also the need to embrace discourses outside traditional psychiatric or psychological frameworks as well as the legal frameworks to which professionals are accountable. However, they have done more than that. By introducing the idea of an MCM, they invested in a collective approach that included a recognition that the states of minds of all those involved was a legitimate and crucial aspect of how help was provided. Their respectful, transparent, and profoundly honest narrative provides an inspiring illustration of what can be achieved when sufficient trust is created between those faced with such intractable difficulties. They have also held a balance between the philosophical and the scientific by embracing the need to use measurement to help support both change and curiosity. The turbulence in the network was steadied by the gentle heartbeat of measurement, of being willing to evaluate the experience of others in working across the network and explicitly making this evaluation part of their method.

Commonly, we describe in AMBIT the importance of enabling team and frontline workers to recognize, support, and accept the place of anxiety as part of the work that they do rather than an indication that things are not going to plan. AMBIT starts with the premise that cases rarely, if ever, go to plan. In the case example described in this chapter, the team recognized anxiety but also showed courage. This is both a feeling and a type of language that mental health teams rarely discuss. With the sort of encouragement that AMBIT provides, teams can begin to reposition anxiety as a 'friend that lives here' rather than a 'threat that lurks outside the door'. Courage is rarely recognized, but it takes courage to contain the anxiety of enabling a profoundly troubled young person to retain control of her life and to find her own way of recovery. The 'treatment' in this case was to not treat, to not take control, and to not insist on removal and assertive care. The proposal of creating the role of a MCM illustrates that taking a position of courage is not an indication of someone discovering a personal attribute but is about creating the conditions in which relational courage could be sustained, that is, that the courage lies in the relationships that are needed to do this work.

References

Ackoff, R. L. (1974). *Redesigning the future: A systems approach to societal problems.* John Wiley & Sons.

Bevington, D., & Fuggle, P. (2012). Supporting and enhancing mentalization in community outreach teams working with hard-to-reach youth: The AMBIT approach. In N. Midgley & I. Vrouva (Eds.), *Minding the child: Mentalization-based interventions with children, young people and their families* (pp. 163–186). Routledge.

Bevington, D., Fuggle, P., Cracknell, L., & Fonagy, P. (2017). *Adaptive mentalization-based integrative treatment: A guide for teams to develop systems of care.* Oxford University Press.

Conklin, J. (2006). *Dialogue mapping: Building shared understanding of wicked problems.* Wiley.

Dykstra, J. A. (2019). Forget 'culture'—focus on operating system instead. *Medium*, 9 August. https://medium.com/culturati/forget-culture-focus-on-operating-system-instead-61d547a34d81

Hansen, F. T. (2018). *At møde verden med undren.* Hans Reitzel Forlag.

Luyten, P., Campbell, C., Allison, E., & Fonagy, P. (2020). The mentalizing approach to psychopathology: State of the art and future directions. *Annual Review of Clinical Psychology, 16,* 297–325. https://doi.org/10.1146/annurev-clinpsy-071919-015355

MacKenzie, K. R. (1983). The clinical application of group measure. In R. R. Dies & K. R. MacKenzie (Eds.), *Advances in group psychotherapy: Integrating research and practice* (pp. 159–170). International Universities Press.

Menon, A., Charumilind, S., Lamb, J., Grahame, J., & Nuzum, D. (2019). *Maximizing the 'value' in value networks and value-based payment*. McKinsey & Company. https://www.mckinsey.com/industries/healthcare-systems-and-services/our-insights/maximizing-the-value-in-value-networks-and-value-based-payment

Mikkelsen, K., & Martin, R. (2016). *The neo-generalist: Where you go is who you are*. LID Publishing.

Porter, M. E., & Lee, T. H. (2013). The strategy that will fix health care. *Harvard Business Review*, October. https://hbr.org/2013/10/the-strategy-that-will-fix-health-care

Prescott, D. S., Maeschalck, C. L., & Miller, S. D. (2017). *Feedback-informed treatment in clinical practice: Reaching for excellence*. American Psychological Association.

Rittel, H. W. J., & Webber, M. M. (1973). Dilemmas in a general theory of planning. *Policy Sciences*, *4*(2), 155–169. https://doi.org/10.1007/bf01405730

Rosa, H. (2019). *Resonance: A sociology of our relationship to the world* (J. C. Wagner, Trans.). Polity Press.

Skårderud, F., & Sommerfeldt, B. (2013). *Miljøterapiboken: Mentalisering som holdning og handling (MBT-M)*. Gyldendal Akademisk.

Stern, D. N. (2010). *Forms of vitality: Exploring dynamic experience in psychology and the arts*. Oxford University Press.

Wampold, B. E. (2015). How important are the common factors in psychotherapy? An update. *World Psychiatry*, *14*(3), 270–277. https://doi.org/10.1002/wps.20238

11
Applying AMBIT to teacher training
Innovations in Germany

Andrea Dlugosch and Melanie Henter

11.1 Setting the scene

This chapter is a very welcome inclusion in the book, as it describes the work of two colleagues from Germany who came to an AMBIT Train the Trainer course with the intention of integrating AMBIT into their modules on a master's degree course for trainee teachers of young people with special educational needs. Not only was the application of AMBIT to a special educational setting new to us at the time Andrea and Melanie attended their AMBIT training; it is also, to our knowledge, one of the first examples of AMBIT being integrated into a core professional training course.

The application of AMBIT to educational settings makes great sense to us, given that education is one of the few 'services' accessed universally by the vast majority of young people, including the subgroup for whom AMBIT was originally designed. Lastly, this chapter also offers an account of the authors' experience of sharing AMBIT with others, following their attendance at an AMBIT: Local Facilitator Training (previously known as AMBIT Train the Trainer) course. Many teams choose this as their method of disseminating AMBIT, but it is rare that there is the opportunity for learning from this process to be captured and shared between teams. It is pleasing to read that Andrea and Melanie's approach to sharing AMBIT with their students has much in common with the ideas outlined in Chapter 12 about how we deliver AMBIT training, in terms of their efforts to offer their students an experience of AMBIT through the design and facilitation of their modules. There are valuable insights not only into the experience of the trainers in facilitating these modules, but also into the responses of the student teachers to this training process. How these responses are considered and managed by Andrea and Melanie are helpful illustrations of AMBIT's adaptive nature in action.

11.2 Introduction

In this chapter we will share our experiences of developing and facilitating an AMBIT-influenced seminar series for student teachers of pupils with special educational needs, as part of their master's degree qualification. We will start by describing why we felt that an AMBIT-influenced approach would be useful, before moving on to share how we designed the seminars, what it was like for the student teachers to implement AMBIT ideas in their work, and, finally, our reflections on the process of working with student teachers in this way.

11.3 The needs of young people in special education settings

The educational experiences of young people with multiple needs (which includes those with special educational needs) are often characterized by significant struggles, including difficulties in managing the academic, relational, behavioural, social, and emotional demands of school settings. Although some schools may have the resources, skills, and flexibility to be able to adapt to these needs, many do not, often resulting in escalating patterns of conflict between young people, their families, and the school; absenteeism; and, in the worst-case circumstances, the young person's permanent exclusion from mainstream education. A 2017 report by the Institute of Public Policy Research in the UK highlighted the scale of this problem, with some 50,000 pupils in England reported to attend an alternative provision for excluded young people (Gill, 2017). These young people were found to be among the most vulnerable in society, with a high proportion having poor outcomes beyond their school years, in terms of experiencing mental health difficulties and being at risk of entering the criminal justice system. The report also highlighted the struggles of school staff and leaders in responding effectively to these young people's needs, with 50% of headteachers reporting that their staff do not feel equipped to identify and address these needs without further specialist input, which 75% of teachers then reported difficulties accessing from external agencies. These bleak findings highlight the pressing need for schools to feel more equipped and supported in their efforts to help these pupils to remain within an educational environment that can adapt to their range of needs. Similar results of qualitative and quantitative research are also being discussed in Germany (Baumann, 2019; Tornow et al., 2012).

11.4 Introducing the pilot project: 'Mentalization-based support for teachers'

The pilot project 'Mentalization-based support for teachers'[1] was instituted in the summer semester of 2018 at the Institute of Special Needs Education at the University

---

[1] We thank the (former) students (Tina Christmann, Laura-Sophie Cronjäger, Debora Gamer, Constanze Geis, Lucca Kisters, Marius Kutscher, Johanna Meller, Anne Ortmann, David Piehl, Lena Rey,

of Koblenz-Landau, Germany, by the AMBIT Local Facilitators[2] Prof. Dr Andrea Dlugosch and Dipl. Päd. Melanie Henter. The aim was to integrate AMBIT-oriented, and thus mentalization-based, elements into the course of study for student teachers of special needs education. The project took the form of a weekly seminar, facilitated by the two authors, for 15 master's degree students, which lasted for two semesters. The students were asked to enter into pedagogical learning and mentoring with a child or adolescent for at least one academic year in parallel to the seminars. In this chapter, we will share how we designed this weekly seminar and our reflections from facilitating it. To help set the context for our work, we will begin by sharing some details about the German teacher training system and the stress levels reported by those in the teaching profession.

11.5 Teacher training and stress levels in Germany

In Germany, teacher training is initially structured in two phases: university studies and then an induction programme, which starts after graduation from university but before the actual teaching career begins. It has a duration of approximately 2 years. During the second phase, the teachers begin to work in schools, where they gradually start to teach. At the same time, they attend weekly courses at seminar schools that emphasize general and subject-specific methods of teaching (Cortina & Thames, 2013; Karing & Beelmann, 2019).

The perception of stress by prospective teachers during the second phase of teacher training, as well as by fully qualified teachers who are in regular work, is particularly high compared with other social occupational groups (Abele & Candova, 2007; Rauin, 2007; Römer et al., 2012). Interventions aimed at addressing the problem of teacher stress have tended to focus on individual stress management strategies, such as mindfulness (Karing & Beelmann, 2019) and multimodal stress management training (Karing & Beelmann, 2016), and have produced only marginal improvements in emotional exhaustion in trainee teachers. Overall, these interventions tended to result in enriched *knowledge* of the topic of stress and how to manage it, but without any meaningful accompanying changes in teachers' *behaviour* in terms of their use of this knowledge (Henter & Dlugosch, 2018).

The findings point to the relevance of mentalization-based approaches for prospective teachers and trainee teachers (Dlugosch & Henter, 2020; Gingelmaier &

Nadine Schmidt, Oliver Seibert, Sabrina Spies, Natascha Stroot, and Vanessa Theobald) for their productive cooperation in the pilot project, and Ms Elena Müller for her support in writing this chapter.

² The AMBIT: Local Facilitator Training was completed by Andrea Dlugosch and Melanie Henter in 2017 at the Anna Freud Centre in London with Laura Talbot and Rebecca Smith. In addition, Melanie Henter accompanied a team to London in July 2018, which completed an AMBIT: Local Facilitator Training with Dr Dickon Bevington and Dr Mark Dangerfield.

Schwarzer, 2019; Henter & Dlugosch, 2018), not least because of the persistence of stress far beyond the induction programme phase (Abele & Candova, 2007; Rauin, 2007). Our pilot project was based on the premise that mentalizing serves, among other things, to (re)create the ability to work in (special) educational fields of work (Dlugosch & Henter, 2020; Henter & Dlugosch, 2018; Kirsch, 2018). In addition, the ability to mentalize is important in the pedagogical work of student teachers with children and adolescents and is relevant to supporting the student teachers' future work in the context of learning and behavioural difficulties, because increased emotional stress is to be expected there too (Dlugosch & Henter, 2020; Gingelmaier & Schwarzer, 2019).

11.6 Using Active Planning to design the seminars

We used an *Active Planning* approach to develop our seminars. This means that we did not decide all of the curriculum and content in advance, but left some aspects open so that we could work with what the students told us they needed. We had some ideas about what might be helpful to them based on our own experience of the education field, but we wanted to make sure that we could also adapt to the strengths, personalities, needs, and ideas of this particular student group. To help us with this, we adapted one of the exercises that is used during the AMBIT Consultation Day and did a card-based activity, which we called 'If training was useful …?' to invite the student teachers to tell us what they felt they needed.

11.6.1 Sensitive attunement—understanding the needs of the student teachers

By doing this card-based activity, we learned a lot about what the student teachers needed. The student teachers were supporting a number of pupils who had complex needs, including mental health needs and special educational needs. They told us that they imagined that working with these pupils would involve often being in conflict with them and their families. They had an understandable worry about progressing from being student teachers to qualified teachers and having to teach a class on their own. They worried about being on their own in front of the whole class and not knowing what to do if there was a problem with a pupil. They wanted to be given a 'toolbox' to help them when they got into difficulties with the pupils and their families, particularly to help them manage behaviour and the 'big emotions' that they imagined they might be confronted with in the pupils and their families.

The student teachers also wanted a space with us to talk about real examples of problems that they were having in their mentoring work and to get some practical help with these problems. Generally, they wanted us to help them 'have a better time with the pupils' but did not have concrete ideas about what this help might look like.

11.6.2 Broadcasting intentions—sharing our own ideas about what might help

In terms of the quadrants of the AMBIT wheel, we noticed that the students were mainly focused on getting help with the *Client* area of their work. It made sense to us that the students were very focused on the pupils and 'what might go wrong' at this early point of their teaching careers, as this is often a time of high anxiety and low confidence for any new professional. In terms of the teachers' ideas about what might help them with the pupils, for us it was not only about them having a toolbox of strategies, but also about helping them to hold a mentalizing stance in their work. This was important to us because we wanted to change their point of view from believing that the solution to a problem is always to immediately *do* something; instead, we wanted to help them see the value in taking time to *understand* behaviour, rather than to immediately respond to it without any reflection on what might be going on. Of course, for a teacher in a classroom it is important to be able to respond quickly sometimes, but we hoped that by sharing a combination of tools and the mentalizing stance, the student teachers might be able to hold a more helpful balance between *doing* and *thinking* in their work with pupils.

We also wanted to help the student teachers zoom out and see the bigger picture, that is, the broader context of their work, which for us included focusing on aspects of team and network functioning. If we were to mentalize the student teachers, it made sense to us that they may not yet be able to recognize these areas as important, given their limited experience of being in a teaching environment. However, in terms of the relevance of a *Network* focus, the student teachers who did have more experience of working in schools spoke of problems that they had noticed in relationships between school staff, external professionals, and the families of particular pupils. This fitted with our idea that it would be helpful for the teachers to be able to apply a mentalizing stance to understanding people in the network around the pupil, as well as having some tools to help them strengthen and improve collaboration in these relationships.

In terms of focusing on the *Team*, we recognize how isolated teachers can be in their roles; they spend so much of their time with their pupils and not much time with other colleagues. If they have a dilemma, there are not many opportunities for help-seeking from colleagues, and when this does happen, it is usually by chance and not necessarily in a planned or structured way, which means that it may not always result in a clear plan. Through our seminars, we wanted to help the student teachers have an experience of being part of a small team of other student teachers, who could work together to help each other with the dilemmas they encountered in their work. We hoped that this might help them to see the value of team support for teachers and to give them ideas about ways that they might develop help-seeking processes for teachers in their schools.

11.6.3 Setting the plan

We used a combination of the student teachers' ideas and our own ideas to set the plan for the seminars, which had several key aims. In the spirit of Active Planning being a dynamic process, we checked in with the students throughout the semester, by asking them 'Is this right? Is this still what you need?', so that we could make sure we were still responding to their needs and could adapt to anything new or different that they thought was relevant. The aim was to achieve a 'dynamic balance'[3] between the individual, the group, the content, and the surrounding conditions, as well as between the cognitive and affective components of mentalizing, and between reflection and action. To summarize, the broad themes of the seminars were to help the student teachers with:

- Taking a mentalizing approach to the work in general (e.g. less focus just on behaviour and on 'fixing' or being solution-focused)
- Understanding the importance of developing epistemic trust in relationships with pupils
- Thinking as a team: having reflective tools to help them explore dilemmas in their work
- Mentalizing networks—the importance of understanding and strengthening the relationships around the pupil.

More detail on the curriculum is provided in Table 11.1.

We used several different methods and processes to facilitate the seminars. First, we wanted the course to be *experiential*, to make sure that the student teachers did not just know about mentalizing but knew how to use it in their work, too. We thought about how we could *model the mentalizing stance* in front of the students ourselves, by making transparent what we were thinking and why, and showing how we were changing what we thought and did because of what we came to understand about their needs, which was a continual process. We reflected that it had been useful for us when learning about AMBIT ourselves to have an experience of the trainers working with us in this way, rather than us just being passive recipients of the AMBIT training content.

---

[3] 'The term 'dynamic balance' contains both a *figure of thought* as well as a concrete *instruction* for leadership. 'Dynamic balance is a very general life concept: the necessity of including opposite poles in life [. . .]. Life is characterized not by static states, but by our being exposed to constant reorientation. The idea of dynamic balance is one way of demonstrating how to favor living learning/teaching and a vibrant life (Farau & Cohn, 1984, pp. 353f.)' (Spielmann, 2017, p. 131, emphasis added).

Table 11.1 Outline of the curriculum

Title of the session	Topics/contents/instruments included in the session
Introduction to mentalization-based support	• *'My personal comfort zone'* (What makes you/me/us upset?) • Meta-level: 'How did I experience the exercise?' 'How did I feel?' ('How was it to be assessed and to assess the other person?') • *ACS* (German version of the revised Attributional Complexity Scale) (Fletcher et al., 1986) • What does 'mentalizing' mean? (Mind map)
Introduction to thinking as a team	• *Four-Player Model* (Kantor, 2012): team exercise • Getting to know the cooperation partner, contracting and beginning the learning mentoring
Understanding mentalizing and stress	• *RFQ* (Reflective Functioning Questionnaire) (Fonagy et al., 2016) • 'Me with you', 'Me with myself', 'Me with you' (as a reflective introduction) • *Role play*: mentalizing and stress in your own educational practice • Additional input: 'Biobehavioural switch model of the relationship between stress and controlled versus automatic mentalizing' (Luyten et al., 2019)
Practising mentalizing myself	• *MASC* (Movie for the Assessment of Social Cognition) (Dziobek et al., 2006) • *Letter to myself*: 'My personal goals, wishes, plans for the next year' (during the course of the year, the lecturers send the sealed envelopes to the students)
Mentalizing tools to support reflection	• *Thinking Together* (Bevington et al., 2017) with regard to selected learning mentorings or challenging situations that were discussed in the previous sessions • Additional input: *RFS* (Reflective Functioning Scale) (Fonagy et al., 1998) and prementalizing modes
Understanding the students' needs	• If training was useful, how do we know? (Collection of cards[a])
Practising using Thinking Together	• Thinking Together—free(ze) style • Describing the case—practising 'Bare Bones' (Stop/freeze and rewind and continue—live) • Additional input: Opaqueness, Quick-Fixing
Mentalizing: what works?	• If training was useful, how do we know? • Excerpt from the video logbook of Dlugosch/Henter (critical reflection on the topic of 'mentalization-based support kit') • Mentalization-based collegial case counselling (reference: Client, Team, Network) • *ASEQ* (AMBIT Service Evaluation Questionnaire) (Bevington et al., 2017)
Mentalizing: what works? Tools and other helpful strategies … CLIENT, TEAM, NETWORKS, and ME	• *'Mentalizing during recess period?'* (How and where has this topic mattered to me during the last weeks?) • Input: *keyworker* (Bevington et al., 2017) • *Pro-Gram* (Bevington et al., 2017) from the perspective of the mentored child—is there a keyworker? • 'What could be possible problems in working with the networks?' • *Dis-integration grid* (Bevington et al., 2017) regarding the learning mentoring

(continued)

Table 11.1 Continued

Title of the session	Topics/contents/instruments included in the session
Reflecting as a GROUP	• Reflection on the videotaped mentalization-based collegial case counselling I • Additional input: *mentalizing stance* (Bevington et al., 2017) • Reflection on the videotaped mentalization-based collegial case counselling II (video) + template mentalizing stance—'Stop and rewind'
We develop assistance for mentalizing for me and others	• 'I express my attitude'—my partner verbalizes this attitude • *Mentalizing myself*: helpful questions for my pedagogical everyday life considering the *mentalizing stance*
Mentalizing in concrete terms	• Group 1: *Thinking Together* and *Trigger Analysis* (Scherwath & Friedrich, 2012) • Group 2: encouraging mentalizing by your partner while taking age, material, and the mentalizing stance into account
One year of mentalization-based support—coming to an end in a good way	• *Mentalization-based collegial case counselling review*: 'Something that I want to take with me'/'Something that I want to leave here'/'Something that I still want to remember 5 years from now' • If training was useful, how do we know? (What did we do in terms of content?) • *APrAT* (AMBIT Practice Audit Tool) (Bevington et al., 2017)

[a] The cards hung visibly on the wall for the entire time. They were used repeatedly during the course of the entire project to check whether one's own concerns had been taken into account, had changed, and/or if a new one had been added.

Second, we used *video logbooks* as a key tool to support learning and reflection. The video logbooks were recordings of the student teachers reflecting together on their mentoring experiences in smaller groups (teams of three), using some of the mentalizing tools. We reviewed the video logbooks as a whole group to highlight examples of mentalizing and non-mentalizing in action. Video logbooks were also used by us as seminar leaders to record our own reflections on the seminar process.

11.7 Reflections on the seminars

In the following section, we describe some of the different aspects of our seminar work with the student teachers. We have included descriptions of what we did together, as well as how the student teachers responded and our reflections on this. We have grouped the descriptions according to different themes.

11.7.1 Using the mentalizing stance and AMBIT tools in team discussions about pupils

A core part of the seminars was supporting the students to reflect on their work as teachers and to get help from their peers with dilemmas that they encountered in the mentoring work that they were all doing with individual pupils alongside the seminars. We noticed patterns in how the teachers talked about and tried to help each other with their mentoring experiences. Typically, their descriptions were long and detailed, often with a focus on seeking out strategies and tools to help them manage the behaviour of their pupils. Group discussion quickly moved into problem-solving and offering solutions, and there was a notable absence of attempts to try to understand more about mental states in self or other (i.e. what might be going on in their own minds as mentors/teachers and in the minds of their mentees or others in the network) to inform their ideas about what might help.

We introduced mentalization-based tools to the students to try to support richer discussion and reflection on their work. As part of this, it was important to us that the student teachers developed a greater awareness of both the emotional impact of their work on them as individuals and how this might be influencing the way they thought about and related to the pupils and their network. We introduced 'Thinking Together' (described in Chapter 2) to help the students reflect on their mentoring work. The video logbooks helped us to understand in more detail how they were implementing this process. Here, we share an example of one group's experience of learning how to use the Thinking Together tool as a group (Box 11.1) to help them with their work. For us, it is an interesting example that highlights the shift in thinking that we were trying to support the student teachers to make, as well as how challenging it is for the students to change their usual patterns of talking and thinking about their work.

11.7.1.1 Vignette—helping a child who is persistently late

A group of students used Thinking Together to discuss 'Anna's' dilemma relating to a child who was persistently late. The group was able to support Anna to use the first two steps of Thinking Together adequately, in terms of her 'Marking the Task' for the discussion (getting help with this child's persistent lateness) and 'Stating the Case'. However, the next step, 'Mentalizing the Moment', in which Anna should have been supported to reflect upon her own thoughts and feelings in relation to the dilemma

---

Box 11.1 Group Thinking Together—a brief reminder

1. *Mark the Task*—the worker is helped to identify a specific task that they want help with from the group.
2. *State the Case*—the worker briefly shares the information that is relevant to the task.
3. *Mentalize the Moment*—the worker bringing the dilemma is mentalized by the group, before being supported to mentalize others involved in the dilemma (e.g. the client, people in the network).
4. *Return to Purpose*—the worker is invited to consider any ideas they have in relation to their dilemma; others in the group can also contribute ideas.

before thinking about those of other key people, was skipped altogether in the process. One of the students commented, 'I think it would be strange to be talking about your feelings ... now', which others in the group unanimously agreed with. The fourth step, 'Returning to Purpose' (where a plan of action is made), occupied a much larger proportion of the entire process. During this step, members of the group began advising Anna on what to do to ensure that the child does not arrive late any more. The dialogue was strongly oriented towards solutions and behaviour management in terms of trying to find a 'fix' for the pupil. Because Mentalizing the Moment was skipped, the mental (emotional) state of the case introducer and the child took a back seat and were not explicitly acknowledged. However, it seemed to us that Anna's feelings were not altogether absent from the process; rather, they appeared to have been picked up by the group in a less conscious way and played out by the discussion taking on an accusatory and punitive tone, which was directed towards the child, in the generation of solutions. For example, one group member advised Anna that she would not ignore the fact that the child is late but would keep bringing it up with the child and asking them why they are always late. She also advised Anna to tell the child directly how his persistent lateness is making her feel and to involve the head of the school, who should inform the parents that they have to make sure their child is punctual. Even when contextual information regarding the family circumstances was offered by Anna that might begin to make sense of the pupil's behaviour (relating to a family bereavement), this was not picked up by the group in the dialogue that followed.

It seemed that the students' thinking was characterized by non-mentalizing modes (teleological, psychic equivalence, and pretend mode), with a sense that supposedly a few quick actions are needed to 'solve the case' (Kotte & Taubner, 2016). Even when invited explicitly by the Thinking Together process to stop and take time to mentalize, this did not happen, with the students explicitly stating that they did not see the relevance of doing this or feel comfortable to do so. The consequences of skipping this step are clear in the quality of the planning that follows in the Return to Purpose; very little had been understood about the child and the suggestions generated by the group continued to focus on 'managing' the child's behaviour, rather than being any closer to understanding it. Although it is easy to imagine that perhaps the group's suggestions came from a place of wanting to ensure that the child attends school on time (which will no doubt benefit his learning), they did not help Anna to broaden her thinking to consider all the factors that might be relevant. As a result, the approach the group suggested Anna should take seems unlikely to help the child feel sufficiently recognized or understood enough by Anna in a way that might lead to a change in his behaviour.

11.7.1.2 Conclusion to section

The student teachers' desire to quickly solve a 'problem behaviour' shown by their pupils was very understandable for us but also made us feel a bit helpless too when we talked about it in our own video logbooks, especially because it was also very present in other students' video logbooks as well as in the seminar itself. Because of this, we had a lot of reflections with the student teachers on this desire to problem-solve.

This helped us to understand it much more from their perspective. Therefore, we tried to 'hold the balance' between the student teachers' desire to have a 'toolbox' to solve problems and our desire to focus on mental states as a way of making sense of behaviour. In order to be able to take both into account, we developed a process of mentalization-based collegial case counselling, which tries to combine solution orientation (i.e. the 'toolbox') and an understanding of the mental states (especially of the colleague who brings the case) with more steps of 'mentalizing the moment' (Thinking Together).

11.7.2 Developing mentalization-based collegial case counselling

We already had an existing method for having more in-depth case discussions about pupils, known as collegial case counselling. In the course of the pilot project, a form of collegial case counselling (Dlugosch, 2006, 2008), which had already been implemented in the course of studies, was taken up again and modified with elements of mentalizing. Collegial case counselling is used in the education field as a method for generating solutions to problems. It consists of a series of questions that a group works through together to help understand and solve an identified problem (as outlined in Box 11.2). This format allows for longer and more in-depth discussions than a typical Thinking Together conversation.

The previous form of collegial case counselling (Dlugosch, 2006, 2008) implicitly referred to different aspects of mentalizing in different phases, but we felt that it could be strengthened, as group conversations could still become focused on sharing or seeking information about the case or prematurely coming up with solutions. To make mentalizing a more explicit focus, two additional steps were added, phase 3 and phase 6. In phase 3, the activity of 'Wearing different hats' was added; this is an exercise from AMBIT training in which people are asked to consider and share aloud what it might be like to be in the position of different people in a network. Similar to the third step of 'Thinking Together', this ensures a closer connection to the affective and cognitive experience of the different people involved in the case and may open up different perspectives for making sense of their behaviour. This is useful in helping to question assumptions that might have been made about others (e.g. moving out of psychic equivalence mode) and helping the group to avoid generating solutions that are based on only one perspective. The addition of phase 6, 'Search for connections', also aimed to counteract a regression (Kotte & Taubner, 2016) to the psychic equivalence (certainty) and teleological (quick-fix) modes by explicitly encouraging the student teachers to form different hypotheses that might help make sense of the behaviour of those involved, before coming up with plans. Overall, the addition of these steps aimed to strengthen the mentalizing attitude of the group and the case introducer, both with regard to the dilemma being discussed and in relation to their own work.

Box 11.2 Procedure of mentalization-based collegial case counselling

A moderator introduces the session and acts as the chair.

Phase 1. Case selection from the group:
- Who has a concern, from a professional educational field with a child or adolescent?
- Consider prioritizing by urgency in case of several case requests.

Phase 2. Case description given by the case introducer (5–10 minutes):
- Presentation should be as concrete and uncensored as possible.
- What is the case introducer's question? ('I would like to ...').
- Moderator repeats/concretizes the question, if needed.

Phase 3. 'Wearing different hats' (5–10 minutes)—a group discussion without the case introducer (who sits outside the circle):
1. What might the case introducer be *feeling* and *thinking*?
2. What might the child be *feeling* and *thinking*?
3. Other relevant people: for example, what might the teacher be thinking and feeling? What might the headteacher be thinking and feeling? What might the parent be thinking and feeling?

Phase 4. Checking back for resonance with the case introducer (2 minutes):
- For example, where was there resonance for me? What did I not agree with?

Phase 5. Factual questions from the group (maximum 10 minutes):
- Opportunity for the group to ask for information, data, facts. Who? When? What? ...

Phase 6. Search for connections (10–15 minutes):
- Different explanatory models are explored (including mentalization-based connections) to help understand the dilemma.

Phase 7. Check back for resonance with the case introducer (5 minutes):
- Case introducer names what seems plausible and understandable, what has been added, and what has opened up a different perspective from listening to the group.

Phase 8. Possible gathering of resources and ideas (5 minutes)—group discussion:
- 'If I was the case introducer I would ...' (each colleague is allowed to share one sentence, without any additional explanation).

Phase 9. Reaction of the case introducer (2 minutes):
- What could I imagine trying out, addressing, initiating...?

Phase 10. Reflecting as a whole group (5–10 minutes) (moving away from the case):
- What was the process of the case consultation like for me? How was I involved?

Or:
- To what extent was I reminded of one of my own cases?

ALWAYS. Closing words from the case introducer (2 minutes):
- In order that the case introducer can move on from the case consultation, any closing thoughts.

What follows is an excerpt from the video logbook transcript of the group attempting the 'Wearing different hats' exercise as part of phase 3 of the collegial case counselling. The moderator has invited the group to mentalize the student teacher, who, as the case introducer, has brought the dilemma of how best to support a particularly disruptive student in the classroom. Compared with the previously described video logbooks, it is clear from this excerpt that the group has moved forward in their willingness to tolerate a focus on states of mind. They are able to draw imaginatively on their own experience as student teachers to think about what it might be like to be in the shoes of the case introducer in relation to this dilemma.

[0:05:24] HANNAH (MODERATOR): Okay ... good ... Then let's just ... do a round. Everybody speak from your perspective first [addressing the case introducer] about what kind of feelings this triggers in them. Whatever comes to mind. Who wants to start [looks around]?

[0:05:48] NORA: Hmm, well, I can start. I think it's particularly at the beginning of the internship or in general, when it's so difficult. If you say, well, I'm not getting anywhere, I'm overwhelmed right now. And yes, I can imagine that you simply didn't feel good about it ... I wouldn't have felt good either.

[0:06:17] VANESSA: I think I'd just be annoyed in that situation because you're trying to calm the class. And you have prepared what you are going to do now for a long time. And ... yes, you think about how the children will react beforehand. And if that doesn't work, or if there's a troublemaker in there, I think I'd mainly be annoyed and frustrated.

[0:06:44] JULIA: I would also have been annoyed in the first place. But also a bit helpless, because you notice, well, when I notice, no matter what you do, it has no effect and does not work. And then I can imagine that the pupils are screaming, why is he allowed to run around and I am not. So that is ... difficult indeed.

[0:07:04] ANNA: Well, I would have felt uncomfortable as well, because I don't know either what I would have done in that situation. But also with a spark of helplessness. Of course, also at the beginning of the … career as a teacher, the uncertainties … So when I let it show, because I notice that I am becoming insecure, it makes me even more nervous. So I would have felt nervous and also … helpless.

These reflections offer a rich account of what it might be like to a student teacher, new to the profession and confronted with supporting students who, for a range of reasons, may struggle in the classroom.

11.7.2.1 Conclusion to section

After the students had these kind of mentalizing discussions as part of the mentalization-based collegial case counselling, we had a lot of reflections on this process with the students to learn more about whether it was helpful and how. An important experience for the students was not to be alone with their feelings of helplessness, which seemed to arise when they did not know how to manage a difficult situation 'correctly'. Feeling mentalized by other student colleagues seemed to be a powerful experience that helped to recover the case introducer's own mentalizing, which had been lost due to high levels of stress (e.g. being new to the profession, being alone with the pupils, feeling a pressure to know how to act). Another important reflection from the student teachers was that taking a mentalizing stance took a lot of practice, because they were more accustomed to trying to help students by giving them advice about how to work better. Therefore, our further intentions for the seminar were (a) to develop (together with the students) an idea of mentalizing cultures (in teams and institutions; see below), in which you are allowed to lose your own capacity to mentalize or to make mistakes; and (b) to think a bit more about other mentalizing techniques, which could help recover the capacity to mentalize.

11.7.3 Reviewing video logs using mentalizing techniques

It was our intention to facilitate the seminars using a mentalizing stance, to ensure that the way that we interacted with the students promoted their capacity to mentalize. The essence of mentalizing is sometimes described as 'seeing ourselves from the outside and others from the inside' (Bateman & Fonagy, 2016, p. 5). The use of video logs provided us with an opportunity to develop the student teachers' capacity to do this. The videotaped case consultations were reflected upon together with the lecturers in the seminar and the students were questioned about their mentalizing potential. To use an AMBIT analogy, watching themselves in the video logs enabled the student teachers to sit at the 'edge of the pond' and take a different perspective on themselves. When examples of mentalizing were noticed in the video log recordings (e.g. not-knowing stance, curiosity, perspective-taking), these were explored and affirmed to reinforce their ongoing use. To address non-mentalizing, we used a mentalization-based technique known as 'Stop, Rewind, Explore' (Bateman & Fonagy, 2016), which is designed for use when someone has lost mentalizing. The interaction is rewound (in this case, literally) to a point before mentalizing was lost and then explored slowly, moment by moment, to make sense of how the loss of mentalizing happened.

It was a new experience for the students to see themselves in this way. They noticed things about how they were impacted by the work and how they interacted as a group. They developed a greater awareness of when their thinking processes might be becoming clouded by certainty rather than curiosity. One very important observation was that they noticed that they were stronger at showing empathy towards the pupils than towards pupils' parents, to whom they were often far less compassionate. Observing themselves in this way helped the students to take a more mentalizing stance towards their pupils' parents in their work. Helping the students to hold the balance between the pupil's and the parent's perspective is something that we would work on addressing more proactively when we run these seminars again.

11.8 Overall reflections on the seminars

11.8.1 The student teachers' perspective

The student teachers told us that they really enjoyed this version of the course. Over time, they came to see how relevant many of the concepts were to their work. Mentalizing became a lens through which they could make sense of their work, rather than just a tool that they could sometimes use. They ended up liking mentalizing in a team.

They also talked about appreciating being part of a group that could help them think about their work; it was a trusted group, where it felt permissible to make and share mistakes. They liked the practical tools that they were introduced to, but they could also see how talking and thinking about their work in this trusted group supported them to do their work better. They enjoyed the interchange of sometimes being the person who was stuck and sometimes being the person who could provide help; both experiences enriched their learning about how to be an effective student teacher for students with additional needs. They commented that they would like to have had the group for a longer time to continue to get help with this.

11.8.2 The facilitators' perspective

We also kept a video logbook throughout the seminar series, to help us with planning and processing the seminars. There are some aspects of the seminars that we wish to keep the same when we run the seminar again:

- The AMBIT wheel as the basis for creating a mentalization-based orientation that does not focus only on the child.
- Sharing AMBIT tools (e.g. Thinking Together, dis-integration grid, Pro-Gram) and mentalizing stance.
- Requiring the work of the students in an educational institution parallel to the seminars.
- Using the 'If training was useful' cards to orient us to the needs of students and using this process to help us with Active Planning.
- Keeping a strong focus on the feelings associated with educational work.
- Using a variety of formats to support reflection (video logbooks of the students, video logbooks of the facilitators, and reflections on the mentalization-based collegial case counselling).

In the spirit of us attending to the *Learning at Work* quadrant of the AMBIT wheel, we want to continuously learn from and improve our seminar offer. There are several other reflections that we wish to highlight about the seminars, in terms of what we felt was important in helping them to be well received by the student teachers and what we would like to improve in the future. We will discuss these in turn.

11.8.3 Creating epistemic trust within the group

Creating trust between the student teachers was key to establishing a learning process in the seminars. Many of our early activities focused on developing epistemic trust between us as facilitators and the student group (e.g. attuning the seminar content to the needs of the students), but next time we would give more attention to supporting the development of trust within the group alongside this. The sense of trust and safety was key to enabling the students to share experiences of their work openly with each other, without fear of judgement. This is similar to the concept in AMBIT of the *well-connected team*, which emphasizes the importance of the quality of the connections between team members and the overall team culture in supporting the work of the individual team members. In particular, embedding a helping culture within the team is seen as critical in enabling workers to sustain and regain a mentalizing stance in their work. This parallels the students' experience of the seminar groups as being a space they grew to trust and value in helping them with their work and, as such, is something that we could nurture more from the outset.

11.8.4 Dealing with emotions in teaching–learning fields

In a university setting, it is rather unusual for emotions, especially those with negative connotations, to be shown and explicitly reflected upon. This applies above all to those in leading positions, but also to students. Instead, the relevance of emotions for learning processes is dealt with on a solely cognitive level. In the introductory round of the seminar, when checking with the students after the recess period, one participant named a bereavement among their immediate family. This led to an emotional response from one of the facilitators, which initially seemed to irritate the other group participants. However, gradually, this emotional response from the facilitator led to similar emotional connections being shared by some of the other students. In retrospect, all participants considered this to be one of the most meaningful moments in the seminars, even if it was still rather unusual for the university context. Here is an excerpt from the video log where we reflected on this:

[0:02:56] AD: I would say for me, it was a situation where I could not adequately regulate my emotions, but that's the way it is in life. And that is a question that still bothers me: how much of it is beneficial and how much of it (isn't). So does it tend to irritate or stabilize the group?

[0:03:29] MH: I had the impression that it was very stabilizing indeed, regarding the group.

[0:04:22] AD: Well ... this is of course a topic that is taboo otherwise. I mean, what was important again, is to show how we deal with emotions; how do I manage to receive something that was said and contain it. And to reflect something back. And also to bring myself back into the state I was in before. So in the sense of my own regulation process ... this time it became visible.

[0:06:12] MH: Exactly, this is the way of dealing with emotions. So what do I do when somebody starts to cry or when I notice that there are very big emotions—what do I actually do then? Well, I had the impression that it was very helpful to them to see this.

11.8.5 How to best capture learning

We reflected that the video logbooks were an extremely useful learning tool and a helpful way of documenting thoughts and ideas throughout the seminars. They were also a very vivid format for doing so. In AMBIT, the online manual (https://manuals. annafreud.org/ambit) is the main tool for recording learning, but it would not have felt appropriate to put the videos in there. However, we could use the wiki manual as a place to record learning that arises from the seminars or video logbooks, as sometimes it would be helpful to have a place to capture important things that we learned from the process, or ideas that we would like to continue with in the future.

11.8.6 How to embed a mentalizing stance: what is good-enough mentalizing?

We were pleased to see the progress that the student teachers were able to make with bringing a mentalizing stance to their work. There was clear evidence of this happening within the seminars. The question is how we help the students take this mentalizing attitude beyond the seminars. To guarantee that this happens in the long run, we feel that something more is needed. It links to the social environments in which the students will be using the skills—the schools themselves—and recognizing that these are demanding environments and that it can be hard to establish a mentalizing culture in institutions. These quotes from our video logs capture some of our reflections on the process of facilitating the seminars as a whole:

[0:01:20] MH: What really comes to mind most concisely again and again is the mentalizing attitude that we have tried to include in the seminar through the increased reflection of the videotaped mentalization-based collegial case counselling. In order to create possibilities to practise there, to see oneself. To observe oneself while mentalizing and not mentalizing and so on. But I think that this is a point that one would definitely have to discuss again, how one can initiate such a mentalizing attitude in the long run. In other words, that the students develop a mentalizing attitude and don't just go out there with their beloved methods kit. I think we had moments when we succeeded. But to really guarantee this in the long run, I think we needed something more [. . .] I wouldn't be able to tell you what.

[0:26:55] AD: I wanted to reinforce this with the mentalizing stance, because I do believe that for people who are used to mentalizing, it is easy to say 'and now it's about these four quadrants'. Therefore AMBIT. But this cultivated form of the mentalizing stance differs from the realities we also come upon. So, this is very full of preconditions. That's what we said, that's actually the core. That would really be an open question, just to think about it. Is it possible to get on with such relative ease without the mentalizing stance? Taking a moment to make oneself the subject of discussion. In certain milieus, that's completely natural. But in some it is also extremely . . . strange. Our idea was to initiate this in the professional biography from the beginning of the career, but perhaps one could also say this is also something that is more compatible in an advanced training sector . . . it is simply demanding. That means [. . .] good-enough mentalizing it should be somehow. Yes, a good-enough mentalizing, like good-enough mothering from Winnicott [. . .] if that's not there, I find it difficult.

Despite the challenges we named, we are interested in how we might extend the mentalizing culture that we established with the students in the seminars beyond the university. We would like to make the group available for the students after they have finished their university programme, so that they can attend when they are working as teachers in schools and the group could continue to support them in taking this stance in their work.

11.9 Implications

This chapter describes a trailblazing project to develop an AMBIT-informed, mentalizing approach to teacher training. One of our visions for the future of

AMBIT is that the core components of the AMBIT approach are incorporated into the core professional training for a wide range of professions so that the approach becomes a part of a shared culture that supports multiagency working for clients with multiple needs. If this were to occur, then it would probably be time for AMBIT to pack its bags and set off for the beach! However, we are certainly a long way from this in the UK, so it is particularly inspiring that the new project described in this chapter has occurred in the context of a different professional system from ours, in Germany. As with other examples in this book, innovations in AMBIT are not confined to the team based in London but are being driven by teams in many parts of the world.

The authors have shared a very interesting account of their efforts to embed an AMBIT-informed mentalizing focus within their seminars for teachers of pupils with special educational needs. They have usefully highlighted the dilemmas of trying to embed an AMBIT-informed approach into a core professional training. The student teachers were trying to use the skills in contexts where this approach was not part of the existing culture. As we have highlighted, AMBIT is a team approach, and it is difficult for workers to implement the ideas fully when they are not supported by a team. The authors recognized the importance of this and created in their seminars the equivalent of a well-connected team to support this work.

The details of how they supported the students to take on this approach usefully highlight the shift in practice that can be required, even when this thinking takes place away from the demands of the working context. They have illustrated that the route to achieving this shift in practice is likely to take place only if it is supported by experiential learning. This theme will be further elaborated in Chapter 12, which describes the evolution of methods of AMBIT training. For us, too, it has become increasingly clear that discussion alone at a broadly conceptual level makes little impact on future practice. It is very encouraging to us that Melanie and Andrea independently reached similar conclusions. And it is to this that we now turn.

References

Abele, A. E., & Candova, A. (2007). Prädiktoren des Belastungserlebens im Lehrerberuf: Befunde einer 4-jährigen Längsschnittstudie [Predicting teachers' stress experience: Findings from a 4-year longitudinal study]. *Zeitschrift für Pädagogische Psychologie, 21*(2), 107–118. https://doi.org/10.1024/1010-0652.21.2.107

Bateman, A., & Fonagy, P. (2016). *Mentalization-based treatment for personality disorders: A practical guide.* Oxford University Press.

Baumann, M. (2019). *Kinder, die Systeme sprengen. Impulse, Zugangswege und hilfreiche Settingbedingungen für Jugendhilfe und Schule.* Schneider Verlag Hohengehren GmbH.

Bevington, D., Fuggle, P., Cracknell, L., & Fonagy, P. (2017). *Adaptive mentalization-based integrative treatment: A guide for teams to develop systems of care.* Oxford University Press.

Cortina, K. S., & Thames, M. H. (2013). Teacher education in Germany. In M. Kunter, J. Baumert, W. Blum, U. Klusmann, S. Krauss, & M. Neubrand (Eds.), *Cognitive activation in the mathematics classroom and professional competence of teachers: Results from the COACTIV project* (pp. 49–62). Springer.

Dlugosch, A. (2006). 'So hab' ich das noch nie gesehen …' Kollegiale Fallberatung auf der Grundlage der Themenzentrierten Interaktion. In G. Becker, M. Horstkemper, E. Risse, L. Stäudel, R. Werning, & F. Winter (Eds.), *Friedrich Jahresheft XXIV 2006. Diagnostizieren und Fördern. Stärken entdecken—Können entwickeln* (pp. 128–131). Friedrich Verlag.

Dlugosch, A. (2008). Ein Fall für 5 bis 8. Mit Kollegialer Fallberatung Lösungen auf der Spur. *Die Grundschulzeitschrift, 22*(214), 4–8.

Dlugosch, A., & Henter, M. (2020). Mentalisieren auf mehreren Ebenen? Zum Fall einer exemplarischen Maßnahmenkarriere in der Kinder- und Jugendhilfe. In S. Gingelmaier, H. Kirsch, & A. Ramberg (Eds.), *Praxisbuch mentalisierungsbasierte Pädagogik* (pp. 204–218). Vandenhoeck & Ruprecht.

Dziobek, I., Fleck, S., Kalbe, E., Rogers, K., Hassenstab, J., Brand, M., Kessler, J., Woike, J. K., Wolf, O. T., & Convit, A. (2006). Introducing MASC: A movie for the assessment of social cognition. *Journal of Autism and Developmental Disorders, 36*(5), 623–636. https://doi.org/ 10.1007/s10803-006-0107-0

Farau, A., & Cohn, R. C. (1984). *Gelebte Geschichte der Psychotherapie: Zwei Perspektiven.* Klett-Cotta.

Fletcher, G. J. O., Danilovics, P., Fernandez, G., Peterson, D., & Reeder, G. D. (1986). Attributional complexity: An individual differences measure. *Journal of Personality and Social Psychology, 51*(4), 875–884. https://doi.org/10.1037/0022-3514.51.4.875

Fonagy, P., Luyten, P., Moulton-Perkins, A., Lee, Y. W., Warren, F., Howard, S., Ghinai, R., Fearon, P., & Lowyck, B. (2016). Development and validation of a self-report measure of mentalizing: The Reflective Functioning Questionnaire. *PLoS One, 11*(7), e0158678. https:// doi.org/10.1371/journal.pone.0158678

Fonagy, P., Target, M., Steele, H., & Steele, M. (1998). *Reflective-functioning manual, Version 5, for application to Adult Attachment Interviews.* Unpublished manuscript.

Gill, K. (2017). *Making the difference: Breaking the link between school exclusion and social exclusion.* Institute for Public Policy Research. http://www.ippr.org/publications/making-the-difference

Gingelmaier, S., & Schwarzer, H.-N. (2019). Die Bedeutung von Mentalisierung und Epistemischem Vertrauen für die Förderung psychischer Gesundheit durch Supervision— theoretische Zusammenhänge und erste Befunde einer empirischen Pilotstudie. In E.- C. Reinfelder, R. Jahn, & S. Gingelmaier (Eds.), *Supervision und psychische Gesundheit* (pp. 125–137). Springer.

Henter, M., & Dlugosch, A. (2018). Das Adaptive Mentalization-Based Integrative Treatment (AMBIT) im schulischen Kontext? Zur Notwendigkeit eines Perspektivenwechsels in der Arbeit mit herausforderndem Verhalten. *Inklusion Konkret. Schriftenreihe des BZIB, 5,* 24– 37. http://www.bzib.at/fileadmin/Daten_PHOOE/Inklusive_Paedagogik_neu/Dateien_ab_ 2018/Inklusion_KonkretBand5gesamt.pdf

Kantor, D. (2012). *Reading the room: Group dynamics for coaches and leaders.* Jossey-Bass.

Karing, C., & Beelmann, A. (2016). Implementation und Evaluation eines multimodalen Stressbewältigungstrainings bei Lehramtsstudierenden. *Zeitschrift für Gesundheitspsychologie, 24*(2), 89–101. https://doi.org/10.1026/0943-8149/a000159

Karing, C., & Beelmann, A. (2019). Cognitive emotional regulation strategies: Potential mediators in the relationship between mindfulness, emotional exhaustion, and satisfaction? *Mindfulness, 10*(3), 459–468. https://doi.org/10.1007/s12671-018-0987-z

Kirsch, H. (2018). Mentalisieren in der Sozialen Arbeit. In S. Gingelmaier, H. Kirsch, & A. Ramberg (Eds.), *Praxisbuch mentalisierungsbasierte Pädagogik* (pp. 208–219). Vandenhoeck & Ruprecht.

Kotte, S., & Taubner, S. (2016). Mentalisierung in der Teamsupervision. *Organisationsberatung, Supervision, Coaching, 23*(1), 75–89.

Luyten, P., Malcorps, S., Fonagy, P., & Ensink, K. (2019). Assessment of mentalizing. In A. Bateman & P. Fonagy (Eds.), *Handbook of mentalizing in mental health practice* (2nd ed., pp. 37–62). American Psychiatric Publishing.

Rauin, U. (2007). Im Studium wenig engagiert—Beruf schnell überfordert [Low engagement during study—quickly overstrained at work]. *Forschung Aktuell, 3*, 60–64. https://www.forschung-frankfurt.uni-frankfurt.de/36050068/Im_Studium_wenig_____12_.pdf

Römer, J., Appel, J., Rauin, U., & Drews, F. (2012). Burnout-Risiko von Lehramts- und Jurastudierenden der Anfangssemester. *Prävention und Gesundheitsförderung, 7*(3), 203–208. https://doi.org/10.1007/s11553-012-0345-2

Scherwath, C., & Friedrich, S. (2012). *Soziale und pädagogische Arbeit bei Traumatisierung.* Ernst Reinhardt Verlag.

Spielmann, J. (2017). Dynamic balance. In M. Schneider-Landolf, J. Spielmann, & W. Zitterbarth (Eds.), *Handbook of theme-centered interaction (TCI)* (pp. 131–136). Vandenhoeck & Ruprecht.

Tornow, H., Ziegler, H., & Sewing, J. (2012). Abbrüche in stationären Erziehungshilfen (ABiE). Praxisforschungs- und Praxisentwicklungsprojekt. Analysen und Empfehlungen. *EREV ABIE Forschungsprojekt zu Abbrüchen in stationären Erziehungshilfen, 53*(3), 1–118. https://aim-ev.de/sites/default/files/2012-3-SR-EREV-Ergebnisse-ABIE-Tornow-Ziegler.pdf

12

Applying AMBIT principles to the training process

Laura Talbot, Rebecca Smith, James Wheeler, and Peter Fuggle

12.1 Setting the scene

All aspects of AMBIT are about learning. Clients learn to develop new helping relationships; workers learn how to mentalize under stress; and teams learn to develop new relationships with other teams. In this chapter, the authors propose that the fundamental process of learning is the same in all these contexts, and that training has many of the same requirements as the process of learning for a client: the participants in the training need to develop a degree of epistemic trust in the trainers if the training is to have a real impact on their working practice. In AMBIT, the principles applied to working with clients are applied in a similar way to the process of training. So, the authors carefully illustrate the way in which AMBIT training is delivered using mentalizing principles and how it pays particular attention to the relationships between trainers and participants. This radical approach to training has taken many years to develop and is based on the experience of training many teams. In many ways, you could say that AMBIT is being applied to itself and that there is no unique special process of learning that we call 'therapeutic' that applies only to our clients: we are all in the mix.

12.2 Introduction

The aim of this chapter is to take you behind the scenes of the AMBIT programme to give you a sense of what it means to apply a mentalizing approach to AMBIT training and to share with you the thinking, methods, and practices that have been developed over the past 15 years that help us to do this.

We have learned both from teams and from evidence to apply three key principles that now organize our whole approach to AMBIT training. These are that:

- Training must attend to the *state of mind of the workers* in order to be experienced as having relevance and value

- Training is a process of change and therefore requires us to pay attention to the *helping process*
- We must attend far more to what is needed to support *implementation in complex multiagency systems.*

It is no coincidence that these principles closely mirror some of the ideas that we set out in Chapter 1; it seems obvious to us now that the ideas that underpin our model should also be core to our training approach. Perhaps what needs explaining is how it took us so long to get here! We hope that broadcasting our intentions about the thinking behind how we design, deliver, and develop AMBIT training will be of interest to those outside the AMBIT programme, perhaps particularly so to those who attend the Local Facilitator Training to be able to share AMBIT with others.

Before going further, we need to take a small detour and place AMBIT training in the context of what is known about how things change in work situations. This is an area of research called 'implementation science' and it raises important questions about what enables training to lead to constructive development for a team or an organization. We know that the simple act of attending training does not in itself necessarily change or improve practice; if only it were that simple!

AMBIT training is part of the Learning at Work quadrant of the AMBIT wheel (see Chapter 2). The tension of this quadrant is between respecting local expertise (the expertise of those we are training) and respecting wider evidence about the process by which training results in changes in practice. Here, we aim to balance our mentalizing approach with the evidence from implementation science. This literature can sometimes make for uncomfortable reading, as the core message is that large-scale organizational transformation, of which training is often a key element, is often resisted and results in little actual change unless certain crucial factors are attended to. In their 2018 White Paper 'A call to action for leaders of health and care', Bevan and Fairman (2014) state that 'people in organisational life will no longer engage in change because they "have to". Increasingly it will be because they "want to"' (p. 13). The key message has been not only to ensure that AMBIT training equips people with the skills, knowledge, and plans to do things differently, but that the overall experience leaves workers feeling motivated enough to put these ideas into practice.

We have learned that it was not just the training itself that we needed to change. Fixsen et al. (2005) have emphasized the critical importance of what happens *before* any new programme is introduced to a local context. In its Implementation Stages Planning Tool, the National Implementation Research Network outlines a four-stage approach to implementation, namely Exploration, Installation, Initial Implementation, and Full Implementation (National Implementation Research Network, 2020). In reflecting on our previous training offer, we saw that the majority of our efforts were focused primarily on the Installation stage (i.e. on the delivery of training). We did not do very much to support teams to prepare the ground for the training or practice change that we hoped would follow, nor did we provide resources within our own team to dedicate the time needed to support all teams with their implementation journey following the training.

Over the past few years, the gradual expansion of the AMBIT programme has enabled us to develop our own version of an Exploration phase (consisting of an engagement call and a consultation day, described below), which are now mandatory for any team considering AMBIT training. We have also strengthened and expanded our post-training supervision offer to assist teams on their journey through the Initial Implementation and Full Implementation stages, although these are areas that we would also like to develop further (as we will discuss in Chapter 14). We make use of AMBIT tools and principles in all stages of this process, and hope that this offers teams not only more 'exposure' to AMBIT ideas but also an experience of how it might feel to be helped in an AMBIT-influenced way.

12.3 An AMBIT-influenced approach to training and implementation support

12.3.1 What do you need? Attending to the state of mind of the workers

Our approach to supporting a team or network through the training process has evolved to align far more closely with one of the central principles of AMBIT, that of paying attention to the state of mind of the worker. In the early years of AMBIT training, teams would book the training days via our website and we would usually know nothing about them until they turned up on the first day. Furthermore, it was quite common for a team to have been 'signed up' for a training by someone in a more senior role who did not always attend the training themselves, meaning that those attending the training did not always know that much about us either. While there were some early success stories of flagship teams who adopted the AMBIT way of working and have remained closely connected to the programme, it may not be a surprise to learn that this training approach also led to some very mixed experiences for trainees and trainers alike. Looking back, we were not following our own principle of adaptation, in that the training would be run in largely the same way irrespective of who attended. Although our understanding of a team would emerge through the training, this happened in an incidental rather than intentional way, and did not necessarily lead to us changing what we did very significantly.

In moving towards attending far more to the state of mind of the workers in our training approach, we are clearer now that teams should attend AMBIT training not with the primary goal of learning about AMBIT, but to *get some help with things that they would like to improve in their practice*. We now invest more time in attending first to the team's state of mind, by seeking to understand what they want or need help with from the outset. Seeking the perspective of frontline workers about what needs to change within a system and empowering them to make these changes has been described as having a beneficial impact on system transformation (e.g. Lankelly Chase, 2016), due to the unique insights that these workers develop daily about the enablers and barriers to effective practice in their local system.

12.3.1.1   How do we help teams to work out what they need?

Putting it in the language of implementation science, we have developed a pretraining exploration phase, which has two aims, namely:

- To support teams to reach a shared understanding of what they need in order to improve their capacity to help well
- To arrive at a shared understanding about whether AMBIT can help with this.

The phase consists of an engagement call (mandatory for all enquiries) and a consultation day (mandatory for any teams considering training following an engagement call). It illustrates what we mean by mentalizing the needs of the team and reframing their training request as a process of help-seeking. What is so prominent in this process is that the team or person seeking help often has not really worked out what they need. Helping a team to become clearer about their needs may be the most important part of the whole training process.

12.3.1.2   Engagement call

We set up a 30-minute engagement call for all new enquirers with a lead AMBIT trainer to better understand their interest in AMBIT and to give them the opportunity to hear more about AMBIT and the possible training options. This has quite a few parallels with a first contact with a client. In the spirit of mentalizing, we invite the enquirer to help us understand more about their team, context, and any ideas that they have for what training might help them with. This can sometimes seem back to front from the enquirer's perspective, as they often come to the call wanting to get some information about AMBIT and the training options. Of course, this information will follow, but starting with them enables us to better adapt our explanation of AMBIT to the team's context. We show curiosity about the team's purpose and what the team members find hard about their work. Some enquirers appear confident in their understanding of this whereas others find this harder to answer, but taking an inquisitive stance can help to kick-start their mentalizing. We have noticed that it is sometimes difficult for the enquirer to separate their own perspective about what the team needs or finds hard from what the team members might say themselves. This is perhaps not surprising from a mentalizing perspective, but the differences that may exist are important to draw out. We do not want training to be experienced by participants as another quick-fix, particularly given how often we have heard of workers suffering with 'training fatigue', having been subjected to several iterations of new initiatives within their organizations. Equally, we do not want the training to be undertaken under the automatic assumption of one or two key people in leadership/

commissioning positions that it is bound to be useful, leaving the frontline workers who attend the training feeling misunderstood and frustrated because it does not fit with what they feel they want or need.

We also encourage the enquirer to think about whether there is anyone in their local network who they may wish to invite into their thinking about having AMBIT training, particularly if there is already a desire to focus on improving network integration.

The trust-building process is in our minds from this first encounter with a team, and our aim to offer an experience where enquirers feel that we have understood something about them and their team, and can recognize themselves in how we explain AMBIT, is a first step towards this. We hope that their state of mind has been attended to, recognized, and responded to more or less accurately, and that they are satisfied with and clear about the plan for next steps.

12.3.1.3 Consultation day

The majority of our engagement calls progress to a consultation day, which is attended by the team(s) who are considering AMBIT training and their managers, leaders, and/ or commissioners. The day involves undertaking a series of exercises to explore the team's perspectives on the challenges in their work and what help they feel they need, followed by a brief presentation about AMBIT. Following this day, a report is produced to summarize the day and, if AMBIT is felt by us to be of potential help to the team, includes recommendations for training objectives and the best training format. This consultation session is offered as either a half day or a full day, depending on the type of training that is being considered and the size of the team. The same session is repeated twice, with the morning session attended by the senior leaders or commissioners and the afternoon session attended by the frontline workers. Good representation from both groups in these separate sessions is important. As we have discussed, frontline workers often have a unique vantage point in a system, and therefore their ideas about what might be needed in order to make improvements to practice are invaluable (although not always taken into account when designing training). Similarly, the inclusion of managers and leaders is important, as they often have the perceived or actual authority to endorse practice change and are invariably involved in supervising staff to implement the model in practice. We have found that facilitating the session in these two separate groups appears to enable both groups to feel greater safety in expressing their needs and ideas. Quite often, what emerges throughout the morning session is a recognition that a difference in perspective may exist between the leadership and frontline groups about how their work is experienced and what is needed. The consultation report reflects the views of both groups.

We have come to recognize that being asked 'How can we help you?' might not be a question that teams are expecting to answer when they are thinking about attending training. In the same way that the process of thinking about what might help often needs to be scaffolded for a client, to help them think about this (rather than simply expecting the client to be able to make sense of their state of mind on their own), we find that it needs to be similarly scaffolded for a team. The process of help-seeking (as described in Chapter 1) applies to both clients and workers and is a useful way of making sense of some of the complexities of the consultation process. Teams can experience barriers to seeking help too, and it is often the case that their help-seeking behaviours need to be nurtured in a similar way to those of our clients.

To be able to ask for help, the prospective help-seeker needs an *awareness* of what they want or need, along with a means of *expressing* this, the perception of the *availability* of a helping source, and a *willingness* to use this source of help (Rickwood et al., 2005). As such, we have designed an exercise called the Four Corners, which invites the team to reflect together on four areas:

1. What do workers need in order to do their job well with clients? What makes the client work challenging?
2. What do workers need from their team in order to do their job well? What makes teamwork hard?
3. What do workers need in order to work well with the multiagency network? What makes networking hard?
4. What feelings does the work bring up in workers, both positive and negative?

This exercise is key in helping us to tune into the state of mind of the workers in the team. The questions deliberately ask about 'workers', so that no one feels inhibited by having to own a response as being true specifically to them in their particular role, which may feel too exposing. For us, the process of this exercise is as important as the content that is generated in helping us to adapt our approach to the team in front of us.

There are usually several familiar themes. First, teams comment that these are not necessarily topics that they have spoken about together before. This is perhaps not surprising, given that there can be relatively little time within the busy working lives of teams to stop, 'zoom out', and take stock in this way. To use an AMBIT analogy, the exercise invites the team to come to the 'edge of the pond' to gain perspective on itself. In doing so, individual workers within a team may be just as unaware of their own perspective on these matters as those of their colleagues. There may be other relational barriers to this awareness not having developed collectively within the team before, including anxiety about what might be uncovered or a lack of trust in how safe it would feel to share (perhaps previously unexpressed) thoughts and feelings with each other. Second, teams often express that they find it reassuring and validating to see similar responses to those they would have given, as well as some curiosity about those that differ. So, as well as us beginning to make sense of the team, the team members are also usually beginning to make sense of each other.

These observations help us to adapt the brief overview of the AMBIT framework that we offer towards the end of the session. Being able to think about how to do this in a relatively short period of time is something greatly assisted by having two trainers, which will be discussed later in the chapter. We hold in mind what we have understood so far from the team about how they experience their work in how we talk about

AMBIT. Where we can see how a challenge they have broadly agreed upon might map on to an AMBIT tool, it is easy to explicitly make a connection to this in order for the team to have a concrete example of how we might be able to help. If they have not acknowledged a difficulty in a particular area, we might introduce this section more tentatively, perhaps focusing more on being interested to understand more about these aspects of their work to see what is already working well and whether there are any of our ideas or tools that might assist them further.

An example of this might be how we manage talking about one of the core assumptions of the AMBIT approach—namely that the work challenges our ability to maintain a mentalizing stance because of the feelings that the work generates. The team's response to the 'feelings' question is therefore highly relevant here. There is little point asserting to the team that the work makes us anxious, if they have not yet connected with this aspect of their experience. We risk being experienced as invalidating, irrelevant, or perhaps too threatening if we appear certain that this must be the case for this team. Instead, we might acknowledge that we heard the team talk about some of the challenges in their work (which are often rather concrete descriptions) but less about how these made them *feel*. We might mark this as something we want to hear more about, as we know that when difficult feelings do come up in the work they are not always easy to talk about and get help with, which can make the work feel even harder.

Throughout the consultation process, we want the team to see that we are keeping our evolving understanding of their state of mind central to the process of designing any 'help' that we might offer (i.e. the training). They are being actively involved in co-constructing with us an idea of what might be helpful for them. It is not simply that we just adapt what we do, but that we try to show the team *how* we are adapting our approach in the light of what we understand about them, and why. We do not want teams to feel that a 'one-size-fits-all' form of help is being imposed on them, but rather that the team can see some links between what is important to them and what AMBIT can offer, so that their act of attending an AMBIT training would make sense to them as an active choice rather than feeling mandated. We end this section with an example of a consultation day with a team (Box 12.1), which illustrates some of the above points.

12.3.2   Training as an AMBIT-influenced helping process

As with working with clients, AMBIT places mentalizing and the creation of epistemic trust at the heart of the training. But it is not without structure. Helping is an inherently stressful task and requires that helpers are supported by others. To this end, AMBIT training is delivered by two trainers, who work as a well-connected team and who use their relationship with each other to model the mentalizing process. The learning that takes place is a social process involving the relationship between the trainers, their relationship with those being trained, and the practitioners' relationships with each other. The content of the training consists of short presentations,

---

Box 12.1 Case example: a consultation day with a team working with adults with complex needs

---

During the Four Corners exercise, when asked to share the positive and negative feelings that the work brings up for workers in the team, the frontline workers quickly named emotions such as anxiety, frustration, pride, and satisfaction. The AMBIT trainers observed that the managers took longer to connect to this question, instead giving examples of situations that were commonly encountered rather than describing feelings that these situations might give rise to. The trainers were (privately) curious about this and wondered how this might influence the kind of support the frontline workers experienced from the leaders in relation to the emotional aspects of the work.

Another interesting difference was noted in the extent to which the two groups connected with and showed enthusiasm for the AMBIT framework. In the morning session, the managers felt certain that AMBIT training would be wanted and needed by the team and were keen to start the afternoon session by telling the team it was going ahead, although the trainers encouraged them to take a more curious position instead and invite the frontline workers to let them know what they made of the approach. The afternoon session revealed that the frontline staff, while seeing some potential benefits in AMBIT, were a little concerned about the rationale for the training being commissioned, and some expressed a worry about it replacing skills or theoretical knowledge they felt were valuable in their work, which they felt the managers might not understand.

The trainers felt that it was important to try to bring together some of these perspectives and asked if one of the commissioning managers would mind returning briefly at the end of the day. The trainers had separately checked out with the frontline workers how best to share their reflections, with the group expressing a preference for the trainers to summarize them on their behalf. Through hearing this feedback, the manager was helped to mentalize the frontline workers more accurately with regard to their worries about what the training might replace, as well as their hopes that the training might attend to them being better supported with some of the emotional impact of their work. The manager received this feedback well and was able to broadcast some of the leadership group's ideas behind their enthusiasm for the training, which was reassuring to the group. The trainers shared with the group that perhaps an important goal for the training would be to increase connection and openness between frontline workers and managers so that they were able to have more of these conversations together, without outside facilitation.

The feedback from the consultation day was positive, with frontline workers showing curiosity and enthusiasm about what was to come. They were particularly keen to know whether the same pair of trainers would be returning to deliver the full training, which perhaps suggests that the team had already started to develop epistemic trust in the trainers.

small and large group reflective exercises, practical exercises to try out techniques, and opportunities to discuss implementation. The aim is to support a process of discovery and experiential learning, rather than just knowledge transfer from trainers to trainees through didactic means. This parallels a similar process of change for a client: with a relational context of trust, the worker seeks to draw on the client's ideas and may also present some of their own ideas, but these are offered in a way where feedback on their usefulness to the client is encouraged and welcomed. In the following section we will describe how we use some of these principles and tools to mirror the helping process in our delivery of training.

12.3.2.1 Who's got your rope? Sustaining a mentalizing stance as a trainer

For us, one of the most critical aspects of delivering AMBIT training is that it is always facilitated by pairs of trainers. Delivering AMBIT training is about building a relationship with a unique group, developing an evolving understanding of their needs, and adapting a set of materials to fit best with these needs. Doing this 'live' in front of a large group is a lot to deal with and requires a constant balance between trying to follow a plan and paying attention to the group to understand when there might be a need to deviate from the plan. This requires the trainers to move flexibly between mentalizing self and other, as they check out—through a combination of both implicit and explicit moves—the degree to which they might be making sense to the people in front of them. It is therefore inevitable that the trainers, no matter how experienced, will find that their mentalizing capacity is at times lost, and it is critical that they are aware of this possibility and able to seek and accept help around it.

There are many different ways in which non-mentalizing might manifest in a training role. Perhaps when starting out in any kind of training role, there is a risk that the trainer's understandable anxiety tips them into a form of pretend mode, where their attention is consumed entirely by the material and the task of delivering it, at the expense of being able to tune in to what is happening in the room, leading them to be experienced by the group as somewhat detached or 'off the mark'. This behaviour might also happen in the context of over-enthusiasm for what is being presented, which leads the trainer into a state of psychic equivalence, where they assume (perhaps erroneously) that the team is as engaged in the material as they are. Check-ins with the group are absent, either because of a fear of what might be uncovered or because the trainer simply assumes that the group is responding positively to the training methods and the material being presented. Any difficulties that arise become sizeable 'elephants in the room', but the trainer ploughs on regardless. At other times, trainers might find themselves overly preoccupied with how they and the material are being received by the group, at the expense of being able to maintain an adequate focus on following the plan for the session. They are too tuned in to the group's state of mind and begin to hypermentalize the group, inevitably yielding some (inaccurate) certainties, which may begin to unhelpfully influence their behaviour. They might manage this by excessively seeking feedback from the group, leading them to become preoccupied with keeping the group 'on side' above all else, or by responding with a series of 'quick-fixes' to try to rescue the group from their own very natural grapples with the material, rather than trusting that these can be resolved (often by the team themselves) through the process of the training.

In our experience as trainers, these are states of mind that we are all vulnerable to falling into when delivering training. These inevitable threats to mentalizing are the reason that AMBIT training is delivered by pairs of trainers, as each trainer needs someone to 'hold their rope' or to be 'on the edge of the pond' to help them feel more secure in the task at hand and to actively help them when they get into difficulty. Working as a training pair allows one trainer to undertake the task of leading on delivering content while the other takes an 'edge of the pond' position, allowing them to mentalize how their co-trainer and the group might be feeling, monitor the interaction between them, and step in when adjustments might be needed. It is important that these roles are undertaken interchangeably throughout the training, which helps to model that seeking and offering help are roles that we move in and out of depending on our position in relation to a stressful task, not because of our relative level of expertise. We make no secret of this being the way that this relationship works to those we are training and aim to make our mutual support of each other visible.

In recent years, we have extended these arrangements further by ensuring that a third trainer is available to the training pair to check in with at the end of each day, usually via WhatsApp. The trainers share an update about the day, including highlights and dilemmas. If the trainers are feeling stuck with something, 'Thinking Together' is used. There are often themes to these conversations. The *task* that the trainers mark often includes issues such as help to understand the group better; one trainer getting 'stuck' and this having an impact on the trainers seeing things differently; the trainers getting drawn into lots of dialogue with the group and falling behind on the content; the group getting stuck with a particular part of the training; or the trainers being unsure how the group are feeling. The trainers then *state the case*, which requires making sense of the day together in order to be able to agree on a summary to share. This in itself can sometimes help with *mentalizing the moment*, where the trainers share how they are feeling in delivering this training, remembering that each may have a different perspective. The third trainer is able to assist with helping the trainers make sense of their respective experiences as well as making sense of where the group might be at. In the *return to purpose*, the trainers arrive at a point where they have had an opportunity to work through how they felt. Sometimes this is enough, or sometimes there may be a need to generate ideas about a plan for the next session, which they are now more able to do. The third trainer may add some ideas if invited to do so. Usually, the trainers share this conversation with the group the next day, in the spirit of modelling the Thinking Together process and highlighting how, through being well connected as a training team, we are able to support each other in these mutual ways.

We feel that these relationships and processes are crucial to the trainers being able to take an adaptive, mentalizing stance in the training. Facilitating training is a complex process, much like client work, and we would expect trainers to need help from each other and from other team members at times if they are embracing these aspects to the fullest. We would encourage anyone delivering AMBIT training to consider how they might be able to set up similar arrangements.

12.3.2.2 Using 'Active Planning' to adapt the training process to the team

In Chapter 1, we described that for help to be experienced as helpful, it needs to be *contingent*. Offering contingent help in the context of training is a challenge and requires holding a number of factors in balance. No two teams are alike, and so nor are two AMBIT trainings. Active Planning (see Chapter 2) has been a useful framework to conceptualize how we navigate the training process in the pursuit of offering contingent help, both during the training itself and in the post-training supervision. In a training context, 'doing the plan' at the top of the Active Planning triangle represents delivering the training content. This needs to be balanced with sensitively attuning to the group, by making ongoing efforts (both implicitly and explicitly) to make sense of them, by inviting their feedback and responding to needs or queries that they raise. Through broadcasting our intentions, we help the group to make sense of our behaviour as trainers. We are transparent about our own state of mind, frequently making our own thoughts and feelings explicit and checking out our understanding with them.

In the next section, we will describe how trainers might use an Active Planning stance to facilitate a helpful training experience.

Sustaining sensitive attunement as a trainer

Paying attention to the group's state of mind alongside delivering the training content is a challenging task. Making efforts to notice how the group is feeling as well as checking this out explicitly is important, rather than relying too much on our own assumptions. For a trainer to do this involves a degree of tenacity, as it requires a genuine willingness to be open to the responses that this might generate, whether positive or negative. Having two trainers allows some of this sense-making process to happen jointly and plans to be made collaboratively, to work out any adaptations that might need to be made.

There are some pitfalls that we might fall into when trying to sustain sensitive attunement. First, while as workers we might feel able to manage these kinds of enquiries in the relative privacy of a one-to-one conversation with a client, we may feel far more exposed doing so publicly in a large group. We may be less likely to actively check out our hunches, especially if we feel we are being received negatively. Allowing this state of psychic equivalence (i.e. feeling certain that our own negative perception of how the training is going is also held by the group) to run on without addressing it is unhelpful, not least because we may be wrong in how we are making sense of the group, but also because it reduces the opportunity for repair. In mentalizing terms, this highlights the importance of a trainer adequately holding the balance between self and other, maintaining as much awareness of their own state of mind as that of the group and recognizing the separateness of these perspectives.

Seeking the help of the other trainer is invaluable at these times. With experience, trainers build up a sense of the 'typical' ranges of responses given by teams to particular exercises and also of the patterns of how teams' responses and reactions develop across the period of training. Having this rough map of the territory can provide a degree of predictability for trainers about what to expect and equip us with the resilience to remain inquisitive about the team's experience and respond to it constructively. Being able to 'trust in the process' of the training is something that we remind ourselves of frequently as trainers. This might feel similar to the experience we have as workers of supporting a client through a helping intervention, where progress might not always be linear and frequent reviews of the relationship help to keep things on track.

Second, showing this level of curiosity towards a group of people can also generate a huge amount of discussion, which is often engaging and stimulating for trainers and trainees alike. Although bringing forth the experiences, ideas, and feelings of the group is fundamental to the process of maintaining an adaptive helping process, it needs to be facilitated well by the trainers to ensure that these discussions remain broadly connected to their intended purpose and allow the progression of the training plan. At times, this may mean taking quite an active stance as a trainer, interrupting to stop and start the flow of conversation, responding succinctly to questions, and 'parking' some things to come back to later.

Third, we have noticed that some groups are able to respond more easily than others to our invitation to share their state of mind with us. This is more likely to occur at the beginning of training, where relationships are new and trust has yet to be established with the trainers, and perhaps also within the group itself. The trainers need to hold a balance between making efforts to facilitate open communication (e.g. making guesses about how the group might be thinking and feeling; having a mentalizing conversation together about this in front of the group; seeking more balanced feedback about what is *not* being shared) and attending to the need to progress with the training plan, which may in itself help increase the group's ability to share more freely.

Being asked to give feedback about whether they are finding the trainers and the training helpful as it is happening (rather than only at the end) is often quite a novel experience for a team. One trainer recalls an example of being asked by one group member if the trainer thought the group was 'dumb' because of the amount of checking-in the trainer was doing, in her attempts to make sense of the group, which was rather quiet. The trainer felt totally thrown by the question and instantly anxious that she had been perceived as thinking of the group in this way, when this was so far from what she intended. Much like in our helping work, our intention to be helpful is often more obvious to us than it is to the client. To avoid these sorts of misunderstandings, trainers must remember to move flexibly between sensitive attunement and broadcasting intentions as to why they might be asking for feedback. Hearing about what might *not* be working well for the group is as important as understanding what *is* working and will help us to adapt our approach rather than causing offence. Sometimes, connecting this process explicitly with how often we invite and expect clients to bring us this kind of feedback can kick-start this conversation with the group. It can also provoke reflection and discussion about just how hard it can be to offer feedback on a helping relationship. The ability to seek out and adapt to feedback is fundamental to the success of any helping process, whether this be with clients, our teammates, or network colleagues. These reflections can generate a more mentalized understanding of others' behaviours in these contexts and ideas about how workers approach these conversations more meaningfully in their practice.

Broadcasting intentions as a trainer

Sharing our own state of mind as trainers is an equally important aspect of building and sustaining a trusting relationship, partly through the way in which it helps to reduce and repair misunderstandings. In practice, this means that trainers frequently think out loud with each other in front of the group, sharing what is in their minds as well as guessing what they think might be going on for the group. Even chats that happen in the coffee break might be shared with the group to let them in on how we might be attempting to make sense of whether or not we are being helpful. In doing this the group gets an opportunity to see the trainers 'from the inside' (i.e. how the trainers are thinking and feeling) and themselves 'from the outside' (i.e. how they are being made sense of). Through these explicit attempts to mentalize, we are inviting the group to build an accurate understanding of our intentions and to check out the extent to which we have accurately understood them. Both of these are key features of developing epistemic trust.

Being transparent about our own state of mind as trainers has another important function, which is to model the inevitability and acceptability of experiencing and expressing vulnerability. This might include sharing when we are not sure we are being helpful, explicitly asking the other trainer for help, or sharing an example from our own practice when we have struggled or made a mistake. As we are keen to promote in AMBIT, part of being a well-connected team rests on being able to ask each other for help when we are in need, which necessarily involves the help-seeker feeling comfortable enough to show their vulnerability to their colleagues. In much the same way as we cannot take for granted that this will be supported by the team's culture, we cannot assume that this is always easy for trainers to do. It may be easily undermined by the trainer's perception of the group, in terms of how much experience, knowledge, and status they perceive them to have relative to themselves. Being from the same or a different professional group as members of the group may be inhibiting for different reasons. Sometimes, the trainer is deterred by strongly held beliefs from the group about what it means to be a good practitioner, which might be tied up in being 'all-knowing' and never uncertain or in need of help. As a training team, we have quite often discussed how to balance being authentic with not being inhibited by worries that we might give an example that is 'bad' and lose the group's trust in our ability as a worker and trainer. More often than not, groups comment that they appreciate our honest and open approach about our experience and practice, as it can aid their understanding of the concepts being discussed and help them feel comfortable to talk more openly with us and each other.

If we are fully committed to putting the helping process at the centre of how we deliver training, we must expect and accept that there will be times where we do not get the balance quite right. As in client work, the point of Active Planning is that it gives us a tool to help us navigate holding all of these important aspects in balance, and some clues as to what we might need to attend to if we have become unbalanced. Through working as a training pair, we hope to model how a team might support a worker to balance these aspects of the helping process as effectively as possible.

12.3.3 Supporting implementation in complex multiagency systems

Our efforts to focus on supporting teams to implement AMBIT after the training have developed in several ways. First, AMBIT is an approach that is implemented not by individual workers but by teams and, increasingly, networks. It therefore makes sense that our training needs to attend to and strengthen team and network functioning in order to support the uptake of AMBIT in these contexts after training. Second, we need to take an active role in supporting implementation *after* the training, not only during it. Third, we must continue to learn about the impact of our training by seeking feedback from workers, in order to be able to improve our capacity to support teams to implement it in a way that leads to meaningful change.

12.3.3.1 Strengthening the well-connected team

It is not only the relationship between trainers and teams that we see as being key to learning. We are equally (if not more) interested in developing a team's capacity to get into learning relationships with each other because it is through these processes that they will be able to create meaningful changes in practice when they are back at work. Furthermore, many of the AMBIT tools and processes rely on the development and maintenance of a well-connected team; in the absence of trust, it is unlikely that anyone will ask a colleague to Think Together or want to do any team manualizing.

For us, using the training process to attend to and strengthen existing connections within a team makes great sense, and in fact some teams have this as one of their training goals. This might be easier to vocalize if there are obvious barriers to this having already happened (e.g. because the team is newly formed or there have been recent staff changes), but trainers should be mindful of the sensitivities that can often exist around team relationships and that discussions around this can risk inadvertently exposing what are often euphemistically referred to as 'team dynamics'. Being concrete about the behaviours that we are keen to promote is useful: that team members will be able to mutually seek, offer, and accept help from each other irrespective of role, and will be able to exchange ideas about the work in order to learn from each other and hence develop the team's (shared) approach to the work.

Establishing safety for the group in the training space is a foundational element of supporting these processes. We want team members to be able to reflect on their own state of mind and be open to hearing about those of their colleagues. As with clients, the capacity for this kind of reflective, flexible, inquisitive thinking is dependent on emotion being sufficiently regulated. The trainers' role in creating and sustaining an emotional context that supports thinking is therefore critical, along with an awareness of the kinds of feeling states that might be triggered when teams are coming together to think and learn in a new space. In recognition of the fact that both the prospect and experience of undertaking exercises together as a team can potentially give rise to a range of negative emotions, we try to design and sequence activities with affect regulation in mind. It is important that the activities generate some degree of feeling in the participants—enough to stimulate mentalizing, but not so much that the experience becomes overwhelming and takes their thinking 'offline'. Although this can be attended to through the design of the activities to a certain extent, it is the trainers' monitoring of the affect of group members and the group as a whole that gives the best chance of this balance being adequately held. Of course, as with clients, different groups are able to tolerate different levels of affect before their thinking becomes compromised. For example, a team that wishes to increase connectedness may benefit from continually changing groups for exercises where they are invited to share dilemmas with each other in order to practise helping exchanges with a range of people. For some teams, this may be too much initially, and it might be more helpful to allow the team to remain in self-chosen small groups and establish safety within these groups before moving on to mixing within the wider team towards the later stages of the training.

Being mindful of issues of diversity, equity, and inclusion within teams is important too, and we acknowledge that there is more we could do to attend to this; we will discuss this issue in Chapter 14. There may be a range of factors affecting the formation of mutually trusting relationships within the team, not all of which the team may be consciously aware of. For example, in attending to issues of power as it relates to job roles, there might be particular times where it is useful to offer managers/leaders and frontline workers separate spaces for activities. Sometimes, this is directly requested by the group, and in such circumstances, it is useful for the training pair to think together and with the group about how best to respond to this issue, given what it might indicate about the development needs of the team, irrespective of whether this is one of their explicit goals. As well as responding contingently to the request by allowing separate groups (assuming all are in agreement with this), the trainers should hold in mind and discuss how to progress to working in more mixed groups during the training. An example of such a situation is given in Box 12.2.

Box 12.2 Example: strengthening help-seeking between leaders and frontline workers

One training exercise invites the group to reflect on their own help-seeking at work and to share with each other what they find easy and challenging about this. In one particular team training, managers and frontline workers expressed quite clearly that they wanted to be in separate groups for this activity, with one manager commenting that it 'did not feel appropriate' for these discussions to take place in mixed groups. The trainers were aware that the frontline workers had talked on the consultation day about not always finding the leadership team supportive, because they did not feel that their work was well understood by them. The trainers respected the request but were also mindful of the need for greater connection between the two groups to be established during the training.

While the groups were undertaking the exercise, the trainers discussed and made a plan, which they shared after the groups had finished talking. The trainers shared their intentions around wanting to use the training to help strengthen the existing connections between the frontline workers and the leaders, as set out in the team's goals. They shared that they had devised an exercise, to be conducted in the existing groups, asking each group to reflect on 'What worries do frontline workers have about seeking help from leaders?' and 'What worries do leaders have about seeking help from frontline workers?' and to then discuss what it would take to feel more comfortable to do this. The groups were receptive to this activity, and representatives from each group were then encouraged to discuss feedback together in a 'fishbowl' with the rest of the group observing.

The exercise was powerful, in that it revealed shared concerns that help-seeking would be perceived by the other group as a sign of incompetence or weakness ('I'm not cut out for the job'), which each group was able to respond to in helpful and re-assuring ways. Comments were shared that actually help-seeking would be perceived positively, as a sign of strength in the frontline workers, and that it would be welcome to see this role-modelled by the leaders. It was also recognized that managers would sometimes need to seek help from their peers rather than from the team. The team agreed that groups should be mixed for the rest of the training to help support these efforts.

12.3.3.2 Using training to promote network integration

We increasingly receive training requests from several teams from a local network that wish to embark on AMBIT training together, rather than as single teams. This has opened up new opportunities to address some of the dilemmas and challenges in the Network quadrant live within the training. Although it is commonplace for workers from different teams to work together to support clients, it seems relatively rare for different teams from a local area to get the chance to meet to reflect on or learn together about their work. In the context of AMBIT, where we are proposing a collective approach to help clients with multiple needs, strengthening the context for trust and collaboration within multiagency networks is key. As well as being approached by groups of stakeholders from a local area who have it in mind to commission training for workers across a number of teams, we now actively encourage teams to consider whether there are other teams that they might wish to invite to join them in AMBIT training, particularly if they express a wish to improve network functioning. These kinds of training tend to result in the network defining two or three key objectives that are shared priorities for all the stakeholders in attendance. Examples of these trainings include those commissioned with the intention to improve outcomes for:

- Young people in need of 'Risk Support' (to use the language of the Thrive Framework (Wolpert et al., 2019))—bringing together teams from the Child and Adolescent Mental Health Service, social care, residential services, and the voluntary sector to support young people who present with a range of complex mental health, educational, and social needs
- Adults with learning disabilities, particularly those with mental health needs—bringing together teams from adult health, adult social care, inpatient, and community teams
- Young people transitioning between child and adult mental health services—bringing together child and adult mental health services, child and adult justice services, youth hubs, and housing pathway provision.

There are a number of different ways in which we adapt the training if we are training a network rather than a single team, to begin strengthening network relationships and developing a shared approach to the work. First, *trust* usually emerges or is deepened by the opportunity for workers from different teams to reflect on the work together, because this usually reveals shared struggles and aspirations in the work. To facilitate this, we ask workers to form groups consisting of a mix of workers from different teams for as many of the exercises as possible rather than carrying these out in their own teams. Workers inevitably report being surprised about the commonalities in their experience, as well as things that they did not know about others or had perhaps misunderstood. It can be useful to give opportunities to practise AMBIT techniques with people from both the same and different teams, to facilitate the process of workers seeking and offering help across the network.

Second, training teams together facilitates the process of finding a *shared language and approach* to understanding and addressing some of the dilemmas that come up when they are back at work. When we are training single teams, they often express how much easier they imagine it would be to make use of AMBIT in their work if other teams in their locality knew about it too; 'How can we use dis-integration grids with people who don't know about AMBIT?', a team might typically ask. Although it is possible to make good use of these ideas as a single team and to bring them into practice with others, the process of training together hugely eases this process. For example, a group of workers from different teams who attended a network training together commented on the relief they feel when attending network meetings with others with whom they had attended the AMBIT training. Even though they still had differences in perspective, AMBIT reminded them not only to expect this as part of the work, but also offered a shared method (i.e. the dis-integration grid) for exploring and understanding multiple perspectives together, which they reported had hugely eased the process of coming up with a shared plan for their clients.

Third, the training is also an opportunity to address some of the *processes underlying the dis-integration* that is so commonly seen in networks. For example, it is only natural for teams and practitioners to hold beliefs about each other, but not all of these promote trust or collaboration. It is nearly always possible to make sense of how these beliefs have arisen, but they can become the default explanation that the team reverts to when making sense of particular workers or services and can powerfully endure even across changes in team membership. It is these beliefs and processes that we have the opportunity to address when training several different teams together.

An example of how we might do this is through the 'Wearing Different Hats' exercise, which invites teams to consider beliefs that they hold about other teams in their network and what beliefs others might hold about them. Doing this with the teams within a network means that teams have the opportunity to share with each other what they think in the course of the exercise. Sometimes the very process of having to face the prospect of sharing beliefs about another team with them kick-starts mentalizing ('Is it really the case that the social care/mental health/housing team are lazy, or might there be another reason that they don't always get back to us?'). Teams usually come to this exercise believing that everything they think about others is accurate but consider most of the beliefs held by others about them to be inaccurate. When it becomes apparent that most of the teams present are making a similar pattern of attributions, it can open up some useful reflection about how often we are lacking curiosity when interpreting the behaviour of others and that we are not always good at making our intentions clear in order to prevent being misunderstood. The opportunity that this affords for teams to make more accurate sense of each other live in the room is invaluable and can make a far greater difference to beginning to reduce mistrust than when a single team does this exercise alone.

The process of training a network is not without its challenges and sensitivities. The trainers' attention to the helping process and facilitation of the exercises is key to ensuring that these are useful learning experiences that do not bubble over into exchanges that become heated or ultimately cement unhelpful perspectives. Overall, we hope that network training offers opportunities for teams to understand each other better, forge more collaborative working relationships, and learn some shared approaches to practice, all of which we hope will increase trust and connection, which in turn positively impact their efforts to offer integrated forms of help to their clients.

12.3.3.3 Keeping a focus on implementation throughout the training

We do not want implementation to be an afterthought or last-minute add-on to the training, given our wish to support the behaviour change needed for teams to meet their goals. To attend to this, we try to thread implementation planning throughout the training by giving brief but frequent opportunities for teams to discuss whether and/or how they might want to make use of each section of training content when they return to work. This prevents material or discussions from earlier parts of the training being forgotten about, which can easily happen when covering a lot of content over 4 or 5 days. We review the team's training goals mid-way through the training and use manualizing to help the team record any ideas that they have for what they might implement in relation to each goal.

As ever, it is important that trainers hold to their mentalizing stance throughout this process, remembering not to rush in too quickly with solutions, either through their own anxiety that a team is not 'getting it' or through their own enthusiasm to contribute to a team's creative process. Similarly, trainers should be mindful not to become too certain that they know what is best for a team. Many of the ideas in AMBIT can be operationalized in many different ways, and it is important to allow a team the opportunity to do some of this working out; as with clients, we need to value the expert knowledge that teams have about their own context. It can be easy to think that something that has worked for one team (or perhaps even in the trainer's own team) might be good for this team too. It can be useful to check out with a team whether it would be helpful to offer examples of things other teams have done, to help stimulate the team's own thinking, rather than conveying these as the 'only' way of doing things—or even generating resistance by pushing ideas on to a team that do not fit.

12.3.3.4 Supporting teams to implement AMBIT after the training

Implementation science is clear that some degree of long-term support is likely to be essential to support processes of change within teams in complex organizations. On the basis of these observations, we now include supervision as standard within the training package, so that all teams have access to this should they choose. The team's supervisor is usually one of the trainers who trained them, in keeping with the relational approach of the model.

The purpose of ongoing support is to provide an opportunity to support the newly trained team to sustain practice in AMBIT methods. Progress with implementing AMBIT post training has been a mixed picture for teams. It is common to find that the existing practices and ways of working in a team easily dominate and for the potential for change to feel much more limited than it did in the training. This partly reflects the reality of trying to implement a different approach within a system that must continue to function—somewhat different from the process of updating technological systems, which can be turned off or paused while the upgrade is applied.

Where we have had more success is when we are able to consolidate a relationship between the AMBIT trainer and a number of key staff in the recently trained team and create a regular supervision space that can be used flexibly, depending on what is helpful to the team. The subject for discussion may not always be 'the implementation plan' but could include a range of activities to develop and consolidate the team's use of AMBIT.

From this starting point the support sessions may take on a range of different functions depending on what is seen as most helpful for the team themselves. The most common patterns have been as follows:

1. *Case discussion.* Some teams use the support sessions to discuss case examples from their service. Often the key theme of these discussions is that the team has tended to get drawn back into focusing exclusively on the work with the clients and has lost sight of the importance of the team and network components of the work. Teams easily become disheartened by the lack of progress with cases and may need to be assured that this is unlikely to be due to their relative inexperience in the AMBIT approach. The acceptance and recognition of achieving only modest improvements for many clients may often be creating significant anxiety within a newly trained team.

2. *Practising AMBIT techniques.* It is commonly the case that teams need some refresher opportunities to practise key AMBIT techniques such as Thinking Together and the use of the dis-integration grid. The support sessions with the AMBIT trainer can provide an opportunity to practise these techniques and consider how they can be integrated into routine team practice.

3. *Encouraging local adaptation and manualizing.* Often the support meetings might focus on consideration of the key principles of the AMBIT approach and how these can be best applied to the team's service context. We routinely encourage teams to manualize these adaptations, even if we might take a lead in manualizing (which has been typically harder to support teams to implement).

4. *Supporting the development of local facilitators.* Teams who have done the Local Facilitator Training use the support space in a variety of ways. We encourage them to hold the balance between ensuring they are focusing on implementing AMBIT in their own practice and planning how to share it with others. Helping larger groups of local facilitators to become a well-connected team features commonly on the agenda, as does helping local facilitators to plan upcoming trainings, share successes, and seek help for any training dilemmas.

12.4 Evaluating our training approach

We measure the impact of training in several ways and have been influenced by Kirkpatrick's Four Levels of Training Evaluation (Kirkpatrick & Kirkpatrick, 2016), which promotes evaluation methods that capture impact at the levels of Reaction (is the training a positive experience?), Learning (do people learn things?), Behaviour (do people change their behaviour at work?), and Results (does this result in improvements for clients?). In this chapter, we will focus primarily on sharing what we have learned in relation to the Reaction and Learning levels. The crucial issue of how we assess the benefit to clients receiving services from teams is covered in Chapter 13. What positive impact looks like at the Behaviour and Results levels will depend on the training objectives that the teams set.

12.4.1 Is the training a positive experience?

The use of session feedback forms models to trainees how the process of gathering and adapting to feedback can usefully guide a helping process. It is also a process that local facilitators can replicate when delivering their own local training.

Since we introduced this system of assessment in 2018, we have collected 860 session feedback forms. Trainees are asked to rate four questions (shown in Table 12.1) at the end of every training day. Ratings are made on a scale from 1 (lowest) to 7 (highest). Although rating scales like this are clearly limited in the information they can provide, the ratings we have gathered from participants indicate very high satisfaction from the training over the period from 2018 to 2021.

Such ratings benefit from additional qualitative feedback. At the end of each training day, trainees are provided with the opportunity to give qualitative feedback on the training so far. The feedback we get from training is extremely positive, and the examples of qualitative feedback that we provide in Box 12.3 have been selected as typical of the majority of feedback we receive. The examples typically focus on the attendees' experiences of both the content and the process of training. We are pleased that our efforts to develop a more explicit focus on process are reflected in this feedback; the approach seems to work well for many who attend, with the obvious caveat that it does not work for everyone.

As we might expect, we do also get feedback that is not so positive. Some people experience the training as too slow and repetitive. Some want more didactic teaching

Table 12.1 Trainee ratings of AMBIT trainings, 2018–2021

Question	Percentage rated 6 or 7	Percentage rated 1 or 2
How engaged did you feel in the session?	82	<0.5
How did you find the quality of the facilitation?	91	<0.5
How helpful was the session in enabling you to learn knowledge, skills, or ways of thinking?	87	<0.5
How much do you feel that you will be able to use the knowledge, skills, or ways of thinking from this session in your work?	83	<0.5

Box 12.3 Examples of qualitative feedback from AMBIT training

---

'The facilitators were amazing at creating and holding a safe and supportive space and I really appreciated that.'

'Great balance of slides, discussion, and exercises; facilitators extremely interested and great at mentalizing.'

'Love the calm approach from both facilitators and an acknowledgement of group needs. Meaningful approaches to tasks in order to help facilitate change positively. Thank you!'

'Thank you so much—it's been brilliant; your facilitation style, sharing of experiences, pace, and support.'

'I found the split staff consultation incredibly helpful to open us up and spot for ourselves exactly why and how this learning is very necessary for us at the moment. All the exercises were absolutely useful and relevant. Very grateful, thank you.'

'I had a great time! I REALLY appreciated the time we had to work as a team to make action steps going forward.'

'I enjoyed the moments when our team could have frank conversations and learn together and even experience a bit of tension with the safety of having the facilitators there.'

'The bit around help seeking was very thought provoking. The sculpting exercise also. Overall the training has been set up in a really helpful way to encourage us to mentalize and work this through. It is an encouraging mindset and approach, as well as providing useful tools.'

'I particularly like the approach of linking learning to implementation throughout—this sometimes gets a bit lost in training, meaning that it has less impact on practice—many thanks!'

'Excellent bringing together of everything. Has been a hugely enlightening course but not only that, we have a clear plan for how we'll try to implement what we've learned.'

'Throughout the training, it made me think of what we currently do and how this could be improved.'

'It is a great shared language to introduce to other agencies.'

'Love the exercises, it feels accessible to all, exercises were really practical and meaningful. Thank you.'

'AMBIT gives a structured way in what can often seem like unstructured times.'

---

and find the tentative style of the trainers frustrating at times. In every team that we train there are usually enthusiasts, but there are also 'doubters' and some who are irritated by the language and feel that we make things more complicated than is needed. AMBIT should never support or strive for uniformity, as this is contradictory to the mentalizing approach. It is important to understand the state of mind of both the 'enthusiasts' and the 'doubters' in any team. Our ambition is not for a team to adopt the AMBIT approach as a new orthodoxy, but that the team comes to understand itself a little better and now has the techniques to continue to discover the team members' own differences, attitudes, and experiences, hopefully within a shared framework of curiosity and support.

12.5 Implications

Over the past 10 years, AMBIT training has changed radically. We have moved from a broadly expert and didactic method of dissemination to a method that is highly informed by the principles of AMBIT itself. It is not just that the training is highly interactive or that it is highly collaborative in style, but it is more that mentalizing the state of mind and the position of those being trained is crucial to the whole method. It has involved the use of explicit AMBIT techniques in working with others around a process of change and development. The principles and techniques that support learning for our clients also support learning in workers. The purpose of this chapter has been to share what this involves in practice, to go beyond the headline phrases and to describe what goes on behind the scenes to bring these methods and principles to life. Going forward, we need more data to enable us to test more accurately whether our speculations and experience of what makes for effective training are supported more fully by evidence. The framework proposed by Kirkpatrick (Kirkpatrick & Kirkpatrick, 2016) is extremely useful and highlights the need for more data to examine the relationship between training experience and changes in practitioner behaviour (the third level in Kirkpatrick's framework). The critical area of development for training is to learn more about how we can improve the degree to which training changes behaviour. We will consider our plans to do this in Chapter 14.

References

Bevan, H., & Fairman, S. (2014). *The new era of thinking and practice in change and transformation: A call to action for leaders of health and care*. NHS Improving Quality. https://www.nat ionalvoices.org.uk/sites/default/files/public/bevan_and_fairman-min.pdf

Fixsen, D. L., Naoom, S. F., Blase, K. A., Friedman, R. M., & Wallace, F. (2005). *Implementation research: A synthesis of the literature*. University of South Florida, Louis de la Parte Florida Mental Health Institute, The National Implementation Research Network.

Kirkpatrick, J. D., & Kirkpatrick, W. K. (2016). *Kirkpatrick's four levels of training evaluation*. ATD Press.

Lankelly Chase. (2016). *'From where I stand': How frontline workers can contribute to and create systems change*. The Lankelly Chase Foundation. https://lankellychase.org.uk/wp-content/ uploads/2017/03/SystemsChangers2016_singlepages.pdf

National Implementation Research Network. (2020). *Implementation stages planning tool*. University of North Carolina at Chapel Hill. https://nirn.fpg.unc.edu/sites/nirn.fpg. unc.edu/files/resources/Implementation%20Stages%20Planning%20Tool%20v8%20N IRN%20only%20Fillable.pdf

Rickwood, D., Deane, F. P., Wilson, C. J., & Ciarrochi, J. (2005). Young people's help-seeking for mental health problems. *Australian e-Journal for the Advancement of Mental Health*, 4(3), 218–251. https://doi.org/10.5172/jamh.4.3.218

Wolpert, M., Harris, R., Hodges, S., Fuggle, P., James, R., Wiener, A., McKenna, C., Law, D., York, A., Jones, M., Fonagy, P., Fleming, I., & Munk, S. (2019). *THRIVE Framework for system change.* CAMHS Press. http://implementingthrive.org/wp-content/uploads/2019/03/THRIVE-Framework-for-system-change-2019.pdf

13
Adopting a mentalizing approach to evaluating outcomes

Peter Fuggle, James Fairbairn, and Anna Oriol-Sanchez

13.1 Setting the scene

In the previous chapters, we have read about the way AMBIT has been applied to a range of service settings and how this approach has been applied to clients with multiple needs. These enthusiastic narratives suggest that the approach makes sense to the workers and has enabled teams to effectively engage with variable client groups (see Chapters 6–8), to support workers across disciplines (see Chapter 9), and to develop collaborative networks (see Chapter 10). We have also worked out methods of providing AMBIT training to very different professional groups (see Chapters 11 and 12). But we need to continue to learn about how AMBIT works for what types of clients. The basic AMBIT framework asserts that AMBIT is an open system that is continually being developed and amended on the basis of the experience of workers and clients. This is a type of learning at work, and is a key part of the approach. There is a need to support AMBIT-trained teams to be curious about the effectiveness of what they do, but this is not always easy. For example, do their clients' lives improve during the period when they are working with them? If so, is this due to the involvement of the AMBIT team? Is it related to the methods used by the workers, or do the clients improve because of other changes in their lives?

Finding out the answers to these questions requires that we measure things. Such measurement is always problematic, incomplete, and in some ways unsatisfactory. The measures we use never capture the full story, the richness of the work, and the multifaceted nature of our clients' lives. The aim of this chapter is to share what we have learned about outcome measurement for workers in AMBIT teams and to make suggestions about creating conditions that support curiosity about outcome measurement in their work. We recognize that readers will be coming to this from very different starting points: some may be very familiar with outcome measurement and how it works whereas others may be less so, and we appreciate that, as with many of the teams that we train, this may not feel close to what they see as important in helping vulnerable clients. We hope this chapter creates curiosity and enthusiasm for this crucial part of the AMBIT approach.

13.2 Introduction

For many frontline practitioners, the question 'Does it work?' may not be that easy to relate to and may appear remote, academic, managerial, or even threatening. Our experience is that practitioners have a belief or conviction that what they are doing is beneficial to their clients. This is a basic stance for the work and this optimistic conviction is adaptive to the work itself. However, this stance may sit uncomfortably with questions about the effectiveness of what they do. If we were to apply this dilemma to football, it would clearly be true that no team wins every match—but every football manager wants their team to believe that they could! It would not be adaptive for a football team to approach a match considering that it was probably time for them to lose a game as they had not lost one for a while. A belief that one can be helpful to all one's clients is a fundamental aspect of positive team culture, even though the evidence suggests that in reality it will not be the case. Clearly, this analogy goes only so far. In football, there are rules and an agreed score at the end of the game, whereas in AMBIT we are faced with working out the rules and needing to agree how to score the result. For many workers, this process may feel quite alien; they are just here for the 'game'.

Coming to understand the impact of the work for the client is part of the AMBIT quadrant of Learning at Work. As described in Chapter 2, holding a mentalizing stance about this aspect of the AMBIT approach is particularly challenging and easily gives rise to non-mentalizing states of certainty ('I know what we do works, we just have to prove it'), evasiveness ('Outcome measures just don't capture what really matters'), or concreteness ('If the measures show improvement, then it works'). Holding a position of doing one's very best to be helpful to a client while at the same time remaining open to the possibility that the impact of the work may not always be what was intended is an extremely hard balance for teams and individuals to achieve. So, we face this problem with humility and, as with all parts of this book, we aim to stay close to the workers' and clients' experience of developing curiosity about the impact of AMBIT on all parts of the system.

The chapter is organized into three main parts. We will first begin by seeing AMBIT outcomes from the inside (from the perspective of lived experience) and propose five methods to create the conditions that enable a team to monitor outcomes in a mentalizing way (Section 13.3). Second, we will look at outcomes from the outside (the need for commissioners to know what they are purchasing) and will describe what we have learned from published studies on outcomes for AMBIT-trained teams (Section 13.4). Based on these two parts, we will finish in Section 13.5 by proposing an outcomes framework, which is being taken forward by a wider collaboration between multiple teams to help develop a richer understanding of the outcomes for AMBIT.

13.3 Looking from the inside: outcomes work for the worker, manager, and client

Let us start by imagining a number of people who are involved in outcomes. We will begin with Jordan, who works in an AMBIT-trained team. Jordan liked his job. He used to work in a special school, but he liked his current team better. He felt they looked after each other more and he always felt supported when he was working with his clients. Once a month, the team had a meeting about outcomes, and he couldn't really understand what this was about. There seemed to be lots of worries about whether the team was doing OK. There was a lot of talk about questionnaires and measures, but he found it hard to see how this connected with his work with his clients. He did not think that measuring outcomes was very important because he had good relationships with all his clients and they were always happy to meet up with him, even when they were missing meetings with other professionals. He felt reasonably confident in how to use the measures but felt that most of his clients would not see filling in the forms as particularly relevant to what they talked about. Overall, he felt it was a burden similar to tasks such as completing risk assessments or session notes, and he tended to avoid doing them.

Usually, when the discussions in the team meetings turned to outcomes, Jordan was quite quiet. The meeting often finished with Lila, the team manager, encouraging everyone to make sure that they completed outcome measures more often. Jordan liked to help out and wanted to be respected within the team, so he did his best with whatever was being suggested. However, he found it hard to see how this connected with the things he really thought about at work. For example, he would think about how his 15-year-old client Julie was having such a hard time with her mother, who was drinking a lot again. Julie really hated her mother's drinking and particularly hated it when her mother shouted horrible things at her younger sister. Jordan related to this a lot because his girlfriend had told him about things that had happened in her own life when she was a child, which were a bit like the things Julie was experiencing now. Trying to help Julie to have something positive to focus on instead of feeling stressed about her home life was what stayed in Jordan's mind—not this stuff called 'outcomes'.

Sally was a team leader. She felt passionately about the work of her team and wanted to show what a great job her team was doing. She was energetic and, when faced with obstacles, would often try to do things herself. It was hard work to get her team to complete routine outcome measures, but they did it. She felt frustrated with the measures because she did not feel that they captured all the things that her team was doing. She felt that the measures sold them short. Sally believed that outcomes were important and felt confident about how to use the measures, but saw them as burdensome and was not sure that they were measuring what really mattered.

Yusuf was 14 and was angry a lot of the time. He had good reason to be angry as, for much of his life, he had been subjected to violence at home. He didn't go to school much and was prone to terrible rages when provoked by men in positions of authority. He had got to know a team worker called Jenny, who had helped him to go to a local boxing club; he liked going to the club because he would do a lot of exercise there and this calmed him down. Jenny would meet Yusuf after boxing most weeks and they would talk about his week. In one session, Jenny had introduced him to the AMBIT Integrative Measure (AIM) cards (see Chapter 4), and he liked them. Using the AIM cards had helped Yusuf and Jenny to identify six key problems, the most important of which was about managing his feelings. He did want some things to be different in his life, and he was OK about starting each session with Jenny by looking through the cards and saying how he was doing with each of these main problems. He didn't find it easy to try to step back and think about his problems on his own; he could only do it when Jenny asked him how things were going, and he used the cards to help him think. He also liked to see how things changed on the cards if he was getting 'better'. This was not an easy process because things were changing very slowly for Yusuf and sometimes he felt that Jenny was exaggerating how well he was doing. For Yusuf, 'outcomes' were very important because, when he met up with Jenny, he wanted things in his life to be getting better; the cards were an easy way to keep track of his progress together with Jenny, so he found them helpful to use.

Jordan, Lila, Sally, Jenny, and Yusuf vary in how they experience using outcome measures. But for all of them it is not entirely straightforward how the process of measuring outcomes fits into their experience of giving and receiving help. This is what we mean by seeing outcome monitoring 'from the inside'—seeing it from the perspective of those engaged in the helping process and applying a mentalizing stance to outcome monitoring for the workers and clients themselves. We do not believe that it is a given that this activity will be something that they initially see as helpful to them.

13.3.1 Mentalizing the worker's experience of outcomes work

At its heart, measuring outcomes is a mentalizing task, although arguably this aspect easily becomes lost in its implementation in services. It is born out of 'not knowing' and a wish to better understand, via a process of inquisitiveness, how another person is currently making sense of aspects of themselves, their experience, or their situation. As we have seen, it should not be a surprise that non-mentalizing states of mind can also permeate (and be triggered by) the task of measuring outcomes (see Chapter 2).

Perhaps unfairly, our experience of encouraging the measurement of outcomes may evoke a sense of certainty for many workers—of knowing that they are being helpful (or not helpful) based on their own thoughts and experience. This is something they know already, and so measuring outcomes is simply a way of proving what they know. The world is how they think it is. Similarly, measuring outcomes may easily drift into pretend-mode thinking, in which the meanings of positive outcomes are debated and questioned in ways that may feel quite disconnected from the difficulties of the clients themselves. Measures may be seen as imperfect, superficial, and partial (which they are), resulting in long discussions about the need for greater meaning and losing sight of the importance of finding out from the clients themselves. Perhaps most of all, outcome monitoring can be vulnerable to teleological thinking: that is, that if the measures show improvement, then the workers have 'done their job'. Here, outcomes become only what is measured rather than the measures being an indication or a marker of wider aspects of a client's life.

These non-mentalizing tendencies may be heightened by the attachment aspects of the work. As described in Chapter 2, the worker enters into a relationship with the client—getting to know them; developing empathy for their situation; listening to their thoughts, feelings, and experiences; taking a positive stance towards their difficulties and trying to figure out how to help; and so on. These behaviours are all aspects of an attachment relationship (although nowhere near the degree to which they would be part of a relationship with a parent/carer), and there is an element of a non-conditional aspect of this. This situation exposes the worker to potential states of certainty that support engagement and commitment to one's clients.

With this in mind, we can see how potentially irritating the whole topic of monitoring outcomes may be for some workers. Their optimistic committed stance to their clients may feel invalidated and 'un-mirrored' by outcome monitoring, leading to feelings of being misunderstood. Outcome monitoring may feel as if it is assessing their work, and they may become fearful of what this may show. It touches a nerve—like being invited to explore how good a parent you are. It is close to a sense of self, a core identity about what sort of person one is. Most people in this area of work do not do it just to earn a living, but because it links to values they hold. Measuring outcomes can be a threat to these identities and can feel uncomfortable and unsettling. However, we do not think this needs to be the case. The task for a team is to allow such concerns to be voiced, respected, and mentalized, so that the team moves away from implicit anxieties about their effectiveness as a team to an explicit recognition that outcomes for clients will be mixed and that this will be true for the team as a whole. Quite strikingly, most training in outcome monitoring focuses almost entirely on how to do it (i.e. what measures to use and how to use them) and devotes very little time to the impact on the mindset of the workers themselves. This absence may contribute to the reluctance of teams to embrace outcome monitoring as a process of exploration. From this perspective, going back to our example, it may be no great surprise to discover that Jordan's lack of curiosity about outcomes may be connected to a sense of his own abilities and confidence in his own skills, that is, to a sense of his own self-identity.

13.3.2 Creating a culture of curiosity about outcomes

As we have described, Jordan, Sally, and Yusuf all have different beliefs and experiences about outcomes. We aim to create a culture of curiosity about variability (i.e. some clients' lives improve a lot and some do not) and also about unpredictability (i.e.

some improve much more than expected, and some do not improve when we predict they might). This is at the core of a mentalized approach to outcome monitoring and, from this starting point, we will propose a number of suggestions about ways of supporting curiosity within teams.

Jordan knows that some of the young people he works with get on with him really well, and he is able to help them make changes to their life. However, there are others where he doesn't feel so good about how things are going; it's not that he doesn't get on with them, but the work never really gets going. There may be avoidance of talking about anything important. For example, he has been working with Simone for 3 months. She sometimes turns up for appointments with him but never responds to his texts. She had made a serious attempt on her life before she started coming to see him, but she never talks about this incident. She says that things are OK, but she often stays away from home and her father often calls Jordan because he is worried about her. Jordan doesn't feel he is helping Simone, but he keeps trying. He doesn't like to think this, but he feels that Simone makes things up and he doesn't feel able to address this. After a while, Simone stops meeting him and Jordan has a final phone call with her father. Jordan explains that Simone can come back to see him in the future if she wants. Jordan agrees with his supervisor to close the case. His experience of working with Simone, however infuriating and inconsistent she may have been, has engaged Jordan in wanting to help her. He is very interested and concerned about the outcome of the work in this particular case, but he does not see his interest in Simone's outcome as being related to the opportunity to make sense of this experience that the process of outcome monitoring might allow. His discomfort and/or irritation with the less-than-positive outcome for Simone, unless explicitly mentalized to some degree, is likely to result in outcome monitoring in the team remaining tokenistic, procedural, and experienced as being of little value to the team itself.

All teams who work with clients with multiple life problems will frequently have experiences similar to Jordan's experience of working with Simone. Jordan's sense of feeling useless is, in our view, highly related to the real process of outcome monitoring. Outcome monitoring needs to include the experience of the worker, and the successes and disappointments that this entails. We know that disappointments will stay more in the mind and that such experiences easily promote non-mentalizing states of mind for workers marked by shame, self-blame, and (perhaps less comfortably) blaming attributions towards the client (e.g. that they are not motivated, that the family is hostile to help, or that they are 'in denial'). Explicit outcome monitoring in a team can provide a way of making sense of variable outcomes (i.e. no one is successful with all cases) and can create opportunities to make sense of such outcomes. Teams that adopt an explicit recognition that outcomes vary for clients and that everyone in the team is responsible for every case are more likely to enable workers to mentalize their experience (disappointment, sense of uselessness, etc.). This would enable workers like Jordan to be able to manage the highs and lows of this type of work better and would help the team to learn collectively about their own effectiveness.

For all mental health interventions (Fonagy et al., 2015), some clients will benefit more than others, and AMBIT is no exception. AMBIT proposes that it is valuable, and perhaps essential, for a team to recognize such patterns in their own caseload. Although such knowledge may be implicit from the routine work of the team (e.g. by knowing how frequently clients attend appointments, from clients' spontaneous feedback about a session), it is easy for this continuous stream of information to never be made explicit and reflected upon. AMBIT proposes that a team will benefit from knowing as much as it can about how and when it is helpful to its clients, and that such curiosity is essentially a mentalizing stance about the impact of the work on those who come for help. From this starting point we will now outline four ways of creating curiosity in outcome measurement.

13.3.2.1 Sharing mental models about outcomes

To support learning at work about outcome measurement, the team may benefit from moving from implicit individual beliefs to more explicit shared ideas about its purpose and practice. Peter Senge recommended that it helps teams to share their implicit assumptions, beliefs, and feelings about the core purposes of their work and what outcomes they expect for the clients with whom they are working (Senge, 2006). Senge calls this *sharing mental models* and suggests that often teams miss this process out. The suggestion is that, rather than being focused on a particular case, a team will benefit from sharing ideas about what should be expected of the team overall.

The following are some suggested key questions that may be helpful for the team to discuss:

- What realistic outcomes would we expect for our clients if a case goes well?
- How do we gauge that things are improving?
- How do we decide that we are not really helping?
- How do we decide when it is time to stop working with a client?
- How often do clients get worse in the course of their work with the team?
- What is it like for the team if a client makes big improvements?
- What is it like for a team member if things deteriorate in a case?
- How do we know if changes are happening, particularly if they are small?
- Sometimes clients do not tell us things when they get better. How can we try to have a balanced understanding of change for our clients?

The assumption behind these questions is that not all clients benefit in the same way from the service that is offered. To use an example from the medical world, staff in a cancer service know that some patients recover and some do not. This may seem like a dramatic comparison, but teams using the AMBIT approach may well have experience of clients who have taken their own lives or ended up in prison having committed serious offences. Where teams are working with high-risk client groups, these outcomes, although undesirable and tragic, will occur, and we are not aware of any service or model of intervention that avoids these outcomes altogether. The idea of the process of sharing mental models is to enable the team to develop a mentalized understanding of the likelihood that not every case will have a good outcome. An alternative mental model is that, if we do things properly, all of the clients will improve, and no tragedies will occur. In our experience (and based on what the research tells us), this will not happen, so it is a mental model that is maladaptive to the context in which the team is working.

These are conversations that may carry a lot of emotion and evoke anxieties about individual responsibility for client outcomes. The purpose of such conversations is not to solve these issues, but to enable implicit anxieties within a team to be expressed and made explicit. This creates a more transparent culture around making sense of the likely impact of the work on clients. However, it is also likely that there will be some recognition that these questions are difficult to answer, and that it is not easy to know whether things are improving for clients unless the workers in the team actively enquire in a systematic way. From a mentalizing perspective, the purpose of these discussions is to enable team members to move from positions of certainty to curiosity. If and when this occurs, it is often not easy to decide how best to monitor change for the clients, and there will be important differences of view about what really matters. One of the first steps for AMBIT-trained teams is to consider the relationship between outcomes and intentional states, and this is what we will consider next.

13.3.2.2 Connecting outcomes to interest in intentional states

Some teams may have a very explicit shared understanding of the purpose of their work as a team (e.g. reducing family breakdown or reducing substance use) whereas other teams may be set up with less well-defined outcomes (e.g. managing crises, improving resilience, or reducing social exclusion). The absence of an explicit, shared sense of purpose may lead workers to gloss over the purpose of the service, and to offer a vague description of their role out of fear that the client may not agree with the purpose. In this situation, the chances of being able to support change are immediately compromised; if workers do not name the type of work done by them/their team and therefore do not offer it as a possible focus, clients may not ask for help with particular problems because they may assume that they are not something the worker can help with. Mentalizing within teams is likely to be strengthened by a team having an explicit shared 'intention' about their work. Teams that lack this shared intention are more prone to workers experiencing the work in non-mentalizing, stressful, and non-adaptive ways, such as being in 'fire-fighting' mode or experiencing a sense of 'drift' in the work. Workers in teams whose overall purpose is clear are likely to have ideas about how to go about collaborating with their clients to achieve their stated outcomes, and may begin to recognize common challenges to their capacity to mentalize when these are being frustrated. For teams that feel the need to further develop their understanding of their core aims and how mentalizing fits with these aims, we now turn to a specific method of approaching this, called *logic models*.

13.3.2.3 Using logic models to determine outcomes that matter

AMBIT teams are often faced with a complex dilemma about what outcomes should be prioritized for the team. A bewildering array of problems and life circumstances may well be very pertinent to the work of the team, and the complexity of the contexts that workers and clients face can be daunting. A method of disentangling some of these challenges, the *logic model*, has been developed by Professor Miranda Wolpert and colleagues at the Anna Freud Centre (Wolpert et al., 2016). We are indebted to their work for this section and for Wolpert's contribution to the AMBIT Study Day in February 2018 (see later in this chapter), where she presented this method of working to a wide range of AMBIT-trained teams.

The purpose of the logic model is to enable a team to identify the core components of its work by inviting the team to specify its work according to four key categories: the target group (who is the intervention for?), the intervention (what are the key components of what we do?), change mechanisms (how and why does the intervention work?), and outcomes (what difference will it make?). The logic model has a standard format, which aims to enable a team to see the relationships between these four components of their work. This format is shown in Figure 13.1.

The aim of the logic model is to encourage a team to come up with concise statements about the core components of each of these categories. However, many teams can find it relatively challenging to develop shared statements that the team generally subscribes to. The value of this process lies in the construction of a model that is seen by the team as genuinely representing the nature of their work. It has less value if it is a document drafted by the service manager as part of routine documentation for the team. It is likely that there will be differences of view between team members about key aspects of the work and, in AMBIT, these differences are seen as important

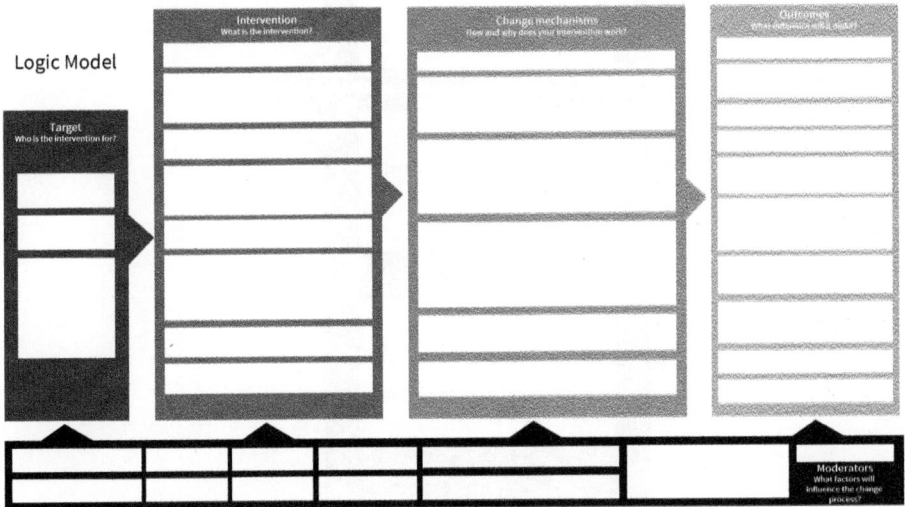

Figure 13.1 The logic model.

in helping the team members to mentalize each other and to develop explicit understandings of each other's perspectives on the work they do. It is expected that, although a team may develop a shared understanding of their work through producing a logic model, it is not consistent with a mentalizing approach to expect a complete uniformity of opinion about every aspect of the shared model.

Here, we will provide an example of building each of the four components of the logic model using some broad parameters that we anticipate would apply to a number of AMBIT-trained teams.

First, the team identifies the target group for the work of the team (Figure 13.2). Perhaps unusually, for an AMBIT approach we would often include clients, workers, and other teams in the network as all being part of the target group for the intervention.

Following the definition of the client group, the team then determines the key components of the intervention. Again, in the AMBIT approach the 'intervention' would not be confined to work with the client but would include team and network components, as shown in Figure 13.3.

Having identified the core components of the intervention, the next step is to determine the processes or mechanisms by which change happens. This is often implicit in the work of many teams, who may have a high investment in relationship building but not necessarily a clear idea of what to do with a relationship once it has been

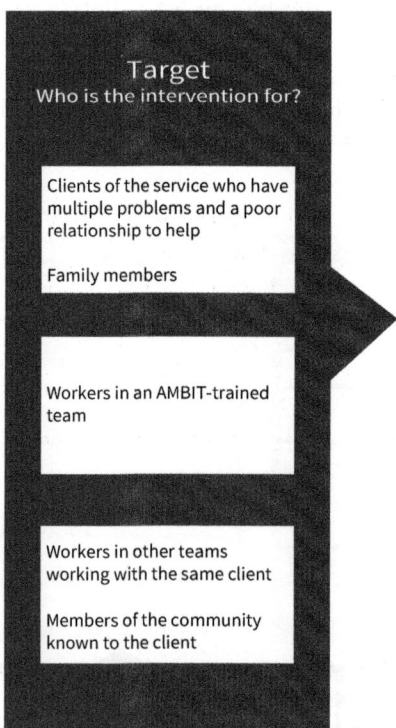

Figure 13.2 Who is the intervention for ('Target')?

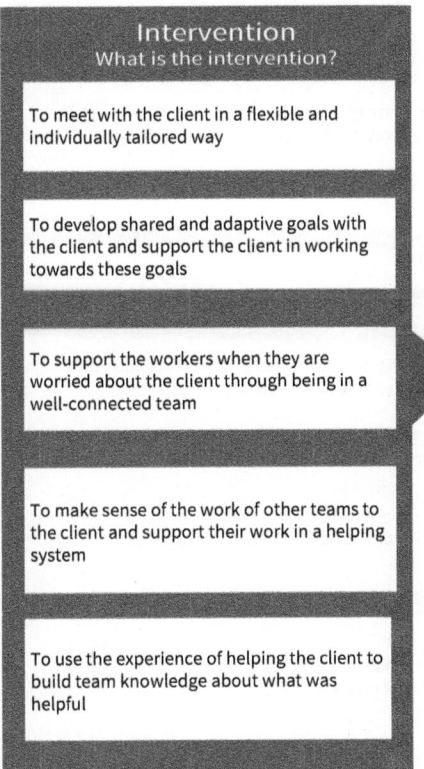

Figure 13.3 What is the intervention ('Intervention')?

established. To counteract this, there is considerable value in workers having explicit and shared goals in the work with a client. For this worked example, this is shown in Figure 13.4.

Having completed the first three sections of the logic model, the task now is to select outcomes that are likely to measure processes that are considered to be relevant in achieving change (Figure 13.5). There may be ready-made standardized measures for some of the identified processes of change, and use of these would be preferable, but sometimes they may not be appropriate, perhaps because they are too complicated or have been developed for research purposes. A key principle at this stage is to identify measures that are simple and easy to complete. For some services there will be what is referred to as a 'primary outcome', which is part of what the service is commissioned to achieve. For example, if a team is commissioned to provide community interventions and avoid hospital admissions, then the number of cases admitted to hospital would be a primary outcome. For teams commissioned to work with substance users, a primary outcome would be some measure of (reduced) substance use.

The logic model anticipates that outcomes will vary across the client group and invites teams to consider what factors are likely to moderate the effectiveness of the interventions offered.

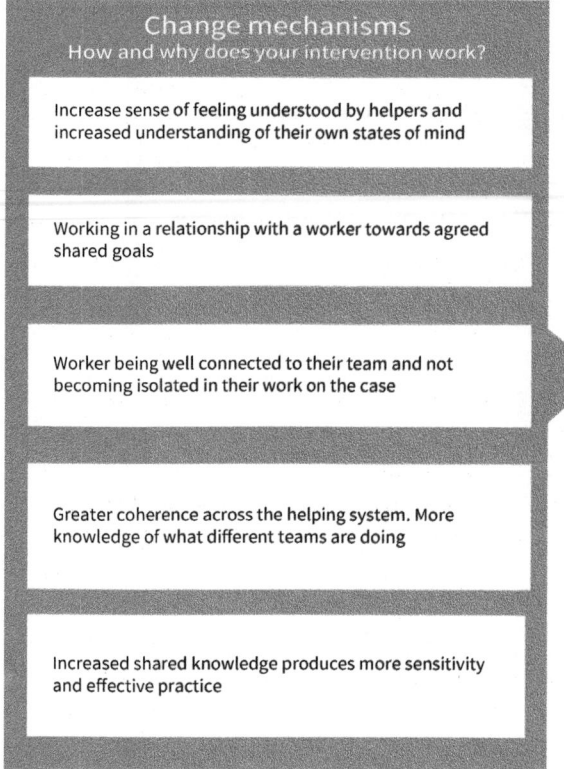

Figure 13.4 How and why does the intervention work ('Change mechanisms')?

Because of the variety of clients or teams using the AMBIT approach, there is no uniform logic model for all AMBIT teams. This is welcomed, as the value of a logic model is in its specificity to the work of a team with a defined target group. In relation to outcomes, the logic model has a very clear purpose in helping the team to focus on outcomes that are related to the change mechanisms that they see as being central to the intervention they are offering, as well as outcomes that are related to the goals of the client group and the requirements of service commissioners and funders. This often results in the need for a number of pragmatic compromises in deciding on an outcomes framework for a specific team. However, alongside this local adaptability of approach, we also believe that measuring functional (rather than diagnostic) outcomes is best suited to the client groups often served by AMBIT-trained teams. There is a balance to be achieved between local adaptability and the capacity to use measures that may be suitable for application in multiple settings. This will be explained more fully in Section 13.5 of this chapter.

It is essential that the process of completing a logic model involves the whole team. The exercise can be completed in an hour-long team meeting, but it is not uncommon for the team to find some aspects of the process challenging,

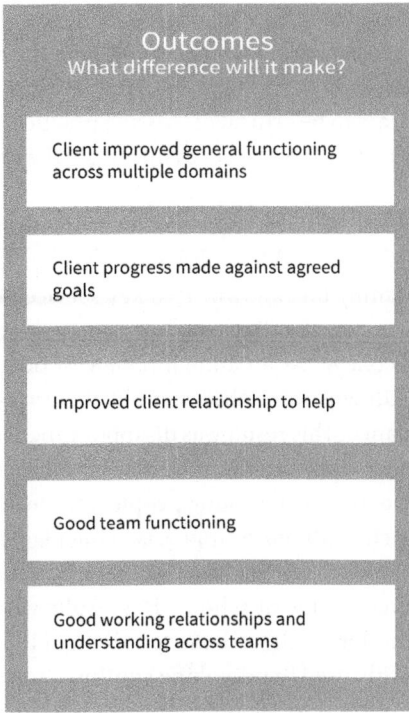

Figure 13.5 What difference will it make ('Outcomes')?

particularly in relation to considering the change mechanisms. Equally important is the degree to which the exercise generates curiosity about these matters, so that the team becomes interested in what type of problems the team is more effective at addressing.

13.3.2.4 Discussing and feeding back outcomes with the whole team

In many teams, outcome measures are completed by team members and no discussions and feedback on these outcomes take place with the team. This means that analysis of their outcomes either does not take place or is reported to the service commissioners and not discussed within the team. Sometimes the reports are simply required to ensure that the service continues to be funded. This is a missed opportunity to stimulate curiosity in the team. For example, before reporting back on the outcomes for a team over a particular time period, the team members can be invited to speculate together on their effectiveness before providing the feedback. Our experience is that teams often estimate the degree of change in their clients to be less than is indicated by the outcomes reported. For one team, this discovery resulted in greater curiosity in the team and discussion about how to include the clients in providing feedback, and even encouraged the team to review the outcomes of their work more frequently.

Such discussions can enable teams to consider what is working well and what is working less well. The discussions may lead to change, but the process may not happen without evoking complex feelings for the team members. It can feel like having an inspection report that appears to be critical of existing practice. As we discussed earlier in this chapter, the conversations may seem to invalidate the efforts and commitments of the team members.

At this point we will describe an example of a situation where outcome monitoring led to both changes of practice and team learning. A team was set up to work with young people at risk of family breakdown. Two key service outcomes were specified by the commissioners: to reduce family breakdown and to increase the young people's attendance at school or college. At an annual review of outcomes for the team, reductions in family breakdowns were observed but there was little indication of an increase in school attendance. This result was disappointing for the team. Lack of progress in returning to school was clearly not the case for all clients, but the overall pattern was not different from before the young people were seen by this team. The team decided on a new approach, with more emphasis being placed on active engagement with school staff, and less focus was given to supporting young people to re-engage with educational curricula outside of school. The results were reviewed a year later and further changes to the approach were made in light of the results. In this process, outcome data were explicitly used in provoking continual revisions of the model.

In this section, we have tried to see outcome monitoring 'from the inside' and to suggest what outcome monitoring may feel like for managers and workers in AMBIT-trained teams. We have made some suggestions about ways of linking outcome monitoring to the real life of the team, so that it is connected to the everyday dilemmas that the team experiences and becomes a part of a culture of learning together at work. We will now turn to looking at outcome monitoring 'from the outside', beginning by providing an overview of what we have learned from local evaluations of work carried out by AMBIT-trained teams.

13.4 Looking from the outside: outcomes for AMBIT-trained teams

As has become clear throughout this book, AMBIT is not a one-size-fits-all approach. In contrast to many approaches, AMBIT supports the integration of its ideas with existing local practice and positively promotes local adaptation of the AMBIT model according to local provision and professional expertise. As we described in Chapter 2, we often use the metaphor that AMBIT is like a computer operating system that is designed to support other evidence-based methods of practice (the 'apps' that run on the system). This should now be familiar ground to the readers of this book.

Because of this local adaptability, local evaluations of the impact of the work of teams trained in AMBIT play a vital role in how we learn about the value of AMBIT and where it conveys benefit to clients. Such studies remain essential for us to ensure that our convictions remain open to challenge, and that our enthusiasms are balanced by what we can learn from others and what we can learn from systematic evaluations of our own work.

From a mentalizing perspective, we have reached a divide in the road between seeing outcomes from the inside and looking at them from the outside. This shift involves a change of focus, moving from the language of relationships, mentalizing, and individual meanings to the language of groups, averages, measures, and scores. Stories of specific individuals, whether clients or workers, rarely cross into this area, and although outcome data lose some meaning on the way, they enable other things to be seen that cannot be seen close up. These evaluations are generally published in academic journals or in local reports where their purpose may be different from the immediate interests of a frontline practitioner such as Jordan, who we mentioned at the start of this chapter. The technical and academic language of these reports has different purposes, such as to ensure that the methods followed are transparent and accurate, and that the data are presented in a clear way. Our aim in this section is to make the conclusions from these evaluation studies as accessible as possible and to avoid technicalities in order to make a connection between what can be seen from the inside and what can be seen from the outside. We will provide an overview of the studies that have been published so far; all the conclusions that we summarize here can be linked back to the referenced documents, papers, and presentations, which interested readers can access to get more detail. As far as we know, we have included all the evaluation reports that had been produced at the time we wrote this chapter.

Eight AMBIT-trained teams have published or reported evaluations of their work. These comprise seven community outreach teams and one inpatient team in Scotland, Australia, Denmark, and England. The teams are mainly run by healthcare agencies but include two teams run by social care and one team working in education. All of them are multidisciplinary, and many use therapeutic methods that are relevant to the specific population they serve in addition to the mentalizing techniques within the AMBIT model. For example, a team working with clients with substance use problems uses motivational interviewing techniques (Miller & Rollnick, 2012) as part of their work within the AMBIT-trained team; one of the teams uses the Assertive Community Treatment approach (Vijverberg et al., 2017). This is consistent with the AMBIT approach. The teams are clearly very different in terms of their service contexts, but they share three crucial factors: all of them work with clients with multiple needs and multiple helpers; they have all been trained in AMBIT; and they all use the AMBIT approach to inform their practice. Putting the reports together enables us to report outcomes for a total sample of approximately 1,800 clients with multiple needs. Even with this large number of clients, we appreciate that we need to tread cautiously with the conclusions we can draw. We need to stay in a mentalizing frame, avoiding non-mentalizing positions such as inappropriate certainty (psychic equivalence), not over-elaborating meaning beyond what is available or missing (pretend mode), and not assuming that reported changes in scores on measures are equivalent to the life changes desired or sought by the clients and workers (teleological thinking). These reports are indications and do not in any way capture the full complexities of the lives of the clients and workers.

All the evaluation studies reported positive results. We are not aware of any reports that describe negative results, but we know that negative results are much less likely to be reported than positive ones, so this is not in itself that surprising. It is clear that these positive outcomes were not solely to do with AMBIT in a narrow sense but were related to the way that AMBIT enables many components of the helping process to come together to *be* helpful. This is suggested by the types of benefits that are reported, as these relate to improvements in the clients' lives and also indicate that more intensive (and expensive!) forms of help may be less often required. We call these *client outcomes* and *network outcomes*, respectively.

What client improvements have been reported? First, some teams reported substantial reductions in mental health symptoms such as anxiety, low mood, self-harm (Daubney et al., 2021; Griffiths et al., 2017; Thomson et al., 2019), behaviour problems (Talbot et al., 2020), and substance misuse (Fuggle et al., 2021). Such improvements do not occur for all clients, but they are frequent enough to meet the commonly used criterion of 'effectiveness', that is, that approximately 50% of clients show a substantial benefit. The evaluations of AMBIT-trained teams that we describe here generally report outcomes similar to this level of improvement.

Also reported are improvements in what are called *general functioning*. This aspect focuses less on specific mental health symptoms and more on how well the client is functioning in general—for example, whether a young person has friends, gets on with their family members, attends school, and so on. Functional outcomes are in many ways the types of outcomes most suited to the AMBIT approach, and several studies have shown substantial improvements in overall client functioning. For example, one study (Fuggle et al., 2021) reported the results of a team working with clients with substance misuse and showed that over 56% of clients showed a significant improvement in their overall life functioning. Interestingly, the team achieved larger improvements in overall functioning than in changes related to substance use alone. This observation suggested that the approach used by the team helped the clients to get back to a more adaptive life pattern even if they continued to use substances some of the time. These evaluations suggested that AMBIT-trained teams achieved improvements for clients with multiple needs and contact with multiple helpers, in terms of both specific problems/symptoms and improvements in overall functioning, and we would suggest that these types of outcomes are highly interconnected—in the same way that the needs of clients are highly interconnected (as we described in Chapter 1). For example, improved peer relationships may contribute significantly to reduced substance use.

These encouraging results were supported by a second range of outcomes, namely changes in network responses to the client's needs. Examples of reductions in the use of institutional, high-cost interventions occurred across all parts of the helping system, for health, social care, and educational agencies. The most frequent finding was a reduction in hospital admissions. In one study (Harmon, 2013), the number of days clients spent in hospital in a 4-year period before the setting up of an AMBIT-trained outreach team was compared with the subsequent 4 years, when the team was in operation. This comparison showed a 60% reduction in the number of bed days between the two time periods and a 40% saving in treatment costs. Similar reductions in the use of hospital admissions were reported in two other studies (Daubney et al., 2021; Griffiths et al., 2017). For young people at risk of family breakdown, one study (Talbot et al., 2020) reported that, after a 1-year intervention by the AMBIT-trained team, 82% of young people remained with their own family (rather than being placed in care) and showed improved family relationships and reduced behavioural difficulties. These results for both hospital admissions and coming into state care are important not only because they avoid the use of highly expensive and intensive interventions, and improve clients' experience, but also because they give some indication of what can be achieved by investing in the relationships that can be developed between teams/agencies to provide networks of multiagency support.

In education, the problem is somewhat reversed. Here, the aim is to support pupils to attend education rather than to reduce their need to attend specialist provision. The work involves supporting pupils who are unable to attend school, enabling them to access education and not become isolated and vulnerable outside this vital aspect of development. For many AMBIT teams, a high priority is placed on supporting young people to return to school, as this is a very common aspect of their multiple needs. In this domain, one study (Stokholm et al., 2019) has reported applying the AMBIT approach to supporting young people who have had long-term school attendance problems. Their study reported that all their clients had achieved a return to some level of school attendance, mainly to mainstream schools but with some young people going to more specialist education settings. The impact of these results has led to the wider application of this approach in their country (Denmark). This is a great example of the AMBIT approach, as the focus of the work was on repairing the helping system, which was not being effective for these clients. Efforts were made to improve the overall system around the young clients rather than focusing exclusively on their mental health difficulties, even where these difficulties were prominent.

One study (Pilling et al., 2014) looked at a specific aspect of network functioning that we highlighted in Chapter 9, where we described the idea of creating a team around the worker as an approach to enabling the helping system to function more effectively. This local evaluation compared the outcomes of families who chose to use the Team around the Worker approach compared with another group of families who chose to have traditional multiagency care. The families who received multiagency care had nine separate teams or agencies working with them concurrently and provided an excellent example of a situation in which families work with multiple helpers. For families who agreed to a Team around the Worker approach, the number of agencies/teams was reduced to an average of four, meaning that the burden to the families in terms of the number of helping agencies they had to interact with was reduced by about half. At the end of the intervention, both groups of families showed improvement (78% in Team around the Worker versus 68% in multiagency care), with outcomes being 10% better for the Team around the Worker group. The experience of families working with the Team around the Worker approach was reported as good.

Overall, these network outcomes suggest that AMBIT-trained teams were able to achieve reductions in high-cost institutional interventions in health, social care, and education settings, as well as in the complexity of multiagency community interventions. The effects of the AMBIT approach were not specific to one type of need, and the teams achieved important improvements in their clients' lives irrespective of the specific presenting problems or life challenges they were facing. The multiplicity of outcomes used in these studies range between domains that are understandable (and appropriate) priorities for those who commission services and those that are closer to the lived experience of the clients. Because of the clients' multiple needs, it is extremely easy for teams to 'slide' between different types of outcomes without being clear about how these aspects fit together. This highlights the potential value of using logic models (as described earlier in this chapter) to help teams to be clear—both for themselves and for their clients—about how they understand the ways that change mechanisms relate to service objectives. For example, the study of Fuggle et al. (2021) suggested that the team was achieving positive outcomes for the service objective of reducing substance use but was also improving clients' overall functioning to an even greater extent. The assumption of this team was that clients' improved functioning was a change mechanism that contributed to their reduced substance use. Empirically, we do not know for sure whether this was how change was happening (an alternative explanation could be that clients' reduced substance use improved their overall functioning), but for the team this is the hypothesis that they followed and, importantly, they were able to show an impact on the mechanisms that they were targeting.

Many of the improvements reported in these evaluations were substantial. More controlled studies will be needed to establish the precise degree to which AMBIT contributes to these promising results. The evaluations indicate that, by looking at AMBIT from the outside, there is much that is encouraging in terms of the achievements made. We see these evaluations as starting points in an effort to embed outcome evaluations as a core component of AMBIT-based practice, to create curiosity rather than certainty, and to give teams the confidence to ask more questions about the approach. To finish this chapter, we will now turn to the work we are doing to try to help teams establish this type of outcomes culture.

13.5 Creating a shared outcomes framework

In February 2018, an international 1-day AMBIT Study Day was held at the Anna Freud Centre to discuss how to evaluate outcomes in AMBIT. We invited mental health researchers, AMBIT practitioners, and AMBIT service leaders from around the world to come together to help us with this problem. It was an act of help-seeking on behalf of the AMBIT development team in London. To our astonishment, an impressively large number of invited professors and therapists turned up to give us a hand. It was a memorable day. The purpose was to consider whether there was a single approach to measuring outcomes for AMBIT teams that took account of the diverse nature of AMBIT teams, the different client groups, the need to integrate with locally required or developed evaluation frameworks, and the need for outcomes to be reasonably robust across the developmental age range. It was clear that focusing on narrowly defined psychiatric symptoms would result in outcomes that were unsuitable for teams working predominantly in social care or educational frameworks. The advice we received from the academic researchers was that we should focus on functional outcomes, that is, outcomes that indicate how the client/young person is functioning in the world rather than in terms of their diagnostic categories. For example: were they going to school? Did they have friendships? Did they have caring family relationships? Were they engaging in positive recreational activities? The view was that, although clients'/young people's presenting problems may be different, all the different AMBIT teams shared the task of trying to reconnect the client/young person to the social, educational, and vocational world from which many of them had become disconnected. Whether the specific purpose of the team was related to drug misuse, family breakdown, self-harm, or violence, the conditions that fostered these difficulties were to some degree shared, namely a process of social exclusion and what we see as a type of developmental isolation (as described in Chapter 3), which placed efforts to repair epistemic mistrust as one of the key change mechanisms of the AMBIT approach. Positive change would be indicated by the client's/young person's capacity to access knowledge from others and by their experience that others had something useful to share with them and enable them to make use of the knowledge and experience of others. The overarching outcome was to increase social inclusion.

AMBIT had already developed a measure of general functioning called the AMBIT Integrative Measure (AIM), which has been used in some teams. This measure was described briefly in Chapters 2 and 4. To briefly recap, the AIM was adapted from the Hampstead Child Adaptation Measure developed by Peter Fonagy and Mary Target (Fonagy & Target, 1996) for their studies of the outcomes of child psychotherapy at the Anna Freud Centre in the 1980s. It was adapted by Dickon Bevington and Peter Fuggle in 2009 to create a more pragmatic measure of functioning for community-based practice (Fuggle et al., 2022). The core constructs of the original measure were retained. The measure consisted of 40 areas of functioning that were rated by the worker or therapist on a five-point scale ranging from 0 (indicating no problem) to 4 (indicating a very severe need). Positive strengths were also captured but did not alter the overall scores generated by the measure. The 40 items were organized into seven domains of functioning, called 'Daily life', 'Socioeconomic conditions', 'Family relationships', 'Peer relationships', 'Mental state', 'Response to the situation', and 'Complexity'. In 2021, a further three items were added to cover discrimination, exploitation, and online life under a new domain called 'Power and control'. The proposal developed out of the Study Day was that this measure should be explored by AMBIT-trained teams as a potential approach to shared outcome measurement. By using the same measures, teams could start to share data and we could begin to understand outcomes across teams.

A second major conclusion of the meeting was that, in addition to a shared functional measure, teams needed to have a method by which they generated an outcome framework that was relevant and consistent with the local context. Measures needed to be linked to explicit mechanisms of change as agreed by those delivering the service (along with input from clients, where this can be included). The use of logic models was proposed by Professor Miranda Wolpert; this method has been covered earlier in this chapter. The use of this method by individual teams would enable them to develop individually tailored outcome frameworks to complement the shared framework provided by the AIM.

13.5.1 An example of a local evaluation using the AIM

As mentioned in the earlier summary of outcomes, one of the local evaluations referred to in the previous section was carried out with a substance misuse team using the AIM as one of their key outcomes (Fuggle et al., 2015, 2021). The study examined outcome data collected between 2013 and 2017 for 499 young people aged between 12 and 20 years (average 16.3 years). Cannabis (81%) and alcohol (63%) were the primary substances used by clients. The study reported an approximately 40% reduction in average cannabis and alcohol use by young people attending the service. Young people were also assessed using the AIM, and average functioning for the whole group showed substantial improvement. A reduction in the total AIM score of 12.9 points indicated a degree of change that was unlikely to be due to chance, that is, it met the criterion for reliable change (Fuggle et al., 2021); 56.5% of cases met this criterion. Of particular significance was that change was not specific or confined to the item of substance misuse but indicated improvements across nearly all areas of the young people's functioning. These results were fully discussed with the team, who were surprised by the positive nature of the outcomes, which were better than they had predicted. The positive affirmation of their work in not focusing on the reduction of substance use as the only legitimate outcome was very validating of the team's whole approach. If we imagine Jordan as being a member of this team, we can imagine that he was encouraged and pleased to be part of this team that was producing positive results. This increased his confidence to focus on the concerns highlighted by his clients rather than just their substance use issues. He could see a bit more how these problems connected up.

13.5.2 Establishing the international AMBIT Study Group

Following the Study Day in 2018, an international AMBIT Study Group was established in 2019 to take this work forward. Many of the authors who have contributed to this book are part of the study group. The ambition of the study group is to support AMBIT teams to develop their own datasets using the AIM, and, in the spirit of learning at work, to generate curiosity about what these datasets can tell us about the characteristics of the clients seen by different AMBIT-influenced teams. Moreover, combining AIM data across international teams would enable us to ask questions about patterns across the data that might directly influence our work. For example, are there similarities and differences in the level of severity of certain types of client problems across teams? Are there particular problems that AMBIT-influenced teams seem to help with, and others that they don't help so much? What can we learn about the characteristics of clients who change, and those who do not change so much, when they are seen by these services?

We are also motivated by the question we posed at the beginning of this chapter: do the lives of clients seen by AMBIT-influenced teams actually improve over the time that we work with them? As we have stated above, a shared AIM dataset will not tell us if it is 'AMBIT's influence' itself that directly facilitates change, but it will allow us to know about the contexts where AMBIT is part of an effective helping system. We can then learn about the settings and adaptations of AMBIT where outcomes are positive or less positive. This will allow us to make more robust comparisons of AMBIT-influenced teams against other quality benchmarks for similar services that do not apply AMBIT principles.

Not surprisingly, building a group of representatives from teams around the world to work together on this goal has not been straightforward. We have learned that teams from different countries bring their own legal frameworks, service contexts, and views about measurement, and do not have the same service infrastructures to support this type of work. As well as practical problems, such as organizational barriers in sharing anonymized client data, there have also been concerns that this type of measurement may lead to non-mentalized conclusions and to scores being treated as certainties (an example of psychic equivalence) rather than opportunities for ongoing curiosity and learning. Manualizing together the steps needed to introduce the AIM 'fresh' into a service has given us a way of learning about the dilemmas and challenges that need to be overcome for this to work. We hope this will serve as a guide for other teams in the future.

The group began its work as the COVID-19 pandemic hit, meaning that planned face-to-face meetings were cancelled and the group's primary task became creating connections between members, moving towards being a working group, while members and their teams managed the challenges of the pandemic. As we might predict, there has been an important process of getting to know each other and an effort to understand each other's contexts. This process involved sharing examples of our client work 'in the field' and asking each other for help with it. It has meant that, as group leaders, we have needed to hold an Active Planning stance, trying to attune to the needs of the group (understandably, the need to connect and think more generally about aspects of AMBIT) while at the same time broadcasting our intentions and holding on to our plan—to develop a shared outcomes framework. At the time of writing, 2 years after the group began working together, the group members are routinely using the AIM in their services and have begun sharing AIM data. This process has already opened up important opportunities for learning together. For example, two teams, both working with young people who are highly socially isolated and often shut off from their social world, have recently shared AIM data in the group and noticed a common pattern in relation to changes in clients' functioning over time. Both teams used the AIM at the start and 6 months and 1 year into client contact. Their data showed almost no change (and in some cases a worsening of severity) over the first 6 months. However, between 6 months and 1 year the picture changed dramatically, and a number of positive changes in functioning could be seen across their clients. This observation has stimulated curiosity about what happens after 6 months to allow this change, and perhaps highlights the significance of the engagement phase of the work for these teams, before measurable changes can be observed. Alongside the importance of workers in the teams having knowledge of these patterns, this information may also be critical for those commissioning these services.

This is the kind of learning that we hope to develop within the international study group. The process of work is ongoing and will continue as we build a sense of 'team' between the collaborators, but we are particularly proud to be working in collaboration with our fantastic international colleagues at a time when the UK, by withdrawing from the European Union, has opted to see its future in rather more isolated ways. In this context, these international relationships have been particularly appreciated by the members of the AMBIT team based in the UK.

13.6 Implications

In this chapter the authors have described a mentalized approach to outcome monitoring and to have as a starting point the mindsets of the key people involved in this work: the client, the worker, and the team leader (or service commissioner). They have recognized the contradictions and challenges that outcome monitoring may represent for workers and managers. As with all of AMBIT, they see the need to understand the mental states of these key people as a major component that supports this work, and they have proposed a number of methods that we believe are likely to create team conditions that enable learning around outcomes to take place without facilitating non-mentalized thinking.

Learning at work is a key component of the AMBIT approach that supports a team to understand their experience of the work that they do, to capture the knowledge gained from lived experience, and to remain fundamentally curious about its impact on their clients. As with mentalizing itself, learning at work enables a team to go beyond the stereotypes of its own practice, whether positive ('outcomes are just about proving that what we do works') or negative ('none of the young people we see get better') to gain access to a more accurate and nuanced experience of individual workers and the benefit of their work with clients. This chapter has aimed to find a balance between including the richness of individually nuanced outcome work and the necessity of developing a measurement approach to assess the utility of the AMBIT approach more fully. It has included a brief review of local evaluation studies, which suggest that AMBIT-trained teams have achieved highly encouraging results so far.

There are still important gaps in our knowledge, though, and the future development of AMBIT will be affected by how well we address these. For example, AMBIT proposes that a well-connected team and well-functioning helping networks will not just enable workers to do their jobs better but will benefit the clients too. The previous chapters in this book have suggested in many different ways that, from the inside of the AMBIT team, this may very strongly appear to be the case. The work ahead is to discover whether this perception can be matched by how it looks from the outside. This leads us on to our last chapter, Chapter 14, where we set out some of the ways in which we see AMBIT developing over the next few years.

References

Daubney, M. F. X., Raeburn, N., Blackman, K., Jeffries, H., & Healy, K. L. (2021). Outcomes of assertive community treatment for adolescents with complex mental health problems who are difficult to engage. *Journal of Child and Family Studies*, 30(2), 502–516. https://doi.org/10.1007/s10826-020-01882-3

Fonagy, P., Cottrell, D., Phillips, J., Bevington, D., Glaser, D., & Allison, E. (2015). *What works for whom? A critical review of treatments for children and adolescents* (2nd ed.). Guilford Press.

Fonagy, P., & Target, M. (1996). Predictors of outcome in child psychoanalysis: A retrospective study of 763 cases at the Anna Freud Centre. *Journal of the American Psychoanalytic Association*, 44(1), 27–77. https://doi.org/10.1177/000306519604400104

Fuggle, P., Bevington, D., Cracknell, L., Hanley, J., Hare, S., Lincoln, J., Richardson, G., Stevens, N., Tovey, H., & Zlotowitz, S. (2015). The Adolescent Mentalization-Based Integrative Treatment (AMBIT) approach to outcome evaluation and manualization: Adopting a learning organization approach. *Clinical Child Psychology and Psychiatry*, 20(3), 419–435. https://doi.org/10.1177/1359104514521640

Fuggle, P., Bevington, D., Fairbairn, J., Talbot, L., Cracknell, L., & Smith, R. (2022). *A practitioner guide to the AMBIT Integrative Measure (AIM)*. Anna Freud National Centre for Children and Families.

Fuggle, P., Talbot, L., Wheeler, J., Rees, J., Ventre, E., Beehan, V., Hare, S., Bevington, D., & Cracknell, L. (2021). Improving lives not just saying no to substances: Evaluating outcomes for a young people's substance use team trained in the AMBIT approach. *Clinical Child Psychology and Psychiatry*, 26(2), 490–504. https://doi.org/10.1177/1359104521994875

Griffiths, H., Noble, A., Duffy, F., & Schwannauer, M. (2017). Innovations in practice: Evaluating clinical outcome and service utilization in an AMBIT-trained tier 4 child and adolescent mental health service. *Child and Adolescent Mental Health*, 22(3), 170–174. https://doi.org/10.1111/camh.12181

Harmon, S. (2013). *Using AMBIT to reduce adolescent inpatient admissions* [Video of a conference presentation]. AMBIT Conference 2013, Anna Freud Centre, London, UK. https://youtu.be/ALvv0yLC68k

Miller, W. R., & Rollnick, S. (2012). *Motivational interviewing: Helping people change* (3rd ed.). Guilford Press.

Pilling, S., Butler, S., O'Brien, M., & Hardy, R. (2014). *Camden Transformation Team evaluation: Interim report*. University College London.

Senge, P. (2006). *The fifth discipline: The art and practice of the learning organization* (Rev. ed.). Doubleday.

Stokholm, M., Andersen, M. J., Bertelsen, L., & Sørensen, S. (2019). U-start: Udviklingsstart til børn og unge med skolevægring i Hvidovre kommune [U-start: Developmental start for children and young people with school refusal in Hvidovre municipality]. In *Skolens fraværende børn—Årsager og indsatser* [*Children absent from school—Causes and efforts*] (pp. 109–138). Dafolo.

Talbot, L., Fuggle, P., Foyston, Z., & Lawson, K. (2020). Delivering an integrated adolescent multi-agency specialist service to families with adolescents at risk of care: Outcomes and learning from the first ten years. *British Journal of Social Work*, *50*(5), 1531–1550. https://doi.org/10.1093/bjsw/bcz148

Thomson, A., Griffiths, H., Fisher, R., McCabe, R., Abbott-Smith, S., & Schwannauer, M. (2019). Treatment outcomes and associations in an adolescent-specific early intervention for psychosis service. *Early Intervention in Psychiatry*, *13*(3), 707–714. https://doi.org/10.1111/eip.12778

Vijverberg, R., Ferdinand, R., Beekman, A., & van Meijel, B. (2017). The effect of youth assertive community treatment: A systematic PRISMA review. *BMC Psychiatry*, *17*(1), 284. https://doi.org/10.1186/s12888-017-1446-4

Wolpert, M., Sharpe, H., Humphrey, N., Patalay, P., & Deighton, J. (2016). *EBPU logic model*. CAMHS Press. https://www.annafreud.org/media/3498/ebpu-logic-model-200416final.pdf

14

What are the future directions for AMBIT?

Liz Cracknell, Laura Talbot, Rebecca Smith, James Fairbairn, Dickon Bevington, and Peter Fuggle

14.1 Setting the scene

For this last chapter, we asked the AMBIT team at the Anna Freud Centre to articulate their ideas about what developments they feel will be needed for AMBIT over the next few years. As the editors of this book, we are part of this team but very much wanted the whole team to have a chance to share their collective vision of what developments in AMBIT would look like for them. We are all clear that AMBIT belongs to the wider AMBIT community of practice and that it needs to be shaped by all those who wish to explore its value in the work they do with their clients. The wider engagement in the development of AMBIT by teams across the world is critical to this process. So, as ever, what we suggest here is just a set of starting points and, as we highlighted in Chapter 1, how they are taken up will depend on how they are seen by those who find this approach useful to them. The future for AMBIT, as the past, needs to be grounded in the realities of its utility.

A number of important developments in AMBIT have been described in this book by different teams. We have seen the extension of AMBIT to adult clients in the Netherlands (Chapter 7), and we have learned how AMBIT has been applied to residential and day provision for young people in Austria (Chapter 8). We have heard about important developments in technique, such as in Sweden, in the linking of psychotherapy to frontline practitioners (Chapter 6); in Denmark, in an exploration of network processes (Chapter 10); and in London, in relation to the Team around the Worker (Chapter 9) and the use of AMBIT Integrative Measure (AIM) cards (Chapter 4). We have also been shown developments in professional training, as in Germany with the training of teachers working in specialist educational settings (Chapter 11). These are some of the examples that illustrate the continuous evolution of the approach. AMBIT should not be seen as a prescription that others should follow, but as an opportunity for others to adapt and develop.

But we are often asked: does that mean that anything goes? Are there developments that we would say are not really AMBIT? How do we determine what is considered to be a positive development of the AMBIT approach, and what may be seen as a diversion or a step backwards? We agree that we need to balance creativity and contextual responsiveness with maintaining an internal coherence for both clients and frontline practitioners. We need to be willing to simplify where we can and take out things that turn out to be over-elaborate or frankly unnecessary. There is no shortage of aspects of the work of the programme that need such attention, but how can we ensure that this takes place in a way that is safe and effective? This chapter aims to illustrate how AMBIT is an open system that places curiosity and efforts towards humility at the centre of its endeavour. In the end, what must temper creativity is attention to outcomes: does this help, and how can we be sure that it does? These principles apply just as much to the development of AMBIT itself as to anything else. We need to stay aware of what we do not know and be curious to find out more to strengthen the helping process, using the starting points we have laid out in this book. This chapter gives you some idea of the ways in which we hope to achieve this.

14.2 Introduction

AMBIT has surprised us. We had not anticipated the degree to which it has resonated with others. As we outlined in Chapter 1, we have discovered that the same issues powerfully emerge for services with different client groups and in different service contexts. This has encouraged us. Particularly during the beginning of the COVID-19 pandemic, we did not know what sort of future AMBIT had. But, paradoxically in this context, AMBIT seems more robust than ever. The interest and enthusiasm of others expressed in this book is a testament to that.

AMBIT is not a finished product. It is an open system designed to continuously evolve in response to the problems and challenges that have been articulated in this book. As described in Chapter 1, AMBIT arose out of concern about the ability of existing services to meet the needs of those with multiple needs—a group of people that often overlapped with the most marginalized and disadvantaged in our society. The dramatic success of medicine and technology in developing new treatments for specific physical conditions has not been matched by improvements in how we address health and social care needs when they are embedded in the complexities of poverty, marginalization, and discrimination—common experiences in the populations targeted by the AMBIT approach. We believe that we are only at the beginning of understanding how to properly address the issues that we raised in Chapter 1. Moreover, it is increasingly (if belatedly) clear to us how crucial it is that we do not fall into the trap of applying a deficit model—either to our clients or to our services—that excludes or, even worse, excuses the oppressive systems within which their struggles emerge. Although AMBIT has offered some useful starting points, these problems need a process of radical continuous development, which will involve collaboration and the integration of many different ideas and approaches, if we are to make important differences to the lives of these clients.

We want to acknowledge the extent to which the world is changing. During the writing of this book the world changed in two important ways. First, we needed to adapt to COVID-19. Our first response to COVID-19 was much like the rest of the world; we could not see how the AMBIT programme of training would continue without the capacity to work with teams in a face-to-face setting. But, like so many, we have adapted to a new world in which transferring much of our training activity into online delivery has been more successful than we initially imagined. The necessity to adapt all aspects of the AMBIT programme (training, client work, and project coordination) to this new reality was unavoidable, and now such adaptations seem to be largely acceptable. There are aspects of training that we believe we could manage better if we were working face to face, but we have been surprised at how readily the participants have adapted to the new world of 'breakout rooms', and of being 'muted' and 'unmuted'! There are benefits, too; remote delivery has helped us to reach teams for whom AMBIT training was previously not accessible or affordable. In all the future directions for AMBIT, we will need to keep in mind how all such developments will work in the context of a (potentially partial) return to face-to-face working, and the adoption of blended ways of working that combine face-to-face and remote (via internet or phone) activities.

Second, the world has changed for us with respect to the much greater highlighting of the role of racism, discrimination, and exclusion in our work and the need to make attention to this more prominent in the AMBIT approach. The important and influential Black Lives Matter movement required us to rethink our approach to racism, and matters of equity, diversity, and inclusion (EDI) more broadly, in a way that we had not previously. We believe that it is important for us to acknowledge this publicly as part of taking the AMBIT model forward. In the themes that we consider in this chapter, we will consider anti-racism and inclusion as crucial themes in their own right and will endeavour to ensure they are included in each of the other themes that we consider.

So, AMBIT needed to adapt in response to these new conditions—and will continue to need to adapt in response to future conditions that we cannot yet predict. In any event, adaptation is required because the challenge of successfully addressing the themes described in Chapter 1 remains far from being met. At its heart, AMBIT requests a profound humility about the challenges of this work, but we now wish to balance humility with ambition (a word whose root, aptly, is ambit). As an open system, we invite others (including you, the reader) to join us to try to identify some of the collective directions of travel for those who make use of AMBIT ideas. Only by working together will we continue to make progress around the issues that have been highlighted in this book.

We have organized our development ideas into three themes:

1. Developing the basic AMBIT approach.
2. Increasing training capacity and diversity.
3. Improving implementation.

In the same way as we invite teams at the end of training to come up with an implementation plan for how they are going to implement AMBIT in their work, here we present our implementation plan for AMBIT for the coming years.

14.3 Developing the basic AMBIT approach

14.3.1 Making AMBIT values explicit and improving our attention to EDI

The need: we have identified a need to broadcast more explicitly the values and ethics that underpin AMBIT as an approach and that guide our work as the AMBIT Programme Team at the Anna Freud Centre. There are a few drivers behind this, which, combined, have brought this issue to the top of our 'to-do list' of development tasks. First, the scale of the AMBIT programme has grown. Where previously we were a very small group of people holding—perhaps only implicitly at times—a shared ethical stance in relation to the work of helping services, the AMBIT programme has grown in size, making it necessary to pay attention to how we develop within the team not only a shared understanding of *what* AMBIT is, but also *how* and *why* we do what we do in the way we do it. Second, and similarly, as we began the process of accrediting international AMBIT Training Centres (see below), we became aware of our wish to ensure that anyone delivering AMBIT training with a badge of accreditation should maintain fidelity not only to the core curriculum but also to the values and ethics that underpin it. Again, in order to do this, we must be able to articulate what those values and ethics are. As is so often the case when we attempt to move from the implicit to the explicit, we realize that there are gaps that require more attention. Finally, the increased attention across much of the world in recent years on issues of social justice, prompted by detailed coverage in print and broadcast media, and on social media, of multiple painful incidents of social injustice across the world, has prompted for us (as it has for so many others) reflection on the contributions of our work to social justice and the perpetuation of social injustices. This in particular has led us to understand, more than we did before, that implicit values are not sufficient to bring about the change that is required. With regard to race, for example, it is not sufficient for one to believe oneself to not be racist—one must be explicitly and actively anti-racist to help bring about systemic change.

The plan: our plan to address this need has three interrelated strands.

14.3.1.1 Articulate AMBIT values and ethics

We will develop and articulate in the core AMBIT manual (https://manuals.annafr eud.org/ambit) AMBIT's underpinning values and ethics. We will make it explicit that, while we encourage local adaption of AMBIT material, the underpinning values and ethics at AMBIT's core must remain. Any changes to that core will be made only following a democratic process involving the AMBIT programme and engagement with the wider AMBIT community of practice. Such values will include the principle that all aspects of AMBIT, even where focused on teams, networks, or learning, exist for the benefit of the clients we serve. AMBIT stands against the social injustice that means that the needs of people who experience multiple disadvantages are often poorly met by traditional helping services or are responded to punitively. Related to this is our open-source principle: AMBIT exists to help clients, and our work of dissemination is to this end rather than for the sake of power, fame, or fortune. We protect our intellectual property for the purposes of ensuring fidelity and academic integrity, and commit to maintaining all our materials and learning freely available online so that they can benefit the largest number of people. We are still working to bring AMBIT in line with some values to which we ascribe great importance—namely, that AMBIT practice should be anti-oppressive and inclusive. The theory underpinning AMBIT must be either cross-culturally generalizable, inclusive of different evidence relating to different cultures, or—where this is not possible—acknowledging and transparent about its limitations.

14.3.1.2 Uphold the values in our work

Just as we follow the principles and practices of AMBIT in the way we operate as the AMBIT Programme Team, we must uphold its values too. A focus on social justice through an actively anti-oppressive stance and intentional promotion of EDI should permeate how we relate as a team, how and from whom we learn, and how we interact with others in our consultation and training activity. We are seeking to learn from the literature and from partners who have greater expertise than us in this area, to strengthen and develop this work. This includes a focus on developing diversity within the programme and the community of practice to ensure the inclusion of multiple perspectives (see Section 14.4.2).

14.3.1.3 Improve how the AMBIT approach promotes EDI

It is our view that the AMBIT approach (and mentalizing generally) has the potential to—and in many cases does—provide tools that help a team to create systems that promote EDI. However, in our writing, AMBIT manual, and training we have not always made this explicit, and so there is work for us to make sure this is foregrounded. There are opportunities in each quadrant of the wheel, of which the following are just examples:

- *Client*: a greater understanding of the impact of marginalization and oppression can help us to better mentalize mistrust in helping services.
- *Team*: mentalizing has the potential to help us to remain curious about difference and to examine unconscious biases, but issues relating to EDI often raise the emotional temperature, making mentalizing more difficult. AMBIT's team practices that support mentalizing can therefore facilitate more effective use of mentalizing to promote EDI.

- *Networks*: AMBIT's tools for expecting, recognizing, and addressing dis-integration can help us to make sense of others, to both invite and value difference, and to exercise cultural humility (Tervalon & Murray-García, 1998).
- *Learning*: a major injustice in our field of work is so-called *epistemic injustice* (Fricker, 2007)—the privileging of knowledge (or evidence) from certain groups over that of others. We must follow our own Learning at Work principles (in which AMBIT encourages an intentional balancing of local practice and expertise with evidence-based practice) to ensure that all voices are heard and the evidence being applied in our work is relevant and generalizable to those we serve.

14.3.2 A deployment-based approach to model development

The need: AMBIT is, by design, perpetually under development; our application of a deployment-focused approach to intervention development (Weisz & Gray, 2008) creates a continual feedback loop (Figure 14.1) in which the model is adapted in response to learning from both research and real-world application. The sources from

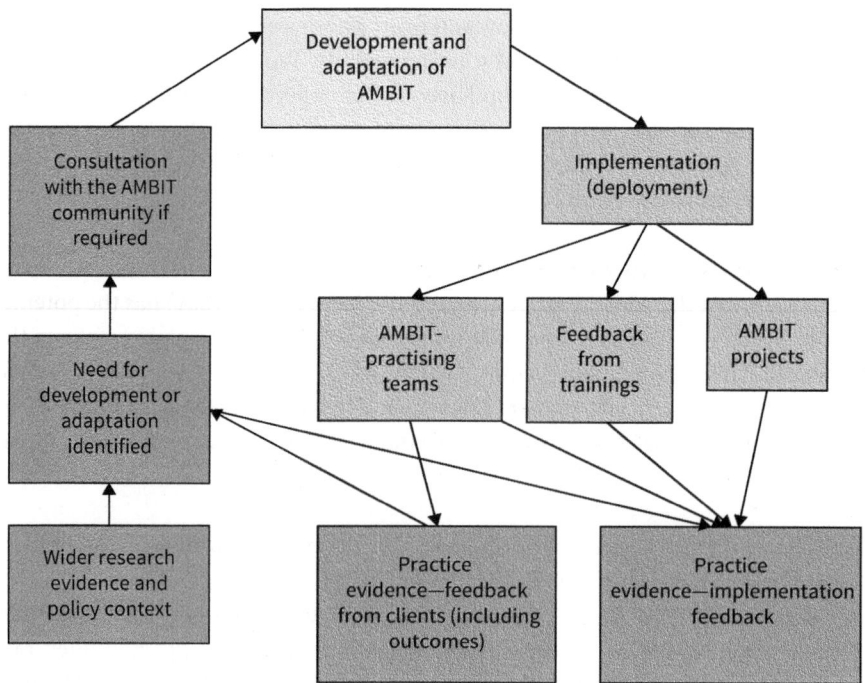

Figure 14.1 AMBIT's deployment-focused approach to development based on continual feedback and learning.

which we receive learning that indicate the need for adaptations to AMBIT are several and include the following:

- Feedback on AMBIT training from teams and systems that we train (particularly those working in different settings, or with different client groups, than those who have traditionally sought AMBIT training).
- Feedback or outcome data from teams and systems who have implemented AMBIT (including feedback from their clients and client outcome data).
- Our AMBIT Programme Team's learning from delivering consultation, training, and supervision.
- Learning from research projects. The AMBIT programme always seeks to have a portfolio of real-world projects in which we can apply and evaluate AMBIT ideas. For example, we are currently working in partnership with a youth organization to design and deliver an AMBIT-influenced peer-mentoring project in which we train young mentors to apply Thinking Together to provide mentorship to younger mentees.
- Learning from the cutting edge of research-based evidence in helping services.

The plan: in Table 14.1 we outline some areas of development that we are currently working on, and the learning that has prompted each area of work. We are sharing this as a way of broadcasting intentions, and hope that by making our process more transparent we are demonstrating our openness to learning from other members of the AMBIT community of practice.

14.3.3 Improving our knowledge of routine client outcomes

The need: evaluating the degree to which AMBIT adds value in complex helping systems is difficult. The adaptive nature of the model and the way it firmly locates itself within complex systems makes this especially hard. Nevertheless, we believe that there is an ethical requirement to ensure that what we are offering is grounded in evidence of effectiveness. As AMBIT develops further, it will be crucial to support ongoing curiosity towards gathering this evidence.

The plan: our ambition is to support a process that produces a regular and consistent stream of outcome data from teams in the AMBIT community who feel motivated to collect, and confident to share and think about, outcomes in relation to various aspects of their work (particularly client work, but also relating to other quadrants of the AMBIT wheel). This would include contributions from the international AMBIT Study Group (see Chapter 13) but could also include contributions from other teams who became interested through using, for example, the AIM. To support this work, we have greatly improved the technical aspects of the online version of the AIM, and we now have versions in different languages that can be scored online with easily

Table 14.1 Current areas of development

Area for model development or adaptation	What learning led to the identification of the need for development or adaptation?	What are our plans?
Developing the process of *manualizing* so that it is more accessible and effective in supporting learning	• Data from the AMBIT Service Evaluation Questionnaire (ASEQ)—most teams do not have a systematized way of recording learning • Feedback from training and implementation: many teams either do not adopt—or cannot sustain—manualizing in practice • There is sound theoretical rationale for manualizing • Feedback on the AMBIT manuals system	Although there is a sound theoretical rationale for team manualizing, it is the least effectively implemented AMBIT practice in the real world. We need to learn more about the barriers to implementation and sustainability in practice before we can know whether we need to entirely revisit the practice of capturing team learning or improve our methods of training teams in manualizing
Developing the method of applying the *Team around the Worker* by looking at how *not* to be the keyworker in the Team around the Worker	• A change in who is requesting AMBIT training and feedback from training and implementation: traditionally, we have trained teams that are likely to contain the most trusted worker. Increasingly, we are training whole systems, including workers who may be better placed in the Team around the Worker than acting as the keyworker	We need to develop and evaluate best practice for teams and workers for contributing to the helping system in ways other than attempting to develop a key relationship with the client. We need to consider guidance for policymakers and commissioners to support the delivery of methods of helping clients other than in face-to-face work
Application of the *mentalizing stance* to client work	• Increased diversity in terms of the types of teams we are training in AMBIT • Feedback from teams implementing AMBIT • Our learning from delivering training and supervision	Perhaps more than with any other quadrant of the AMBIT wheel, the principles and practices of Working with your Client are applied differently in different settings, and we have adapted our training to accommodate this. However, this has resulted in some ambiguity about how the mentalizing stance should be applied to client work that is not best characterized as 'therapy'. We plan to work on methods of operationalizing the stance in non-therapy settings to support our training and to support teams to assess progress in implementation

exportable data. The plan is to bring together outcome data from a group of teams and create opportunities for reflection and model development linked to the findings that emerge.

14.3.4 Developing a research programme on the core model

The need: in the core AMBIT model, a number of specific causal hypotheses are proposed that we believe need to be tested empirically. Perhaps the most prominent is the prediction that client outcomes are moderated by the quality of team functioning (including team learning) and the degree of connectedness that exists in key network relationships. This is the cement that binds together the AMBIT wheel, and it needs to be examined and tested. At present, these are reasonable conjectures. Studies of how to categorize the variations of the relational patterns (social network analysis (Kadushin, 2012) might offer one pathway towards this, for instance) and their impacts on a range of core outcomes are required. Alongside this, studies of the core mechanisms of change in (and achieved by) AMBIT-trained teams are crucial if we are to determine the elements that are critical to successfully adapting key factors that affect outcomes for clients.

The plan: this level of research requires funding and collaboration between researchers and practitioners beyond what can be achieved in small-scale local evaluations. The mechanisms of change are not controversial. It is likely that well-connected teams will enable their workers to function better, and there is existing research (e.g. Glisson et al., 2010) showing that a positive team culture improves client outcomes. However, we still do not know enough about the nature of the elements that promote 'well-connectedness' in a team, how 'well-connectedness' could be sensitively measured, and how it affects client outcomes. Similarly, with respect to networks, we have some data that suggest that AMBIT-informed services may have an impact on the type of help that might be offered to clients (e.g. less institutional interventions such as hospital admissions) and may reduce referral rates between services. Despite all our efforts, AMBIT-informed care is not going to work for everyone (there is no intervention in the world that does that), and we do not know enough about which clients benefit from, and may prefer, what could be called 'collective care' compared with those who prefer specialist services. For example, an important question for us is whether AMBIT is useful in more collective cultures. A person in such a culture might be less likely to seek professional help at all because their needs are met within their family and community, or because there is massive stigma related to help-seeking, or because it would be perceived as a shaming comment on the functioning of the family/group (because an individual's problem would be viewed as a group problem).

14.4 Increasing training capacity and widening diversity

14.4.1 Setting up international AMBIT Training Centres

The need: as described in Chapter 1, AMBIT was designed initially in response to the challenges of offering effective help in service contexts in the UK, where the AMBIT programme began. Over the past decade, however, we have increasingly been invited to work with organizations around the world and have discovered that, despite social, political, and cultural differences and significant variations in helping-service ecologies, those challenges are more universal in nature than we had imagined. That contributions to this book come from teams in several different countries is testament to the promise that AMBIT shows internationally, and requests for consultation, training, and supervision continue to come in from around the world—increasingly so, in fact. This is very encouraging to us, but it has raised two important questions: how can we most efficiently expand AMBIT's reach from our base in the UK, and how can we ensure that AMBIT, and AMBIT training, are most effectively adapted to local contexts that are unfamiliar to us?

The plan: our response to these questions has been to develop a process for accrediting international AMBIT Training Centres. AMBIT material has always been freely available under a Creative Commons licence, which allows sharing and adaptation of our content as long as it is attributed to us as its original authors and that there is no commercial gain. Our accreditation process is designed to allow eligible individuals within organizations meeting certain criteria to deliver and charge for training and associated activity with supervision from the AMBIT programme in London. The process was created following a consultation with members of the AMBIT community around the world. At the time of writing, we are in the process of signing off our first accredited AMBIT Training Centre, and expect more to follow.

14.4.2 Widening diversity within the AMBIT Programme Team and in the community of practice to improve learning and adaptation

The need: core to the AMBIT approach is *learning and adaptation*. It is our view that offering the most effective help requires a judicious balancing of (external) evidence-based practice and (local) practice-based evidence (see Chapter 2, in Section 2.7 on Learning at Work). This principle applies as much to the AMBIT programme as to the work of AMBIT-trained teams. Yet learning is, arguably, inherently biased. The knowledge that is accessible to, and privileged by, our small team in London is inevitably influenced by our professional and personal backgrounds. Although it is our responsibility as individuals to resist so-called epistemic injustice, in which some groups' knowledge is heard and accepted while others' is silenced or discredited, we believe it is harder to do this while we remain a relatively small and homogeneous group. AMBIT theory and practice will develop most effectively with contributions from a broader range of perspectives. We also feel that we have had mixed success in our efforts to facilitate different forms of communities of practice (often online groups), with the AMBIT Study Group being an example of where it has worked well, but other initiatives have not really taken off. We have learned that we need to invest the necessary time and effort, that it needs to be purposeful, and that we need to be clear about who is taking the lead/some responsibility in facilitating it.

The plan: we are working towards increasing diversity within the core AMBIT Programme Team here in London as well as within the most engaged and influential members of the AMBIT community of practice across the world. In this context we refer to diversity in its range of forms, in terms of professional, educational, and sociocultural backgrounds. We are fortunate at the time of writing to be in a position to expand the AMBIT Programme Team in London, and are keen that as part of this our team becomes more representative of the teams to whom we provide training. Additionally, we hope that the creation of accredited international AMBIT Training Centres and the shared learning that this work enables will introduce a broader range of perspectives while also to some extent decentralizing influence over the development of AMBIT. We are also keen to continue to explore ways of supporting communities of practice; in particular, we are developing the idea of a Local AMBIT Community of Practice Facilitator as a way of supporting the development of local networks with shared understandings and encouraging mentalization-based practice.

14.4.3 Widening methods of dissemination through training and consultation

The need: one of our core strategic objectives is to improve help for those with multiple needs by disseminating AMBIT broadly to those involved in commissioning, managing, and delivering that help. While our training tends to be evaluated positively (see Chapter 12) and outcomes for teams implementing AMBIT are encouraging (see Chapter 13), we continually work to develop our methods of dissemination with the goal of positively influencing helping services by the most efficient, economical, and equitable means. It is important that we remind ourselves continually of the intention of this objective—which is to improve the effectiveness of help for those disadvantaged by multiple needs, and *not* the endless expansion of the AMBIT programme for its own sake or our own sense of pride. Indeed, a true sign of success would be that AMBIT was no longer required because its principles and practices had become 'treatment as usual' (or that it had become obsolete due to other improvements).

The plan: we remain of the belief that, currently, whole-team training is our most effective method of dissemination; this seems to be almost as much about the *process* of a team learning together, which we help to facilitate, as it is about the AMBIT *content* that we share (see Chapter 12 on our methods of training). The types of dissemination work we would like to consider include influencing at scale through national initiatives such as, in the UK, the training of young people's mental health crisis teams, and contributing to pre-qualification professional training courses (as described in Chapter 11) for groups such as youth workers, social workers, doctors, and teachers, thus increasing the reach of AMBIT training. We also aim to increase the depth of AMBIT training by developing advanced AMBIT workshops for teams or individuals in relation to specific areas of practice, and for policymakers, commissioners, and senior leaders of statutory and voluntary sector services. There is already a fairly rich array of freely available, short web-streamed videos that provide basic introductions for individuals or groups, but these, too, could be improved.

14.5 Improving implementation

14.5.1 Supporting implementation after training

The need: not all teams that engage in AMBIT training find it easy to implement AMBIT afterwards. The systemic problems described in Chapter 1 reassert their power and make implementation hard. The homeostatic power (or inertia) of existing practice in individuals, in teams, and in networks is huge, so it is easy to revert to very familiar and well-established patterns. This is because they have a kind of logic—a logic that AMBIT is endeavouring to challenge. This type of experience is disheartening but not unpredicted. We need to develop ways of creating resilience in teams that supports the gradual establishment of aspects of AMBIT practice that are not immediately swept away by such forces. This process will require leadership, the application of implementation science, and knowledge on how to learn ways to achieve quick wins to gain traction and confidence in the challenging business of change. We know that teams can achieve this, but we need to find methods that enable it to happen more frequently for teams whose existing systems are less favourably disposed to the adoption of AMBIT methods.

The plan: after most AMBIT trainings, the newly trained team has the opportunity to have ongoing 'supervision' of their implementation of AMBIT. We need to learn more about how to use this valuable time in the most effective way. We need to develop a more systematic way of understanding both the facilitators and the barriers that teams experience and, based on this knowledge, to develop more specific interventions that will enable 'quick wins' during the fragile first stages of implementation. We believe that we need to move away from the traditional language of 'supervision' and adopt a more collaborative language so that the purpose of these meetings is explicitly to support local mentalizing-based work and local implementation plans. We want to avoid teams being positioned as passively implementing AMBIT. We feel that we need a more collaborative frame for this follow-up work and would like to consult others about this.

14.5.2 Improving the wiki manual

The need: the value of the wiki manual (https://manuals.annafreud.org/ambit/) to the AMBIT developers and training team at the Anna Freud Centre is beyond doubt. Its value to teams trained in AMBIT is less clear. We have given a high value to enabling teams to have adaptable versions of the core AMBIT content and to making this material freely available. However, as highlighted in Section 14.3 on developing the basic AMBIT approach, we are less sure of how effective it is in supporting ongoing implementation of AMBIT in a local team.

The plan: the current AMBIT manual is large (running to thousands of pages) and has many functions. Fundamentally, it is the depository of all aspects of the AMBIT model and related knowledge, research, and practice made freely available to all. In consultation with AMBIT teams, we would like to create a more focused web-based resource targeted at supporting teams, particularly during the early stages of their implementation of AMBIT.

14.6 Conclusion

Around 70 years ago, Leonard Bernstein and Stephen Sondheim wrote the famous musical *West Side Story* about two gangs in New York. The show includes a song that imagines a conversation between a police officer (Officer Krupke) and the young people in the gangs, in which they try to work out who should help the young people to get a better life. The song is playful but conveys with astonishing clarity society's confusion as to whether the young people should be given treatment, employment, better care, or punishment. The muddle and contrasting views of the different agencies involved with the young people is brilliantly illustrated. But the overall tale remains tragic, as characters in the story die in ways that are depicted as pointless and despairing. Over half a century on, these dilemmas and realities remain an elusive challenge with continuing tragic outcomes.

The AMBIT programme (and this book) is our humble contribution to trying to address this profound and enduring difficulty. In the time since *West Side Story* was written, there have been multiple initiatives, new government programmes, and evidence-based interventions that have been presented as the new solution, as the standard that all other programmes should follow. In our view, many of these initiatives have been fragmented, relatively short term, and do not address the profound challenges of this work: the need for well-connected teams and a sophisticated approach to network functioning, a more collective approach. The hypothesis that AMBIT proposes is that effective help is unlikely to come from some new idea (that nobody has considered previously) but that it is dependent on the creation of complex difficult collaborations between adults, helpers, carers, teachers, therapists, and others to provide individualized meaningful and effective help. This cannot be achieved by managed systems alone but needs to recognize the profound psychological challenges this presents for clients and workers alike to achieve change. Whether mentalizing is the crucial fuel that can drive this bus remains to be established, but our experience over the past 15 years is that it may provide one piece of the complex jigsaw that we need to make progress with this puzzle. For now, we are backing non-heroic, team-based, psychologically sensitive, and individually tailored help provided by multiple teams working in collaboration together. If this becomes 'treatment as usual', we will be very pleased when the world gets there, and it will surely be time for us to go out of business.

References

Fricker, M. (2007). *Epistemic injustice: Power and ethics of knowing.* Oxford University Press.

Glisson, C., Schoenwald, S. K., Hemmelgarn, A., Green, P., Dukes, D., Armstrong, K. S., & Chapman, J. E. (2010). Randomized trial of MST and ARC in a two-level evidence-based treatment implementation strategy. *Journal of Consulting and Clinical Psychology, 78*(4), 537–550. https://doi.org/10.1037/a0019160

Kadushin, C. (2012). *Understanding social networks: Theories, concepts and findings.* Oxford University Press.

Tervalon, M., & Murray-García, J. (1998). Cultural humility versus cultural competence: A critical distinction in defining physician training outcomes in multicultural education. *Journal of Health Care for the Poor and Underserved, 9*(2), 117–125. https://doi.org/10.1353/hpu.2010.0233

Weisz, J. R., & Gray, J. S. (2008). Evidence-based psychotherapy for children and adolescents: Data from the present and a model for the future. *Child and Adolescent Mental Health, 13*(2), 54–65. https://doi.org/10.1111/j.1475-3588.2007.00475.x

Index

For the benefit of digital users, indexed terms that span two pages (e.g., 52–53) may, on occasion, appear on only one of those pages.
Note: Tables, figures, and boxes are indicated by an italic *t*, *f*, and *b* following the page number.

accreditation of AMBIT Training Centres 342, 348, 349
action mode *see* quick-fix; teleology
active listening 93
Active Planning 41
  AIM cards 86–87
  AMBIT Study Group 335–36
  child and youth social service institution 191, 192–93, 195, 196, 197, 203–4, 211, 213–14
  Map ('Egg and Triangle') 41, 42*b*–43*b*, 42*f*
    AIM cards 88–89, 94–95, 98
  psychotherapy outreach work 153, 163–64
  teacher training 272–76, 284
  training process 301–4
Adolescent Multi-Agency Support Service (AMASS) 239
  bridging professionals into relationships where epistemic trust already exists 233–35
  building relationships with the young person 232–33
  family's perspective on helpfulness 227–29
  requesting help versus making a referral 226–27
  service design 224–26
  supporting development of helping processes 229–32
  supportive team processes 235–38
adverse relationship experiences (AREs)
  ECID project 110, 116–19
  as impediment to relationships 112–16
  parental 110, 112, 113, 114–16, 117
  personality disorders, adults with 167–68
  psychodynamic psychotherapy 141–42
  psychotherapy outreach work 143
affect
  characteristic of mentalizing 22, 27
  Working with your Client 36
AIM 42*b*, 55–56, 250
  cards *see* AIM cards
  child and youth social service institution 187, 205–6
  Excel sheet 163–64
  outcomes 333–35, 336, 345–47
  psychotherapy outreach work 163–64

Questionnaire 85–86
  Version 1: 57*b*
  Version 2: 57
AIM cards 41, 42*b*, 83, 104–5
  child and youth social service institution 190, 205–6
  client feedback 103–4
  description 85–86
  mentalizing 86
  outcomes 318
  use 102
    in ambivalent help-seeking 101–2
    step 1: introducing the cards 87–88
    step 2: client agreement to use the cards 88–89
    step 3: client decides how to look through the cards 89–90
    step 4: client labels the piles of cards 90
    step 5: client sorts the cards into piles 91–93
    step 6: worker attunes to client as they sort the cards 93–94
    step 7: worker and client explore how they have sorted the cards 94–97
    step 8: exploring what the client might want to be different 97–100
    step 9: exploring who can help with the chosen cards 100–1
AIM Questionnaire 85–86
Altrecht 168–79
AMASS *see* Adolescent Multi-Agency Support Service
AMBIT community of practice 57*b*, 339, 342–43, 345, 348–49
AMBIT Development Group 210
AMBIT Evaluation Day 205–6
AMBIT implementation wheel 211–14, 212*f*
AMBIT Integrative Measure *see* AIM
AMBIT Local Facilitator Training course 269, 292, 310
AMBIT manual *see* wiki manual
AMBIT Practice Audit Tool (APrAT) 57*b*, 275*t*
AMBIT Programme Team 342, 343, 345, 348–49

AMBIT Service Evaluation Questionnaire
(ASEQ) 57b, 253–54, 346t
AMBIT Study Day 323, 332–35
AMBIT Study Group 205–6, 254–55, 334–36,
345–47, 348–49
AMBIT Train the Trainer course 148, 183, 204,
249, 269
AMBIT Training Centres 342, 348, 349
AMBIT wheel 23–24, 23f, 28
child and youth social service
institution 187, 195
ECID project 108–9, 126–27, 134–35
equity, diversity, and inclusion 343–44
networks, working with 249
outcomes 345–47
personality disorders, adults with 176–77, 178
psychotherapy outreach work 148–49, 150
research programme 347
teacher training 273, 284
see also Learning at Work; Working with your
Client; Working with your Network;
Working with your Team
anger, and psychotherapy outreach work 143–
44, 146
Anna Freud Centre, London 1, 145
AIM cards 163–64
AMBIT Programme Team 342, 343,
345, 348–49
AMBIT Study Day 323, 332–35
AMBIT Study Group 254–55
future directions 339
Hampstead Child Adaptation Measure 85–
86, 333–34
logic model 323
training 108, 146, 148, 178, 183, 248, 249
wiki manual 351
anti-racism 341, 342
anxiety, and help-seeking process 11–12
Assertive Community Treatment 329–30
assertiveness, graded 196–97
attachment relationships
adverse relationship experiences 112, 115–16, 118
ECID project 111, 131
networks, working with 247–48
outcomes 319
personality disorders, adults with 170
psychotherapy outreach work 150–51, 155–
56, 164
attachment theory
helping process 12–13
psychotherapy outreach work 140, 141, 142,
145, 156, 159
attention deficit hyperactivity disorder (ADHD),
and psychotherapy outreach work 158–
59, 160–61

attunement see sensitive attunement
autism, and psychotherapy outreach work 158–59,
160–61, 162

Black Lives Matter 341
borderline personality disorder, parental 187–88
broadcasting intentions 41
AIM cards 87–89, 98, 99–100
AMBIT Study Group 335–36
child and youth social service institution 199,
203–4, 209
deployment-based approach to model
development 345
'Egg and Triangle' 42b–43
NET-Aim-Questionnaire 252, 253
teacher training 273–74
Team around the Worker 227–29
training process 292, 301, 302–4
bullying, and prevalence of multiple needs 4

case screenings 195–96
case triangles 193–95, 199–201, 205
certainty see psychic equivalence
Child and Adolescent Mental Health Services
(CAMHS)
ECID project 108, 127, 130–31
networks, working with 242–43, 247–
58, 260–65
prevalence of multiple needs 4
unequal relationships 122–23
Choice and Partnership Approach (CAPA) 199
clients see Working with your Client
coexistence, and psychotherapy outreach
work 154–55
cognitive behavioural therapy 149
collaboration between agencies, difficulties in
achieving 8–9
collective cultures 347
collegial case counselling 275t, 279–82, 280b,
284, 286
co-mentalizing (relational mentalizing/we-
mode) 68–69, 77–79
breakdowns 74–75
epistemic trust 69–70
teleology 67
community/community-based work
AMBIT community of practice 57b, 339, 342–
43, 345, 348–49
Assertive Community Treatment 329–30
Functional Assertive Community
Treatment 168, 169–70, 175–76, 178
see also outreach work
compassion 76–77
Learning at Work 54
teacher training 283

compassion fatigue
    child and youth social service institution 184
    networks, working with 259
complex needs
    child and youth social service
        institution 185, 193
    training process 298b
    Working with your Network 46
    see also multiple needs
complex systems 77–78
    child and youth social service institution 181,
        184, 193, 202–3, 214
    development of AMBIT 15
    joint attention 68
    long-term team support 309
    networks, working with 256–58, 260, 265–66
    outcomes 345
    Team around the Worker 218–19, 225–26
    training process 292, 304–10
    wicked problems 244–46, 248, 250, 255, 257–58
    Working with your Network 44
consultation day, training process 294, 295–
        97, 298b
continuity of help 30
corrective emotional experience 141–42, 155–56
counter-transference 157
COVID-19 pandemic
    AMBIT Study Group 335–36
    child and youth social service institution 195,
        199–200
    future of AMBIT 340, 341
Creative Commons 348
criminal justice system see justice system
curiosity
    AIM cards 88, 98, 99
    characteristic of mentalizing 22, 30
    child and youth social service institution 186
        AMBIT implementation wheel 213
        current situation 210–11
        evaluation 206–7, 208, 210
        Learning at Work 204–5
        Working with your Client 188, 189–90
        Working with your Network 200, 202
        Working with your Team 194, 196
    ECID project 118–19, 121, 122, 123–26, 133–34
    future directions 339–40, 345
    Learning at Work 51, 52
    networks, working with 249, 265–66
        case example 262, 264–65
        mentalizing case managers 256–57
        NET-Aim-Questionnaire 250, 253, 255
        outpatient milieu therapy 247–48
        resonance of young people and their helping
            systems 259–60
    outcomes 315, 316, 336–37

from the inside 318, 319–28
from the outside 332
shared framework 334–36
personality disorders, adults with 175, 177, 178
teacher training 283
Team around the Worker 222
training process 294–95, 296, 298b, 302, 305,
    308, 311–13
Working with your Client 36, 40–41
Working with your Network 45, 48
CUSS (Concern Uncertain, Safety, Stop)
    model 196

delicate problems 244, 245
deployment-based approach to model
    development 344–45, 344f, 346t
discrimination 341
dis-integration
    child and youth social service institution 200,
        201–2, 213
    grid see dis-integration grid
    networks, working with 245–47, 248, 249
        mentalizing case managers 256
        NET-Aim-Questionnaire 252, 255
        resonance of young people and their helping
            systems 259–60
    personality disorders, adults with 175
    Team around the Worker 225–26
    training process 308
    Working with your Network 43–44, 48–49
dis-integration grid 50f, 50b
    child and youth social service institution 196
    personality disorders, adults with 175
    psychotherapy outreach work 150
    teacher training 275t, 284
    training process 307–8, 310
dissemination, widening methods of 349–50
diversity see equity, diversity, and inclusion

eating disorders
    interconnectivity 4–5
    multiple helpers 6–7
    networks, working with 242–43, 260–65
    single difficulties vs multiple needs 3–4
ECID project 107–10, 134–35
    Learning at Work 132–33
    Working with your Client 110–26
    Working with your Network 130–32
    Working with your Team 126–30
education
    child and youth social service institution 182–
        83, 184–85, 200–1, 210
    ECID project 110, 123, 125–26, 132, 133
    networks, working with 242–43, 264, 265
    outcomes 328, 330, 331

education (*cont.*)
    psychotherapy outreach work 146, 147, 153–54, 160–61, 162–63
    special needs *see* special educational needs
    Team around the Worker 226, 228–29, 234–35, 238
    see also teacher training
'Egg and Triangle' 41, 42*b*–43*b*, 42*f*
    AIM cards 88–89, 94–95, 98
'elephant in the room' 66, 299–300
emotions in teaching 284–85
empathy
    characteristic of mentalizing 22
    and compassion fatigue 184
    ECID project 117
    epistemic trust 71, 72
    networks, working with 248
    teacher training 283
engagement call, training process 294–95
epistemic injustice 72, 344, 348–49
epistemic isolation 72, 75–76
epistemic trust 24, 58, 61, 64–65, 73–76, 77–79, 85
    adverse relationship experiences 112–14
    AIM cards 83, 87
        use 88–89, 92, 93–94, 96, 97, 98, 99–100, 101
    child and youth social service institution 192–93, 203, 210
    co-mentalizing 69–70
    defined 64
    ECID project 108
        Working with your Client 110–11, 113–14, 117, 118–19, 120, 123, 124, 125
        Working with your Network 130, 131
        Working with your Team 126–27
    helping process 10–11, 13, 15
    Learning at Work 51–53
    mentalizing 86
    networks, working with
        case example 261–62
        mentalizing case managers 256
        NET-Aim-Questionnaire 251, 252, 253
        outpatient milieu therapy 247–48
    non-mentalizing helping system 14
    outcomes 332–33
    personality disorders, adults with 170–72, 175, 176
    Pro-Gram 49*b*–50
    psychotherapy outreach work 139, 141, 142, 144, 146, 147, 148, 150–52, 156, 157, 164
    severe personality disorders, adults with 169
    teacher training 274, 284
    Team around the Worker 218–19, 238–39
        AMASS 229–35, 236–38
        supports 220, 223, 224
    teleology 67
    training process 291

helping process 297–99, 302, 303
    implementation in complex systems 305, 306–7, 308
    workers' state of mind 295, 296, 298*b*
    Working with your Client 38, 39, 40, 42*b*–43
    Working with your Network 46–48
    Working with your Team 29–30, 31–32, 34
epistemic vigilance 36, 61, 69–70, 74, 83–84
    ECID project 110, 113–14
equity, diversity, and inclusion (EDI) 305, 341, 342–44, 348–49
ethics 342–43, 345
EVAS 206
evidence, respect for 53–54, 292
exclusion 341
expertise, local *see* respect: for local practice and expertise

family therapy 140, 141–42, 144
Feedback-Informed Treatment (FIT) 163
Four Corners exercise 296, 298*b*
Four Levels of Training Evaluation 310–11
Four Voices model 259–60
Functional Assertive Community Treatment (FACT) 168, 169–70, 175–76, 178
functional outcomes 330, 332–33, 334, 335–36
future directions 339–42, 351–52
    developing the basic approach 342–47
    diversity, widening 348–49
    implementation improvements 350–51
    training capacity, increasing 348–50

graded assertiveness 196–97
groupthink 77–78

Hampstead Child Adaptation Measure (HCAM) 85–86, 333–34
helpers *see* workers
helping systems
    adverse relationship experiences 114
    AIM cards 97, 98–102, 104
    attachment theory 12–13
    child and youth social service institution 184–85, 187–88, 197, 203–4
    collaboration 67–73, 77–78
    continuity of help 30
    early relationships 83–84
    ECID project 110–11, 115, 117, 122, 123, 130–31, 134
    fragility 11–12, 15
    future directions 339–40
    importance 10–11
    integrating the help 45, 46–47
    mentalizing 67–73
    networks, working with 243–47, 258–60
        case example 264–65

mentalizing case managers 256–58
   outpatient milieu therapy 247–48
non-mentalizing 14–15, 73–74
outcomes 62–63, 330, 331–32, 345
personality disorders, adults with 167–68, 172–
      73, 175, 179
psychotherapy outreach work 150–52
scaffolding 63
teacher training 273–74
Team around the Worker 48, 218–19, 223–24,
      226–32, 234–37, 239
training process 292, 294, 295–96, 297–304
Working with your Client 40
Working with your Network 48
Working with your Team 33–34, 37b
homosexual people, and prevalence of multiple
      needs 4
hospital admissions 330–31
humanity 76–77
humility 134–35
   AIM cards 94
   characteristic of mentalizing 22–23
   child and youth social service institution 181,
      187, 201–2, 208
   ECID project 118, 121, 122, 124–25, 126, 130,
      132, 134
   future directions 339–40, 341
   networks, working with 256–57
   outcomes 316
   characteristic of mentalizing 22
   child and youth social service institution 188,
      190, 210
   ECID project 121
   Learning at Work 54

identity
   AIM cards 103
   development 70–71
implementation
   child and youth social service institution 181,
      185–87, 206–7
      AMBIT implementation wheel 211–14
      Learning at Work 204–5
      lessons learned 208–10
      Working with your Client 187–90
      Working with your Team 191–200
      Working with your Network 200–4
   ECID project 109, 116–17, 119–24, 127–29,
      131–32, 133, 134
   future directions 350–51
   Implementation Stages Planning Tool 292–93
   personality disorders, adults with 176–77
   psychotherapy outreach work 145, 146, 153
   Team around the Worker 223b
   training process 292, 304–10, 312b
implementation science 292–93, 294, 309, 350

inclusion see equity, diversity, and inclusion
individualized approach, as overarching
      theme 2
integrating the help 45, 46–47
intellectual disabilities see learning disabilities
intellectual property 342–43
intentional states, connecting outcomes to
      interest in 322
international AMBIT Training Centres 342,
      348, 349
intersubjectivity, and psychotherapy outreach
      work 154–55
Inventory of Life Quality in Children (ILK) 206

joint attention 68, 77–79
   ECID project 120, 121, 123
justice system
   mentalizing group for violent prisoners 61–
      62, 63–64
   juvenile 4
   special educational needs 270

KASAM 163
keyworkers see workers

Learning at Work 52f
   basic practice 55–56
   child and youth social service institution 204–
      5, 213–14
   development of AMBIT framework 315
   ECID project 132–33
   equity, diversity, and inclusion 344
   mentalizing and non-mentalizing 51–53
   openness to 63
   outcomes 316, 334–35, 336–37
   personality disorders, adults with 176–77
   psychotherapy outreach work 148–49
   stance features 53
      respect for evidence 53–54
      respect for local practice and expertise 54
   teacher training 284
   tools and techniques 56b–57b
   training process 292
learning disabilities
   network integration, training to promote 307
   professional expertise 134–35
   psychotherapy outreach work 162–63
listening, active 93
Local AMBIT Community of Practice
      Facilitator 349
Local Facilitator Training course 269, 292, 310
local practice and expertise see respect: for local
      practice and expertise
logic model, to determine outcomes that
      matter 323–27, 323f, 324f, 325f, 326f, 327f,
      332, 334

looked-after children, and prevalence of multiple needs 4

manual, AMBIT *see* wiki manual
manualizing 55, 56
    child and youth social service institution 186, 203–5
    deployment-based approach to model development 346*t*
    ECID project 133
    outcomes 335
    personality disorders, adults with 177–78
    psychotherapy outreach work 148–49
    Team around the Worker 236–37
    training process 304, 309, 310
Maslow's Hierarchy of Need 42*b*–43
mental health services
    ECID project 108, 110–11, 114, 119, 122–23, 127–33
    personality disorders, adults with 167–79
    see also Child and Adolescent Mental Health Services
mental models about outcomes, sharing 321–22
mentalization *see* mentalizing/mentalization
'Mentalization-based support for teachers' project *see* teacher training
mentalization-based treatment (MBT)
    child and youth social service institution 208–9, 210
    personality disorders, adults with 168, 169–70, 172–73
mentalized affectivity 121
mentalizing case managers (MCMs) 255–58, 259–62, 263–64, 265–66
mentalizing/mentalization
    adverse relationship experiences 113–14, 115
    AIM cards 86, 87–89, 90, 91–93, 95, 99, 101, 102
    AMBIT wheel 23–24
    characteristics 22–23, 30
    child and youth social service institution 181, 186, 187, 214
        AMBIT implementation wheel 212
        current situation 211
        evaluation 208–9
        Learning at Work 204–5
        Working with your Client 187–90
        Working with your Network 200–3
        Working with your Team 191–93, 194, 195, 196
    and collaboration within helping systems 67–73
    collegial case counselling 275*t*, 279–82, 280*b*, 284, 286
    defined 21–22
    dimensions 40–41, 121
    ECID project 108–9, 134
        Learning at Work 133

        Working with your Client 111, 117, 118–19, 120–21, 122, 124, 125
        Working with your Network 131–32
        Working with your Team 127, 128–29
    focus on 74–77
    fragility 25–27
    future directions 351–52
        deployment-based approach to model development 346*t*
        equity, diversity, and inclusion 343
        implementation improvements 350
        Local AMBIT Community of Practice Facilitator 349
    interventions based on 24
    Learning at Work 51–53
    networks, working with
        case example 260, 261–63
        mentalizing case managers 255–58
        NET-Aim-Questionnaire 249–55
        outpatient milieu therapy 247–48
        resonance of young people and their helping systems 259–60
        values 245–46
    neurology 25
    outcomes 316, 336–37
        from the inside 318–20, 321–22, 323–24
        from the outside 329–30
    parents 115–16, 117–18, 125, 158–60
    personality disorders, adults with 167, 168, 169–70, 178
        Learning at Work 176–77
        Working with your Patient 170, 171–72
        Working with your Team 172–75
    psychotherapy outreach work 141–42, 143–45, 147–49, 164–65
        Working with your Client 150, 153, 154, 155, 156–57, 158–60
    in real-world settings 61–65
    relational *see* co-mentalizing
    stance 40–41
    as strength and vulnerability 65–67
    teacher training 270–71, 286–87
        broadcasting intentions 273
        curriculum 275*t*
        reflections on seminars 276–83, 277*b*, 284, 285–86
        setting the plan 274–76
        stress management 271–72
    Team around the Worker 217–18, 219, 238–39
        AMASS 225–26, 228–30, 233, 234–35
        supports 220–24
    training process 291, 292, 313
        evaluation 311–13, 312*b*
        helping process 297–302, 303
        implementation in complex systems 305, 308, 309

workers' state of mind 294–95, 297, 298*b*
trauma-related 115–16
Working with your Client 36–38, 40–41
Working with your Network 43–45, 48–49
Working with your Team 28–31, 32, 33–34
milieu therapy 247–48, 251, 261–62
mindfulness 271
'mind-reading' 158
mistrust *see* epistemic trust
misunderstandings, as characteristic of
    mentalizing 22–23
motivational interviewing 53–54, 97, 220, 329–30
multimodal stress management, teachers 271
multiple needs
    AIM cards 91, 92
    defined 1
    interconnectivity 4–5
    and multiple helpers 5–10
    as overarching theme 2
    prevalence 3–4
    Working with your Network 45–46
    see also complex needs
multiple perspectives
    as characteristic of mentalizing 30
    Working with your Network 45
multiple teams, as overarching theme 2

National Health Service 7–8, 16
neo-generalists 257
networks 241–42, 243, 260–66
    AMBIT approach 248–49
    case example 242–43, 260–65, 266
    helping system 243–47
    mentalizing case manager 255–58
    NET-Aim-Questionnaire (NET-Aim-Q) 249–
        55, 256, 262, 263
    NET-Stat-Questionnaire (NET-Stat-Q) 255
    outpatient milieu therapy 247–48
    resonance of young people and their helping
        systems 258–60
    training to promote network integration 306–8
    see also Working with your Network
New Public Management 245–46, 265
NHS 7–8, 16
non-heterosexual people, and prevalence of
    multiple needs 4
non-mentalizing/non-mentalization
    AMBIT 77–79
    characteristics 30, 66–67
    child and youth social service institution 189,
        191, 196, 202, 208–9
    ECID project 120, 129, 132
    fragility of mentalizing 25
    helping systems 14–15, 73–74
    inevitability 28
    Learning at Work 51–53, 54

networks, working with 247–48, 249, 250, 253,
    258–59, 262
outcomes 316, 318–19, 320, 322, 329–30, 335
parents 115, 117–18, 125, 155, 189
in real-world settings 62, 64–65
states of mind 25–26
teacher training 276, 282–83, 286
Team around the Worker 222
training process 299–300
vicious cycles 125
Working with your Client 36–38, 40–41
Working with your Network 43–45, 48, 49
Working with your Team 28–31, 32–33
not-knowing, tolerance of
    characteristic of mentalizing 22
    child and youth social service institution 188
    ECID project 122, 126, 130
    networks, working with 260–61
    personality disorders, adults with 178
    Working with your Client 40–41

online training 341
open-source principles 342–43
ostensive cues 69, 70
outcomes 315–16, 336–37
    AIM cards 86
    American Psychological Association
        report 62–63
    child and youth social service institution 205–
        7, 207*f*
    ECID project 132–33
    from the inside 317–28
    from the outside 328–32
    future directions 339–40, 345–47
    Learning at Work 55–56
    NET-Aim-Questionnaire 254–55
    psychotherapy outreach work 144–45, 163–64
    scaffolding of help 63
    shared framework 332–36
outpatient milieu therapy 247–48
outreach work
    child and youth social service institution 182–
        83, 184, 211, 214
    co-mentalizing 68
    ECID project 111, 115, 116–17, 119–24, 127–28
    epistemic trust 69–71, 72–73
    mentalizing 65–66
    outcomes 329–31
    psychotherapy 139, 164–65
        AMBIT 148–63
        beginnings 145–46
        evaluation 163–64
        first clients 146–47
        first meeting 142–44
        origins 140–42
        team formation 147–48

outreach work (*cont.*)
    team today 139–40
    thought processes 144–45
    Team around the Worker 233

Paedakoop *see* social services: multiprofessional
    cooperation in child and youth institution
parents
    of adults with personality disorders 171–72, 177
    adverse relationship experiences 110, 112, 113,
        114–16, 117
    AMASS 226, 227–29, 231–32, 234–35, 238
    with borderline personality disorder 187–88
    child and youth social service institution 187–
        90, 192–93, 199, 200–1, 203–4
    ECID project 110, 113, 116–18, 119–20, 125
    mentalizing 115–16, 117–18, 125, 158–60
    networks, working with
        case example 242–43, 261–62, 263, 264
        NET-Aim-Questionnaire 251, 252, 254
    non-mentalizing 115, 117–18, 125, 155, 189
    psychotherapy outreach work 139–40, 141, 144,
        146–47, 151, 158–63, 164–65
personal narratives, and epistemic trust 70–
    71, 72–73
personality disorders, adults with 167, 178–79
    borderline, in parent 187–88
    context of work 168–70
    Learning at Work 176–77
    working with 167–68
    Working with your Network 175–76
    Working with your Patient 170–72
    Working with your Team 172–75
plans, making and carrying out 41
    AIM cards 88–89, 94–95, 99–100
    child and youth social service institution 195,
        196, 209
    networks, working with 245–46
    non-mentalizing helping system 15
    personality disorders, adults with 171–72, 173–
        75, 176, 177, 178
    psychotherapy outreach work 152–53, 163–64
    teacher training 274–76
    see also Active Planning
pond metaphor *see* 'ripples in the pond' metaphor
power issues, and fragility of mentalizing 26–27
practitioners *see* workers
pretend mode
    AIM cards 89
    characteristic of non-mentalizing 26, 30, 31, 66
    child and youth social service
        institution 189, 198
    Learning at Work 52
    outcomes 318–19, 329–30
    personality disorders, adults with 169–
        70, 172–73

psychotherapy outreach work 141, 156–57, 158,
    159, 160
teacher training 278
training process 299–300
Working with your Client 36
Working with your Network 45
prisons/prisoners *see* justice system
professional triangles, child and youth social
    service institution 193–95, 199–201, 205
Pro-Gram 49*b*–50, 49*f*, 100
    child and youth social service
        institution 196, 203–4
    teacher training 275*t*, 284
psychic equivalence (certainty)
    AIM cards 87
    characteristic of non-mentalizing 25–26, 30,
        31, 67, 74
    Learning at Work 52
    'mind-reading' 158
    outcomes 318–19, 322, 329–30, 335
    psychotherapy outreach work 141, 156–57,
        159, 161
    teacher training 278, 279, 283
    Team around the Worker 222
    training process 299–300, 301–2
    Working with your Client 36
    Working with your Network 44
'psychobabble' 158
psychodynamic psychotherapy 140, 141–42,
    144–45, 156
psychoeducation 172, 176
psychological scaffolding 63
psychosis 168
psychotherapy
    NET-Aim-Questionnaire 251
    outreach work 139, 164–65
        AMBIT 148–63
        beginnings 145–46
        evaluation 163–64
        first clients 146–47
        first meeting 142–44
        origins 140–42
        team formation 147–48
        team today 139–40
        thought processes 144–45
    personality disorders, adults with 168–70
purposefulness 83–84, 85
    AIM cards 101
    child and youth social service
        institution 210

quick-fix
    characteristic of non-mentalizing 30, 31, 67
    child and youth social service institution 192–
        93, 198
    Learning at Work 52

personality disorders, adults with 169–70, 175–76
psychotherapy outreach work 153–54
teacher training 279
training process 294–95, 299–300
Working with your Network 44
see also teleology

racism 341, 342
redesign of services *see* systems change
reflection
  AIM cards 87–88, 91–92, 103
  characteristic of mentalizing 30
  identity development 70–71
  mentalized affectivity 121
  networks, working with 245
  parents 115–16
  psychotherapy outreach work 145, 146, 152, 153, 154, 155–58
  teacher training 273, 274, 275t, 276–86
  training process 296, 297–99, 298b, 302–3, 305, 306b, 307, 308
  'Wearing Different Hats' exercise 50b–51
rejection 75–76
remote training 341
research programme on core AMBIT model 347
resonance 258–62, 263, 265
respect
  for evidence 53–54, 292
  for local practice and expertise 54
    child and youth social service institution 200–2, 204–5, 210–11, 213–14
    networks, working with 262
    personality disorders, adults with 177–78
    Team around the Worker 234
    training process 292, 309
'ripples in the pond' metaphor 34
  child and youth social service institution 196
  psychotherapy outreach work 144–45, 150
  training process 296, 300
risk management
  child and youth social service institution 190, 196–97
  personality disorders, adults with 171, 173–75, 177–78
  Working with your Client 39–40
rope metaphor 35
  training process 299–301

salutogenesis 74, 150, 163
scaffolding
  AIM cards 104–5
  ECID project 109, 124–25
  helping systems 63
  personality disorders, adults with 170
  psychological 63

Team around the Worker 223b
  training process 295–96
  Working with your Client 39, 41
  zone of proximal development 62
schools/schooling *see* education
sculpts 175
self-harm
  child and youth social service institution 190, 200
  outcomes 330
  personality disorders, adults with 171, 173–76
  psychotherapy outreach work 143–44
self-reflection *see* reflection
sensitive attunement 41
  AIM cards 88–90, 92, 94–95, 96, 98–99, 102
  child and youth social service institution 199, 209
  teacher training 272–73
  Team around the Worker 230–31
  training process 301–3
service redesign *see* systems change
severe personality disorders *see* personality disorders, adults with
shared attention *see* joint attention
shared caseload 175–76
shared language and understanding 307–8, 312b
shared outcomes framework 332–36
sharing mental models about outcomes 321–22
social inclusion 332–33
social justice/injustice 342–43
social network analysis 347
social services
  multiprofessional cooperation in child and youth institution 181–83, 214
    current situation 210–11
    evaluation 205–10
    help needed 183–85
    implementation 185–205
    initial contact with AMBIT 183
    AMBIT wheel 211–14
  psychotherapy outreach work 139–40, 144–45, 146, 147–48, 150–54, 155, 158, 162
special educational needs
  needs of young people 270
  prevalence of multiple needs 4
  teacher training *see* teacher training
status
  child and youth social service institution 193–94
  Team around the Worker 219
Stop, Rewind, Explore technique 282–83
stories about other services, resisting unhelpful 50b–51
stress
  and mentalizing 76
  teachers 271–72, 275t, 282
  workers 29–30, 31–32, 33–34

substance misuse
  outcomes 329–30, 332, 334
  prevalence of multiple needs 4
suicidality
  child and youth social service institution 190,
    200, 204
  mentalization lapses 76–77
  personality disorders, adults with 171, 173–
    75, 177–78
systemic therapy 141–42
systems change
  child and youth social service institution 182–
    83, 191, 200, 211
  ECID project 109, 116–17, 127, 129–30, 131–32
  limitations 10
  networks, working with 248
  outcomes 331
  training process 293–94, 295

teacher training 269–70, 286–87
  in Germany 271–72
  pilot project 270–71
    Active Planning for seminar design 272–76
    curriculum 275*t*
    reflections on seminars 276–86
    special education settings, young people's
      needs in 270
    and stress levels 271–72
teachers as keyworkers 199–200
Team around the Client 47, 47*f*
Team around the Worker 47–48, 47*f*, 217–
  18, 238–39
  case example 224–38
  deployment-based approach to model
    development 346*t*
  described 218–19
  implementation examples 223*b*
  outcomes 331–32
  responses to the idea 221*b*
  supports 220–24
  see also Working with your Team
teleology
  characteristic of non-mentalizing 26, 67
  child and youth social service institution 192–93
  Learning at Work 53
  outcomes 318–19, 329–30
  psychotherapy outreach work 141, 151, 153–
    54, 156
  teacher training 278, 279
  Working with your Client 41
  see also quick-fix
therapeutic relationship
  American Psychological Association
    report 62–63
  ECID project 109–11, 127
  psychotherapy outreach work 144–45, 146,
    147, 155–56

Thinking Together 35, 37*b*
  child and youth social service institution 192–93
  ECID project 127, 128–29
  networks, working with 260–61
  peer-mentoring project 345
  personality disorders, adults with 172–73
  psychotherapy outreach work 149–50
  teacher training 275*t*, 277*b*, 277–79, 284
  Team around the Worker 231–32
  training process 300, 304, 310
THRIVE model 198–99
Train the Trainer course 148, 183, 204, 249, 269
training 1–2, 20
  active listening 93
  AMBIT principles applied to 291–93, 313
    evaluation 310–13, 311*t*, 312*b*
    helping process 297–304
    implementation in complex systems 304–10
    workers' state of mind 293–97, 298*b*
  AMBIT Service Evaluation Questionnaire 57*b*
  Anna Freud Centre, London 108, 146, 148, 178,
    183, 248, 249
  broadcasting intentions 87–88
  capacity, increasing 348–50
  child and youth social service institution 183–
    84, 185–86, 188–89, 196, 208–9, 210
  deployment-based approach to model
    development 345
  ECID project 108, 109, 126–28
  fatigue 294–95
  and implementation improvements 350
  individual vs collective help 9–10
  international AMBIT Training Centres 342
  Learning at Work 52–53
  Local Facilitator Training 269, 292, 310
  mentalizing case managers 256
  networks, working with 241
  online delivery 341
  in outcome monitoring 319
  personality disorders, adults with 177, 178
  psychological scaffolding 63
  psychotherapy outreach work 146, 148, 149–50
  respect for local practice and expertise 54
  response to 107
  supporting implementation after 350
  teachers *see* teacher training
  Team around the Worker 220–22, 223–24
  Train the Trainer 148, 183, 204, 249, 269
  'Wearing Different Hats' exercise 50*b*–51
transference 141–42, 200–1
transgenerational transmission
  of attachment 115
  of relational trauma 112, 113, 115, 116
trust *see* epistemic trust

value-based management (VBM) 245–47,
  248, 265

values, making explicit 342–44
video logbooks, in teacher training 275*t*, 276, 277, 278–79, 281, 282–83, 284–86
Vorarlberger Kinderdorf *see* social services: multiprofessional cooperation in child and youth institution

'Wearing Different Hats' exercise 50*b*–51, 308
well-connected team 86
   child and youth social service institution 181, 210
   ECID project 126, 128, 129–30, 133
   need for 351–52
   networks, working with 245, 248, 249, 251, 256, 259, 263
   personality disorders, adults with 172
   psychotherapy outreach work 150
   research programme 347
   teacher training 284, 287
   training process 297–99, 300, 303–5, 310
   Working with your Team 32–33, 34, 37*b*
we-mode *see* co-mentalizing
wicked problems 244–46, 248, 250, 255, 257–58
wiki manual 56*b*
   future directions 342–43, 351
   psychotherapy outreach work 148–49, 163–64
   teacher training 285
workers
   individual keyworker relationship 31–32
   isolation 31–32
   multiple
      child and youth social service institution 193–95
      and multiple needs 5–10
      as overarching theme 2
   retention 30
   state of mind 220
      child and youth social service institution 184
      as fundamental to help 14–15
      as overarching theme 2–3
      training process 291, 293–97, 298*b*
   stress Team 29–30, 31–32, 33–34
   teachers as keyworkers 199–200
   turnover
      child and youth social service institution 183–84
      effects 30
   well connected to team 32–33
   well-being 183–84
Working with your Client 38*f*
   basic practice 40
      Active Planning 41
      epistemic trust 40
      mentalizing stance 40–41
      scaffolding relationships 41

child and youth social service institution 187–90
   ECID project 110–26
   equity, diversity, and inclusion 343
   learning 55
   mentalizing and non-mentalizing 36–38
   personality disorders, adults with 170–72
   psychotherapy outreach work 149–64
   stance features 39
      managing risk 39–40
      scaffolding relationships 39
   teacher training 273
Working with your Network 46*f*
   basic practice
      mentalizing approach to address dis-integration 48–49
      Team around the Worker 47–48
   child and youth social service institution 200–4, 213
   ECID project 130–32
   equity, diversity, and inclusion 344
   learning 55
   mentalizing and non-mentalizing 43–45
   personality disorders, adults with 175–76
   psychotherapy outreach work 149, 152–53, 158–62, 163–64
   stance features 45
      integrating the help 46–47
      meeting multiple needs 46
   teacher training 273
   tools and techniques 49*b*–51*b*
   training process 306–8
Working with your Team 29*f*
   basic practice
      helping processes in teams 33–34
      'ripples in the pond' 34
      'who's got your rope?' 35
   child and youth social service institution 191–200, 213
   ECID project 126–30
   equity, diversity, and inclusion 343
   learning 55
   mentalizing and non-mentalizing 28–31
   personality disorders, adults with 172–75
   psychotherapy outreach work 147–48, 149–50
   stance features 31
      individual keyworker relationship 31–32
      keyworker well connected to team 32–33
   teacher training 273–74
   tools and techniques 35, 37*b*
   see also Team around the Worker

young people's and adult services, interaction between 7

zones of proximal development 62, 63